HEALTH CARE ETHICS

HEALTH CARE ETHICS

A CATHOLIC THEOLOGICAL ANALYSIS

FIFTH EDITION

Benedict M. Ashley, O.P.
Jean K. deBlois, C.S.J.
Kevin D. O'Rourke, O.P.

Georgetown University Press
Washington, D.C.

As of January 1, 2007, 13-digit ISBN numbers will replace the current 10-digit system. Paperback: 978-1-58901-116-8

Georgetown University Press, Washington, D.C.

Nihil Obstat
Reverend Patrick J. Boyle, S.J., Ph.D.
Censor Deputatus
November 16, 2005

Imprimatur
Reverend George J. Rassas
Vicar General
Archdiocese of Chicago
November 23, 2005

The *Nihil Obstat* and the *Imprimatur* are official declarations that a book is free of doctrinal and moral error. No implication is contained that those who have granted the *Nihil Obstat* and *Imprimatur* agree with the content, opinions, or statements expressed. Nor do they assume any legal responsibility associated with publication.

Library of Congress Cataloging-in-Publication Data

Ashley, Benedict M.
    Health care ethics : a Catholic theological analysis / Benedict M. Ashley, Jean K. deBlois, Kevin D. O'Rourke. — 5th ed.
        p. cm.
    Includes bibliographical references and index.
    ISBN-13: 978-1-58901-116-8 (pbk. : alk. paper)
    ISBN-10: 1-58901-116-3 (pbk. : alk. paper)
    1. Medical ethics—Religious aspects—Catholic Church. 2. Medicine—Religious aspects—Catholic Church. I. DeBlois, Jean. II. O'Rourke, Kevin D. III. Title.
    [DNLM: 1. Ethics, Medical. 2. Delivery of Health Care—ethics. 3. Catholicism. 4. Bioethical Issues. 5. Religion and Medicine.
    W 50 A817h 2006]
    R724.A74 2006
    174.2—dc22   2006003222

This book is printed on acid-free paper meeting the requirements of the American National Standard for Permanence in Paper for Printed Library Materials.

13 12 11 10   9 8 7 6 5 4 3

Printed in the United States of America

CONTENTS

Introduction   ix

List of Abbreviations Used in the Text and in Citations   xv

Part I: Health Care Ethics and Human Needs

1 **Bioethics in a Multicultural Age**   3

   Overview   3

   1.1   The Emergence of Secular Bioethics   3

   1.2   The Foundations of the Ethics of Health Care   5

   1.3   Current Methodologies in Bioethics   9

   1.4   Faith and Reason in Health Care Ethics   19

   1.5   Conclusion   30

2 **Ethics and Needs of the Common Person**   31

   Overview   31

   2.1   An Ethics Based on Innate Human Needs   31

   2.2   Jesus Christ, Healer, as Ethical Model   40

   2.3   Character and the Major Moral Virtues   42

   2.4   Prudent Decision Making   50

   2.5   Moral Norms Especially Relevant to Health Care   53

   2.6   Conclusion   60

Part II: Clinical Issues

3   Sexuality and Reproduction   63
Overview   63
3.1   The Meaning of Human Sexuality   63
3.2   When Does Human Life Begin?   69
3.3   Ethical Issues in Reproduction   73
3.4   Pastoral Approach to Ethical Problems Arising from Sexuality   88
3.5   Conclusion   89

4   Reconstructing and Modifying the Human Body: Ethical Perspectives   91
Overview   91
4.1   Modifying the Human Body   91
4.2   Genetic Intervention   94
4.3   Genetic Screening and Counseling   98
4.4   Organ Transplantation   103
4.5   Reconstructive and Cosmetic Surgery   108
4.6   Experimentation and Research on Human Subjects   113
4.7   Conclusion   122

5   Mental Health: Ethical Perspectives   125
Overview   125
5.1   What Is Mental Health?   126
5.2   Medical/Surgical Therapies   130
5.3   Psychotherapies   136
5.4   The Christian Model of Mental Health   145
5.5   Ethical Problems in Mental Therapy   148
5.6   Conclusion   160

6   Suffering and Death: A Theological Perspective   163
Overview   163
6.1   Mystery of Death   163
6.2   Fear of Death   166
6.3   Defining Death   169
6.4   Truth Telling to the Dying   173
6.5   Care for the Corpse or Cadaver   175
6.6   Suicide, Assisted Suicide, and Euthanasia   178
6.7   Allowing to Die: Withholding or Withdrawing Life Support   182
6.8   Care of Permanently Unconscious Patients   194
6.9   Treatment of Pain   197
6.10 Conclusion   198

Part III: Social and Pastoral Responsibilities

7 **Social Responsibility   203**

   Overview   203

   7.1   Professions: Depersonalizing Trends   204

   7.2   Characteristics of Medicine as a Profession   206

   7.3   Health Care Counseling   210

   7.4   Professional Communication and Confidentiality   212

   7.5   The Political Situation of Health Care Today   215

   7.6   Principles of Health Care Policy   218

   7.7   Health Care Ethics and Public Policy   225

   7.8   Responsibilities of Catholic Health Care Facilities   227

   7.9   Conclusion   233

8 **Pastoral Care   235**

   Overview   235

   8.1   The Goals of Pastoral Ministry   235

   8.2   Pastoral Care of the Health Care Staff   239

   8.3   Pastoral Care and Ethical Counseling   241

   8.4   Spiritual Counseling in Health Care   244

   8.5   Celebrating the Healing Process   249

   8.6   Conclusion   255

Glossary   257

References   265

Index   305

INTRODUCTION

PURPOSE OF THE BOOK

IN THE MID-1970s, BENEDICT ASHLEY, O.P., a fellow of the Institute of Religion at the Texas Medical Center, Houston, Texas, and Kevin O'Rourke, O.P., vice president for Medical Ethics at the Catholic Hospital Association, St. Louis, Missouri—both former presidents of the Aquinas Institute of Theology then located in Dubuque, Iowa—sought to produce a volume that would explain *The Ethical and Religious Directives for Catholic Health Care Facilities* of the United States Catholic Bishops Conference (ERD). We had a twofold purpose: (1) to present a study that would consider the basic principles underlying the Catholic understanding of health care ethics and (2) to assist Christian, and especially Catholic, health care professionals and health care facilities in their task of offering service and witness in the Christian tradition, in a milieu influenced by diverse and conflicting value systems. Thus we sought to consider the nature of the human person seeking to fulfill human needs under the influence of grace, explain the principles of Catholic theology that are pertinent to the practice of health care, and present individual clinical issues in health care from this perspective.

As we present this fifth edition of *Health Care Ethics,* our purpose remains the same as it was when we prepared the first edition. We proceed from the theological perspective of the Catholic Church, and this theological perspective is founded upon sacred scripture but also depends upon human reason, usually referred to as natural law. Hence, as indicated in chapters 1 and 2, we believe that the Catholic theological perspective has much to contribute to the discussion of bioethics in the twenty-first century.

We welcome a third author to this edition, Sister Jean deBlois, C.S.J. Jean was a registered nurse before pursuing studies in moral theology and ethics. She received a Ph.D. in moral theology from the Catholic University of America in 1987, and she was a faculty member of the Center for Health Care Ethics at Saint Louis University Health Sciences Center for a number of years before going to the Catholic Health Association. There she served as ethicist and vice president for mission and sponsorship for a number of years. Currently Jean is on the faculty of Aquinas Institute of Theology in St. Louis, Missouri, where she is associate professor of moral theology and director of the Master of Arts in Health Care Mission program. She is also sponsor liaison to Ascension Health for the Sisters of St. Joseph of Carondolet. In that capacity, she serves on the board of trustees of Ascension Health.

NEW EDITION

The fourth edition of *Health Care Ethics: A Theological Analysis* was published almost ten years ago. Since that time there have been many new clinical innovations and theoretical issues that have arisen in the field of health care, which necessitate another edition of our work. To name just a few of the recent developments in medicine, we consider in this most recent edition of this book the completion of the Human Genome Project and its potential for radically changing the practice of medicine, recent efforts at controlling sexual selection of infants, efforts at genetic modification of the human genotype and phenotype, cloning, development of palliative care as a medical specialty, the acceptance of persons without beating hearts as organ donors, the retrieval and cultivation of embryo and adult stem cells as a source of therapy, development of reconstructive and cosmetic surgery, the use of pharmacology to treat mental illness and awareness, and the weakening of managed care as a method of controlling costs of medical care. In addition to these developments in clinical practice, the role of the federal government in regard to funding health care has increased and technology has proliferated, as has the influence of health management organizations of one kind or another. Because these changes in the health care environment tend to weaken the bonds of the patient-physician relationship, we once again devote attention to personalizing the health care profession.

After the many encyclicals of Pope John Paul II in the early 1990s, such as *The Gospel of Life, The Splendor of Truth,* and *Faith and Reason,* which have relevance for the study of health care ethics, and since the publication of the last edition, the Church did not offer any new encyclicals influencing the ethics of health care. However, there were two significant allocutions issued by Pope John Paul II that merit our attention: one concerning the care of patients in a persistent vegetative state, and the second considering palliative care for dying patients. In addition, the Catholic Bishops of the United States revised a few norms of the ERD. The complete text of these important directives is found on the U.S. Catholic Bishops website (see ERD 2001).

GENERAL OUTLINE

In the course of twenty-five years and five editions of this work, this is the most thorough revision that we have undertaken. We have long maintained that health care ethics is "everybody's business." It is not an esoteric topic reserved for a few. Realizing that many people with a general interest in health care ethics, as well as health care professionals, have used our book for reference and education, we have sought to make it more "user-friendly." With this in mind, we have limited some of the theoretical considerations and engaged as soon as possible in the main discussion clinical issues that are of interest to our readers. We have retained, however, considerations of the various methods of engaging in the study of bioethics and the ethical responsibilities of social organizations such as the federal government and the Church.

We believe that each person bears primary responsibility for personal health and the right to retain ultimate control over his or her health. We also believe that each person has the right to help from the community in achieving personal health, as well as the reciprocal obligation to assist other members of the community in the same search. Fulfilling these personal and social responsibilities is a value-centered, ethical endeavor. For this reason, in part I, we devote attention to the various methods of ethical discourse utilized in the United States today, explaining why these methods do not fulfill our purpose, and present the method of ethical decision making utilized in Catholic tradition, with Jesus Christ as the model for human well-being.

One of the unique features of our study is the question "What does it mean to be human?" In answer to this question, we consider the needs of the human person and the quest to fulfill these needs. In this consideration of what it means to be human, we consider persons as individuals—but also as members of a community—an essential factor of human identity and fulfillment. We conclude this section with a consideration of the virtues that are needed to develop a habit of Christian ethical decision making.

Next, in part II, we consider the more common ethical questions and dilemmas occurring in clinical care. When considering these questions we offer, first of all, arguments from human reason, sometimes called the natural law. We confirm natural law reasoning with the teachings of the magisterium of the Catholic Church, whether contained in papal statements or in the ERD promulgated by the United States Conference of Catholic Bishops (USCCB, 2001). Because the teaching of the Church often is open to various interpretations, we seek to present the various responses that have been offered by different voices from within the Catholic community. For example, the *Directives* concerning Extra Uterine Pregnancy (D. 48) and Treatment of Rape Victims (D. 36) prohibit any therapy that would be a direct abortion. But which method of therapy in these clinical situations is truly a direct abortion is open to discussion. Hence we seek to provide options that will further this discussion. When discussing clinical issues, and in other places throughout the text, we often refer to *physicians*, but we really wish to include in that word all other medical personnel engaged in serving others in their quest for health. If sometimes we seem to devote more attention to physicians than to other members of the health care team, it is only because they are more visible and their responsibilities are more clearly defined by professional standards. However, what is predicated for physicians should be applied to other health care professionals as well.

Having considered the various particular ethical issues that arise in the study of health care ethics in part III, we conclude our study by presenting the major social concerns and investigating the nature and responsibility of health care professionals involved in pastoral care. Social concerns are the responsibility of the health care profession, the federal government, and the health care facilities sponsored by juridical persons within the Church. Because of our conviction that social concerns are an important part of our study, we have chosen the term *health care ethics* rather than *bioethics* to designate the matter under study due to the former's wider connotation. Pastoral care concludes our study because it is an integral element of health care ethics, insofar as it focuses on spiritual development, which in a certain sense is the goal of all human activity.

DIVERSE VALUE SYSTEMS

Too often, bioethical controversies are confusing and frustrating because participants do not define their value system or have little idea of the ethical system they are using and its theoretical implications. Many today assume that there is an accepted neutral system of bioethical decision making. Many also assume that any discussion of issues in bioethics will be made in light of this neutral and often value-free system. We take a different view and believe that the Roman Catholic system of moral decision making has much to offer a public discussion of these issues. To give a privileged position to a humanistic perspective from the outset only frustrates honest debate and prevents cooperation in our pluralistic society. Now, the humanistic or value-neutral method of decision making is considered self-evident in our society. The President's Commission on Bioethics (PCB) shows some signs of mitigating this presumption by openly considering values presented by different religious communities.

Catholics reason ethically in terms of a value system rooted in a view of reality contained in the Christian Gospel interpreted by the Church in its life of faith and authoritatively formulated by the Pope and the bishops. Catholics believe in this teaching founded upon the Gospels with a commitment of faith, and they accept its ordinary formulation and application by the Pope and bishops with "religious assent," even when these statements lack the authority of a final definition. This commitment to authoritative teaching, as well as respect for a long tradition of theological reflection, however, cannot exempt educated Catholics from listening honestly to other systems of belief nor from comparing their beliefs with the findings of science and history and with the personal experience of life (Vatican Council II 1965). For Catholics, therefore, faith and reason are complimentary, not contradictory sources of truth and value (John Paul II 1998b).

Because our ethical discussion of concrete issues is presented within the Catholic value system, we have subtitled this book *A Catholic Theological Analysis*. We define *analysis* as an effort to solve concrete ethical problems in terms of principles rooted in sacred scripture and tested by the experience of individuals and communities motivated by and rooted in faith. We hope that in doing so we are in line with intellectual independence, combined with respect for authority and tradition that, to us, is one of the chief characteristics of a Catholic and Christian ethical system.

GRATITUDE

As in the past, we have been aided in the production of this work by many different medical, nursing, and hospital administrative personnel and ethicists too numerous to mention. We thank them for their willingness to read and critique sections of our book that pertain to their specialties. We also offer our grateful thanks to Mark Kuczewski, Ph.D., director of the Neiswanger Institute for Bioethics and Health Policy at the Stritch School of Medicine, Loyola University, Chicago, who provided support and encouragement for the production of this work; to Catherine Gacek, Robbin Hiller, and Laura Bartosik, also of the Stritch School of Medicine, who calmly and industriously helped as editorial assistants; to Donna Troy of the Catholic Health Association, who generously assisted in the transfer of material between St. Louis and Chicago; to the Mission and Ethics Department of the Catholic Health Association; and to several friends who listened patiently and encouraged us as we discussed the intricacies of our work. In recognizing the patient and generous people who have helped us, we also assume responsibility for any shortcomings in the work.

Abbreviations Used in the Text and in Citations

AA	Alcoholics Anonymous
ADHD	attention deficit/hyperactivity disorder
AHA	American Hospital Association
AHN	assisted hydration and nutrition
AID	artificial insemination donor
AIDS	acquired immunodeficiency syndrome
AIH	artificial insemination by the husband
AMA	American Medical Association
APA	American Psychiatric Association
ART	assisted reproductive technology
CBT	cognitive behavior (or behavioral) therapy
CCBI	Canadian Catholic Bioethics Institute
CCC	*Catechism of the Catholic Church*
CDF	Congregation for the Doctrine of Faith
CHA	Catholic Health Association
CIC	Code of Canon Law
CPE	clinical pastoral education

CT   cognitive therapy

D & C   dilation and curettage

DNA   deoxyribonucleic acid

DSM-IV   *The Diagnostic and Statistical Manual of Mental Disorders, 4th edition*

EAB   Ethics Advisory Board

ECT   electroconvulsive therapy

EEG   electroencephalogram

ERD   *Ethical and Religious Directives for Catholic Health Services*

ESB   electrical stimulation of the brain

FIAMC   World Federation of Catholic Medical Association

GAD   U.S. General Accounting Office

GIFT   gamete intra-fallopian transfer

IRB   institutional review board

IUD   intrauterine device

IVF   in vitro fertilization

JCAHO   Joint Commission for Accreditation of Health Care Organizations

MCS   minimally conscious state

NBAC   National Bioethics Advisory Commission

NCBC   National Catholic Bioethics Center

NCCB   National Conference of Catholic Bishops

NFP   natural family planning

NHBD   non-heart-beating organ donation

NIH   National Institutes of Health

OAR   oocyte assisted reprogramming

OHSR   U.S. Office of Human Services Research

OPTN   Organ Procurement Transplantation Network

PCB   President's Council on Bioethics

PCEMR   President's Commission for the Study of Ethical Problems in Medicine
              and Biomedical and Behavioral Research

PGD   preimplantation genetic diagnosis

PKU   phenylketonuria

PVS   persistent vegetative state

SAMHSA	Substance Abuse and Mental Health Services Administration
SCNT	somatic cell nuclear transfer
UDDA	Uniform Definition of Death Act
USCC	United State Catholic Conference
VS	vegetative state
WHO	World Health Organization

Part I

HEALTH CARE ETHICS AND HUMAN NEEDS

Chapter One

BIOETHICS IN A MULTICULTURAL AGE

OVERVIEW

HEALTH CARE ETHICS ORIGINATED IN THE Christian concern for healing using a medical science developed by the Greeks and advanced by Jews and Muslims. But recently health care has become increasingly secularized, and its ethics is often named more inclusively "bioethics." Current bioethics, however, is fragmented into a variety of ethical methodologies. Because Catholic medical professionals and health care facilities serve persons of various ethical views, and must work in this multicultural environment, it is imperative that Catholics understand the basis of their own Christian ethics of health care well in order to engage in a constructive way with other points of view. Christian ethics of health care has its foundations both in faith and in human reason.

1.1 THE EMERGENCE OF SECULAR BIOETHICS

The rapid medical advances in the last fifty years have raised a multitude of difficult problems in the field of bioethics and have produced an ever-expanding literature on the subject. To understand why these issues are so controversial and to propose effective strategies for their solution, it is first necessary to recognize that in our multicultural age there is no agreement on a common value system. We confront this problem in part I, chapter 1. In chapter 2 we seek a working solution to this basic question before proceeding, in parts II and III, to discuss in detail the main bioethical questions that are now urgent.

The term *bioethics* began to replace the term *pastoral ethics,* or medical ethics, early in 1971, after the biologist Van Rensselaer Potter, in his book *Bioethics: The Bridge to the*

Future, introduced it to include the many new interrelated biological issues arising from life sciences and their social implications (Potter 1971). This terminological change was fostered by the realization that health care decisions are not the monopoly of the medical profession, nor are ethical questions the monopoly of the clergy. New questions are constantly arising, and the media quickly and often sensationally opens them up to public debate. The use of this new term *bioethics* also signaled that new ethical methodologies were becoming influential in these debates, methodologies that were no longer, as they had been formerly, based on religious traditions (Guinan 2001).

In the United States, Catholic hospitals and medical schools, along with some other religiously sponsored health facilities in the United States, play an important role, although as a minority, in the secularly dominated network of such institutions. Secular medical schools seldom, until recently, gave courses on medical ethics. Percival's *Medical Ethics* (Percival 1803), often cited as the first American work on the subject, was hardly more than a treatise on professional etiquette. Although as early as 1847 the American Medical Association (AMA) adopted its Code of Medical Ethics, this too did little more than provide guidelines against malpractice suits.

As the term bioethics came into general use, secular centers for this newly secularized field began to spring up such as The Hastings Center, founded in 1969 at Hastings on Hudson, New York. In 1971 the Kennedy Institute for Ethics was established at Georgetown University. These two institutes were originally under Catholic influences but soon opted for a secularist approach (Stevens 2000). To respond to this situation, The Catholic Bishops of the United States issued its *Ethical and Religious Directives for Catholic Health Care Facilities* (ERD) in 1971. In 1973 the Catholic Hospital (now Health) Association sponsored the foundation of the John XXIII Medical-Moral Research and Education Center in St. Louis (since 1997, the National Catholic Bioethics Center [NCBC], Philadelphia) that provides consultation and workshops on bioethics for Catholic bishops and others. Today there are numerous such centers and publications, religious or secularist in mission. It was with this widening of the field that controversy about ethical theory and methodology became prominent.

The literature on bioethics is now enormous and in large part purely secular in orientation. In the past, Catholic health care professionals and facilities seldom had to face this division of views, but today the formation of "joint ventures" between Catholic and non-Catholic medical facilities, the education of professionals in secular institutions, the spread of health care plans with general membership, and the promotion of ecumenical openness by Vatican II have forced Catholics to confront this ethical diversity (Hamel 2002; Kenny 1997).

Today's secular humanism originated in the Age of Enlightenment in the eighteenth century (Ashley 1996a, 2000b). In Europe the religious wars between Catholics and Protestants and among Protestant denominations in the seventeenth century had disillusioned many of the intellectual elite with Christianity and led at first to a widespread skepticism. To replace Christianity, whether Catholic or Protestant, certain thinkers began to propose a "religion of reason" that would replace dogmas of faith. Thus they no longer placed their hopes in God, but in the power of natural science and its technological applications, which had made such remarkable advances in the seventeenth century.

This co-option of science by the Enlightenment, because it is only one perspective on science, can be called "Scientism" and is characterized by its claims that natural science must be "value free," a conception that was foreign to the founders of modern science such as Galileo, Newton, and Harvey, who always supposed that the ultimate purpose of science is "to manifest the glory of God," the Creator. John Paul II, in his encyclical *Fides et ratio* (1998c, no. 88), characterizes this view as follows:

> *[S]cientism* . . . is the philosophical notion which refuses to admit the validity of forms of knowledge other than those of the positive sciences; and it relegates religious, theological, ethical and aesthetic knowledge to the realm of mere fantasy. . . . Science would thus be poised to dominate all aspects of human life through technological progress. The undeniable triumphs of scientific research and contemporary technology have helped to propagate a scientistic outlook, which now seems boundless, given its inroads into different cultures and the radical changes it has brought. . . . And since it leaves no space for the critique offered by ethical judgement, the scientistic mentality has succeeded in leading many to think that if something is technically possible it is therefore morally admissible.

A worldview without a value system, however, would not have satisfied the determination of the Enlightenment to replace religion as a guide to life. Consequently, while one face of secular humanism is value-free Scientism, the other face is Romanticism, a movement that sought to create or construct values aesthetically, much as a work of fine art is created. This dichotomy between the objectivity of value-free Scientism and the subjectivity of value-creative Romanticism is reflected in the modern university by what C. P. Snow (1999) called "the two cultures," the "hard" sciences versus the "soft" humanities. Thus it is to the humanities that ethics is assigned, and some medical schools are now giving courses in what are called "the medical humanities" that interrelate medicine with history, literature, and ethics. No wonder, then, that our created value systems have become so diverse! To understand this diversity of current secular bioethics, however, it is first necessary to look back at its roots in an older tradition. Only when these roots are understood can these divergent ethical systems be compared and evaluated.

1.2 THE FOUNDATIONS OF THE ETHICS OF HEALTH CARE

The medical profession as we know it today originated in Greco-Roman culture. The first known code of medical ethics is the Hippocratic oath to which most physicians still commit themselves. This oath probably originated with the pagan Pythagorean sect, but was transmitted to our age in Christianized form (Edelstein 1943). Roy Porter, editor of *The Cambridge Illustrated History of Medicine*, writes, "It is no accident that the triumph of the Christian faith (after Constantine made Christianity legal in 313) brought the rise of nursing and the invention of hospital as an institution of health care" (2001, 213; cf. also Kelly 1979). The Christian religious orders founded the first hospitals, and Christian theologians developed an ethics of health care as a feature of medical traditions to which Jews (Zohar 1997) and Muslims (Daar and Khitamy 2000) had made important contributions.

In the Bible two contrasting yet related ethical methodologies are evident. In the Old Testament the dominant ethics is that of the Torah, or Law, contained in its first five books (Harrelson 1980; Kaiser 1983; Birch 1991; Janzen 1994). It is of the *deontological* (Greek *deontos*, duty) type, because it chiefly evaluates behavior ethically as to whether it is dutiful and obedient to the laws of God revealed to Moses. Because, however, in current writing the term *deontology* is understood in different ways, we will henceforth refer to this ethical methodology as "duty ethics." It is also called "voluntarism" because it bases moral obligation on the will (the Latin *voluntas*) of some lawgiver, either God or some legitimate human lawgiver. This type of ethics, still evident in Jewish and Muslim works on bioethics (Feldman 1986; Meier 1986; Rosner 2001; Zohar 1997; Kenny 1997), can be called "divine command ethics."

In other books of the Old Testament, however, a different type of ethical wisdom is elaborated. In the wisdom literature (Murphy 1990), an ethics is presented that is based largely on ordinary human experience of what kinds of behavior lead to a happy life and what kinds lead to unhappiness. Furthermore, the biblical prophets deepen this experience accessible to human reason by teaching that no merely external practice of laws is truly moral unless motivated by genuine love of God and neighbor. This makes evident that the principal weakness of any legalistic, duty methodology is that it does not give any ultimate reason why the will of the lawgiver is right or wrong, and hence how the laws promulgated by authority are to be reasonably interpreted and applied to special circumstances. Even God, as Job complained, sometimes seems to be unfair. Laws are useful and indeed necessary guides for our ethical decisions, but we must still ask whether a law is really just before we can ethically obey it. If we obey it on trust, as sometimes we need to do, then we must at least know the legislator to be morally trustworthy. Therefore the more profound type of ethics is one that is based not on law made by the will of the legislator but on the motivation of the law and its observance. This is called *teleological* (the Greek *telos*, goal) ethics, which judges the morality of a decision in terms of the relation of an action taken as a means to happiness, the true goal of life. Just as we use the term "duty ethics" in preference to "deontology" to avoid certain confusions, we will henceforth speak not of "teleology" but of "ends–means ethics."

Jesus as Model

As shown in the New Testament, Jesus Christ, who for Christians is not only the wisest of teachers but also the best model of human living, faced these two views of ethics (Schnackenburg 1973; Schrage 1988; Farley and Cahill 1995). During his time and in later Orthodox Judaism, the rabbis, although they certainly understood the importance of ethical motivation, saw themselves primarily as interpreters of the Mosaic Law (Torah) in its complicated provisions. In the Torah, moral and ritual laws tended to be regarded as equally important, because ritual observance was thought to enforce ethical observance. Jesus, however, taught in the line of the prophets. He by no means permitted violation of the Mosaic Law (Mt 5:17–20), but put far more emphasis on its ends–means motivation. God's purpose in creating human beings was to share his love with them, and he asks us to return that love by loving our neighbor. Thus what is central to ethics is not just obedience to law, but love. Jesus in a special way manifested this by his miraculous healing of the sick. Hence, in the Christian tradition, health care ethics, while not neglecting moral laws or norms, should be principally and profoundly an ends–means, love ethics. This does not mean, however, that it is altruistic in the sense that the moral person must neglect his or her own happiness, as Jesus said, "Love your neighbor *as you love yourself*" (Mt 22:39). Rather it is a social ethics that teaches that no individual can be truly happy except by sharing that happiness in a truly happy community.

In this book we have preferred the term *health care ethics* and subtitled it "A Catholic Theological Analysis" precisely because for us the ultimate ethical norm is not a set of ethical rules or values but a historical person, Jesus Christ—God become truly human. Therefore he is our model of what it is to be human and the only source of grace that can empower us to overcome our sinful inhumanity and in him become truly human as God created us to be. Thus, in a search for consensus with all those of goodwill, we join with fellow Christians and with other religious people in prayer, meditation, fraternal dialogue, and cooperation, but we can also honestly join with secular humanists to make the world more truly human. To lose hope in the possibility of this union of heart and mind in Christ (1 Cor 1:10) would be to lose hope in Jesus as savior of all humanity.

In the first millennium of the church, ethical questions were generally treated separately in biblical commentaries, sermons, penitential guides for confessors, or in canon law rather than in systematic treatises. Yet the great Western church doctor, St. Augustine of Hippo (354–430 A.D.), in his many works of different types proposed an organized ethical theory that is of the ends–means type and centered on Christian love (O'Donnell and Fitzgerald 1999). At the same time Augustine, in a way more realistic than previous theologians of the Eastern and Western traditions, addressed the problem of why God's good creation seems so distorted by sin. Augustine's writings on the doctrine of original sin and the consequent need of divine grace for the restoration of the creation made it clear why ethical decisions are often so difficult. His teaching had little influence in the Eastern Church, but it became the basis of all subsequent theology in the West. After the division of the Eastern Orthodox Churches from the Catholic Church under the Bishop of Rome in 1054, the further development of moral theology was largely the work of the medieval universities in Western Europe, with their three professional schools for clergy, lawyers, and physicians.

Thus it was in this type of Christian theological ethics that the rising medical profession was first trained. In the thirteenth century this theological ethics received its most systematic treatment by the Dominican, St. Thomas Aquinas (1225–1274; see Weisheipl 1974; Torrell 1996; O'Meara 1997), who used the ethical writings of the ancient Greek Aristotle (384–322 B.C.), a pioneer in scientific biology, embryology, and psychology, to provide a strictly end-means system of ethics. At the same time, he assimilated to this theory elements derived from the ethics of Plato and of the Greek and Roman Stoics. In particular he adopted the Stoic term *natural law,* meaning accessible to human reason, but gave it an ends–means interpretation. He also made use of both Jewish and Islamic thought. Thus Aquinas synthesized the Greek ethics based on reason with the New Testament ethics based on revelation and pictured Jesus Christ, the Healer, as the perfect historical model of both human and divine virtue.

In the late Middle Ages, however, this synthesis began to fragment as a result of disputes between the university theologians and the university philosophers who were committed to the interpretation of Greek thought given by the Spanish Muslim scholar Averroes (Ibn Rushd, 1126–1198; Rubenstein 2003, 20). The central issue concerned whether God created and governed the world freely or fatalistically, which had major ethical implications, because human freedom and hence human ethical behavior are only a participation in God's freedom. The theologians of the Franciscan order, beginning with John Duns Scotus (1266–1308) and more radically with the nominalist movement headed by William of Ockham (1280–1344) vigorously defended the freedom of God. Unfortunately, in defending God's freedom, these writers thought it necessary to adopt an ethical *voluntarism* according to which morality is simply faithful obedience to God's freely willed laws, a divine command ethic, or religious legalism (Gilson 1955; Wolter 1997; Maurer 1999). How extreme this could be is shown by Ockham's assertion that if God were to command us to hate him then to love him would be a sin!

Luther and Calvin

Luther, the father of the Protestant Reformation, who was educated as a nominalist, experienced the Law of God as a crushing imposition that tempted him to rebel against God. Only when he read in St. Paul of justification by "faith alone" was he reassured that Christ had paid the price for our sins (Lohse 1999), and what remains for us is simply to accept that vicarious atonement in faith.

Yet the authentic Catholic doctrine, which nominalism had obscured, is that God's Law is not an imposed burden but a loving guide on the path toward happiness with him. Jesus has indeed atoned for our sins, but by doing so has also made us a "new creation" (2 Cor 5:17; Gal 6:15), so that we live by a "faith working through love" (Gal 5:6; Jas 2:14–17). Thus by grace we truly cooperate in faith with Christ's saving work, so that St. Paul can say, "Now I rejoice in my sufferings for your sake, and in my flesh I am filling up what is lacking in the afflictions of Christ on behalf of his body, which is the church" (Col 1:24).

Calvin, by stressing even more than Luther had done the sovereign freedom of God and the corruption of human reason by original sin, pushed voluntarism in ethics still further (Bouwsma 1988). Hence Protestant theologians have seldom attempted to develop an ends–means type of ethics. As the author of the article on "Moral Theology" in *The Oxford Dictionary of the Christian Church* (Cross and Livingstone 1997, 298), puts it, "Protestants have tended to dissociate themselves from attempt to produce detailed systems of duties binding on all Christians, on the ground that good works are a free and grateful response to the completed work of justification in Christ. Thus for Martin Luther, Christians are freed from self-concern implicit in 'works-righteousness' to serve their neighbors in love." Yet among Protestants the tendency to rely on ethics exclusively on biblical precepts has led to a moral rigorism that leads them to accuse Catholics of moral laxism as a result of their reliance on forgiveness of sins in the confessional.

In reply to such accusations, Catholic theologians in the period after the Council of Trent encouraged the laity to use the sacrament of confession more often and more conscientiously. To facilitate this, many very detailed manuals for confessors were published that included numerous questions about the ethics of health care (Kelly 1979). Members of the new religious Society of Jesus, the Jesuits, wrote the most widely employed of the manuals for confessors. Although committed to the theology of St. Thomas Aquinas, these authors were influenced by the attempt of Francesco Suarez, S.J. (1548–1617), to synthesize Thomism with the thought of John Duns Scotus. Thus their manuals had a markedly voluntaristic and legalist tendency.

Hence arose the long "moral systems controversy" between the Dominicans loyal to Aquinas and the Jesuits loyal to Suarez. The debated issue was how to resolve a difficult moral decision when the application of a moral law was doubtful. The voluntarists based their position on the principle that "a doubtful law does not oblige," because it is the obligation of the lawmaker to make his will clear. Thus one can conscientiously prefer an easier interpretation of the law if that interpretation can be shown to be at least probably true (probabilism). Dominicans, trained not in a duty ethics but in an ends–means ethics, argued that on the contrary one should follow the interpretation that was the more probable (probabiliorism), as the purpose of law is to guide us in choosing the best means to arrive at our true goal. If you want to get somewhere, why take a path that will less probably get you there?

St. Alphonsus Ligouri, C.Ss.R., founder of the Redemptorist order, finally calmed this dispute in his famous revision of a popular Jesuit manual. His compromise was to accept probabilism but to insist that the more lenient interpretation of the law could be followed only if it has "solid" probability, that is, is supported by several "standard authors" generally recognized as faithful to church teaching. This position has prevailed in practice, but the Catholic Church has never passed judgment on the theoretical issue between duty ethics and ends–means ethics. Since Vatican II, however, the diversity of the proposed revisions of duty ethics makes it difficult to say who is a "standard author."

Up until the rise of modern science in the seventeenth century that was to make modern medicine and health care possible, it seemed sufficient to treat questions of medical ethics in various contexts, such as the treatment in manuals for confessors of the fifth, sixth, and ninth commandments. Although as early as 1477, the Dominican archbishop Antoninus of Florence, in his *Summa Theologiae Moralis* (Kelly 1979), had provided a special section on the ethics of the medical profession. It was only in 1621 that the physician of Pope Innocent X, Paolo Zacchia, provided a model for later special treatises on the subject in his three volume *Medical-Legal Questions*. In 1666 the Belgian theologian Michael Boudewyns in his *Ventilabrum Medico-theologicum* further developed this kind of treatise, and numerous similar works continued to be written through the eighteenth and nineteenth centuries, culminating in the very influential four volume *Pastoral Medicine* of Giuseppe Antonelli in 1891 (fifth edition, 1932).

In the United States, the first of these special treatises to appear in English was *Pastoral Medicine,* by German Karl Capelmann (1878), to be followed by such American works as Gerald Kelly, S.J., *Medico-Moral Problems* (1958) and Charles J. McFadden, O.S.A., *Medical Ethics* (1967; cf. Kelly 1979). A need for such treatises also began to be felt in Protestant circles, and Joseph Fletcher, in his 1954 *Morals and Medicine,* proposed an approach based on his theory of situation ethics that will be explained later. In 1970, Paul Ramsey, in his more substantial *The Patient as Person: Explorations in Medical Ethics,* acknowledged that he had been strongly influenced by the Catholic tradition. There are also important Jewish publications on the subject, notably by Rabbi David Feldman, *Health and Medicine in the Jewish Tradition* (1986), and Fred Rosner, M.D., an expert on the great medieval physician, philosopher, and theologian Maimonides, in his *Medicine in the Bible and Talmud* (1994) and *Biomedical Ethics and Jewish Law* (2001). Only recently have writings on Muslim (Kenny 1997), Indian, and Chinese health care ethics and those of indigenous peoples such as those of Africa and, in the United States, of Native Americans begun to appear in English.

1.3 CURRENT METHODOLOGIES IN BIOETHICS

The current methods of reaching bioethical conclusions may be divided into duty ethics and ends–means ethics. We shall treat the systems in each method separately.

The Varieties of Duty Ethics

Because, as we have seen, bioethics in its present secular form originated in the Christian tradition, and in that tradition there was always a tension between duty ethics and ends–means ethics, it is no surprise that this same tension is still present in current bioethics. We must therefore consider the current forms of duty ethics and the current forms of ends–means ethics. René Descartes (1596–1650) is called the "Father of Modern Philosophy," but, as a believing Catholic, he was not a secular humanist. It was the most influential Enlightenment thinker, Immanuel Kant (1724–1804), who proposed a duty ethics independent of revealed religion known as formalism, quite different from the religious legalism of the Old Testament tradition (Guyer 1992; Kant 1999; Timmons 2002).

He had carefully considered the controversy between biologists who reduced living organisms simply to their chemical parts and other biologists who saw them as functionally designed. He resolved this dilemma by supposing that it is the biologists themselves who in a creative way project such purposeful design on the biological data (Zumbach 1984). Similarly, he thought that we cannot know human values as intrinsic to external acts, but instead project them on such acts. Hence, for Kantians, it is our preferences that provide us with values, but these preferences must not be based on desires, but on pure reason. Influenced by his Protestant background and perhaps by ancient Stoicism, Kant emphasized the irrationality of human emotions and of subjective self-interest and thereby insisted that behavior be purely altruistic, not motivated by desire for one's own happiness. Thus, for Kant, duty ethics was irreconcilable with an ends–means ethics (*eudaimonism*, Greek for an ethics of happiness).

Hence, if these values are to form a consistent system convincing to all reasonable persons, they must be checked against certain rational standards of a purely logical, formal kind. These standards must be grounded in what Kant called the "categorical imperative," namely, "One should oneself follow those norms and only those norms that one would be willing for others to follow," or as he sometimes puts it, "Treat others as ends, not means." For example, the reason I should not tell lies is that I would prefer that others would not lie to me.

Kant

Unlike most voluntarists who thought of morality as obedience to laws imposed by the authority of another, Kant urged the categorical imperative precisely because he thought it freed a person from obeying others (heteronomy) and thus gave each person moral autonomy in following his or her own conscience. In current bioethics, the theory of justice developed by a confessed Kantian, John Rawls (1921–2002), is highly influential. This theory revolves around the adaptation of two fundamental principles of justice that are required, Rawls claims, to guarantee a just and morally acceptable society (Rawls 1971). The first principle guarantees the right of each person to have the most extensive basic liberty compatible with the liberty of others. The second principle states that social and economic positions are to be to everyone's advantage and open to all. A key problem for Rawls is to show how such principles could be universally adopted. Hence he introduces the concept of a theoretical "veil of ignorance" in which all the "players" in the social game would be placed in a situation that is called the "original position." Having only a general knowledge about the facts of "life and society," each player is to make a "rationally prudential choice" concerning the kind of social institution with which they would enter into contract. By denying the players any specific information about themselves forces them to adopt a generalized point of view that bears a strong resemblance to that of Kant. Critics of Rawls have pointed out that such a method, although it aims at altruism, actually accentuates the individualism of modern society, in which the equality of persons obscures the unique contribution each member of a community makes to the common good.

Moreover, Kantian duty ethics is open to serious criticism because it is purely formal, that is, it states the logical form of moral rules but not their specific content. It is true that he proposed four applications forbidding suicide and lying, and commanding the development of one's talents and striving to help others, but his arguments for the first two are dubious and the positive commandments remain entirely abstract. Hence, after Kant but contrary to his view, ethicists found that in order to descend from Kant's universal, very abstract principles to actual moral decisions in concrete cases they were forced again to resort to Romanticism, with its aesthetic construction of values on the basis of essentially subjective and emotional preferences. This became the ethical methodology called emotivism. Each culture or community or even each individual constructs a lifestyle based on certain emotional attitudes of approval or disapproval, which then becomes the standard for ethical judgment of what is good or bad behavior. Though Kant distrusted the emotions, he admired the work of Jean-Jacques Rousseau (1712–1778), who argued that most people have naturally good emotional instincts when these have not been distorted by bad education.

A British friend of Rousseau, the empiricist philosopher David Hume (1711–1776), against whose skepticism Kant defended the claims of science to objective truth, supported emotivism for another reason, namely, that it is a logical fallacy ("the naturalist fallacy") to argue from "is" or factual statements to "ought" or value statements. The views of both Rousseau and Hume have greatly influenced American culture. When politicians appeal to the "wisdom of the American people," they are assuming with Rousseau that the moral instincts of most people must be sound, or with Hume that public opinion or preference is the only criterion of morality. In debates about medical ethics, it is not uncommon to meet physicians who think that the decency of reputable doctors is the best way to settle any ethical question. Others settle the abortion question by saying, "It is legal, but most good doctors don't like to perform abortions." The difficulty with this approach is that it provides no method of public, objective discussion, but leaves problems to rhetoric and prejudice. Whose instincts are sound? Whose feelings are "decent"? Today we are haunted by the recollection of how the very decent German nation supported Hitler's genocide (Lifton 1986).

Thus Kantian formalism paradoxically reduces to emotivism when it has to provide concrete values or practical rules, as in the example given, one refuses to lie only because one does not like to be lied to. The problem with this is that, although I may have negative feelings about others lying to me, I may very well have positive feelings about lying to them! To meet such criticisms, however, Kant also formulated the categorical imperative as "Always treat other persons as ends not means." While most ethicists would accept this principle, Kant fails to explain why this is morally obligatory. Do we only respect other persons because we have fellow feelings for them, or because they are objectively of great value?

That Kant's duty ethics is very influential in current bioethics is evident from the fact that, as bioethics became secularized, the most widely used textbook in the field, Tom L.

Beauchamp and James F. Childress, *Principles of Biomedical Ethics* (2001), was based on what is often called principalism (Evans 2000). According to this theory, the categorical imperative to follow the course of action that one wants everyone else to follow is the supreme principle of ethics. Concrete moral decisions, however, cannot be deduced form this supreme principle without certain "middle principles" that are not as concrete as actual cases but that may at least give consistency to concrete ethical judgments. This reflects Kant's rejection of the older correspondence theory of truth as "conformity of the mind to things," because he believed the nature of things (*Ding an sich*) is inaccessible to us. Consequently he replaced this definition by a consistency or coherence definition of truth.

To avoid the lack of ethical foundations from which concrete ethical norms can be deduced, however, Beauchamp and Childress propose four "middle principles." These are (1) autonomy, the right of persons to care for themselves; (2) nonmalfeasance, that is, "do no harm"; (3) beneficence, or seeking the patient's benefit; and (4) justice to all concerned (to which can also be added the special trust required by the professional-patient relationship). In a later edition of their influential work, the authors, without abandoning these principles, concede to critics of principalism that these principles are so abstract as to admit of very different interpretations. Hence they now propose a more "eclectic" approach using a variety of methodologies. The contractualism of another eminent bioethicist, Robert M. Veatch (1981), which grounds moral obligation simply on the wills of the contracting parties to make and keep their contract, is also a duty ethics. Finally, positivism maintains that the only norms of morality are law and custom and hence is strictly voluntaristic because for it morality depends on the will of the legislator or of the majority.

Casuistry

Because such abstract principles can in application be so differently interpreted, others, such as Albert Jonsen, Baruch Brody, Stephen Toulmin, and James Keenan, S.J., supplement principalism with casuistry. Such a casuistic methodology was long traditional in the Catholic Church in the post-Trent manuals already mentioned. It begins not with generalities but with concrete cases from which it is hoped a better agreement on general norms can be worked out. Yet, in a pluralistic community, it is precisely on certain concrete issues such as contraception and abortion that diversity is most conflictual. The existentialism so popular a few years ago has little influence in bioethics. Existentialism is, however, like casuistry, a kind of act duty ethics in contrast to the other forms of rule duty ethics we have mentioned because it did not propose any general norms. It pushed Kant's notion of autonomy to its limits by claiming that by our free acts we produce ourselves. This notion was formulated as "the priority of existence over essence," that is, our acts, because their reality makes us what we are. Of course, this is true in a sense because our acts form our character; however, the idea is absurd if it denies that our acts are rooted in our nature and our needs.

It may seem strange to group with the previously mentioned duty ethicians Germain Grisez (1983, 1993, 1997) and his colleagues Joseph Boyle and John Finnis (1987), William E. May (1995), and John Finnis (1980), as they are staunch defenders of Catholic orthodoxy and present their methodology as a refinement of the ends–means ethics of St. Thomas Aquinas. Yet we agree with Kevin M. Wildes, S.J., who in his *Moral Acquaintances: Methodology in Bioethics* (2000) sees in these authors' methodology a significant resemblance to Kantian principalism, because it emphasizes the autonomous, deductive structure of ethics, the need for middle principles, and a consistency in ethical judgment attained by a harmonizing (weighing or balancing) of values.

Grisez does not agree with Aquinas that every free and deliberate human act must intend an ultimate goal. He agrees with Aristotle and Aquinas that "Do good and avoid evil" is the first formal principle of ethics, stating that all human acts should aim at "happiness." However, he prefers the term *integral human fulfillment* or *human flourishing* as the goal of ethical activity. Aristotle and Aquinas, for reasons we will present in chapter 2, held that the content of this formal goal—happiness—is chiefly the "contemplation of truth." Grisez considers this too elitist and Aquinas's acceptance of it too clerical, because most people engage in an active life in which contemplation can play only a relatively minor role. Moreover, he holds that Aquinas's emphasis on the virtues fails to provide the middle terms needed to pass from the first formal principle to concrete moral judgments. Hence, instead of Aquinas's one ultimate end, he proposes seven "incommensurable goods" as such middle terms. Thus this system can be designated plurifinalism, although its proponents do not use that term. Three of these incommensurable goods are "substantive": (1) "Life itself, including health, physical, integrity, safety and the handing on of life to new persons"; (2) "knowledge of various forms of truth and appreciation of various forms of beauty or excellence"; and (3) "activities of skillful work and of place, which in their very performance enrich those who do them." The other four are "reflexive" (also "existential" or "moral"): (4) "Self integration, which is harmony among all the parts of a person which can be engaged in freely chosen action"; (5) "practical reasonableness or authenticity, which is harmony among moral reflections, free choices, and their execution"; (6) "justice and friendship, which are aspects of the interpersonal communion of good persons freely choosing to act in harmony with one another"; (7) "religion or holiness, which is harmony with God, found in the agreement of human individual and communal free choices with God's will" (1983, 124, 205–22).

Incommensurable Goods

Plurifinalists think that because these goods are "incommensurable" they furnish an irrefutable defense against those who deny that there are concrete moral norms that can never be morally violated, because each of these ends is absolute, and acts contrary to them are intrinsically evil. Yet, because they are incommensurable, these seven goods cannot be ranked hierarchically, as Aristotle and Aquinas did, by their subordination to the supreme good of truth (contemplation). Thus plurifinalism maintains the unity and consistency of moral life through the "harmony" among the three substantive incommensurable goods established by the four reflexive goods. Because Grisez holds that these incommensurable goods are self-evident (Grisez 1983, 195–96) and hence do not depend on an anthropological analysis of human nature, his theory, like that of Kant, is marked by a certain apriorism. Moreover, this multiplicity of unranked goods makes it difficult to class his theory as a true ends–means ethics, because in actual concrete decision the reconciliation of these seen goods remains so problematic.

Thus if we ask what are the strengths and weaknesses of duty ethics, we can say first that for much of our lives and for most people moral decisions are made in terms of laws or norms learned from their parents, their peers, or the culture in which they live. It would be too much to expect people to work out a detailed value system for themselves. This, of course, raises a question about the practicality of Kant's dismissal of heteronomous ethics. While ultimately every person must make her or his own decisions, can these ever be entirely autonomous, as we all have to rely on the guidance of others? Second, duty ethics provides a consistent and rationally ordered pattern of behavior within which particular decisions can be made to fit changing circumstances. But Kant, under the influence of Descartes and Leibniz, was fundamentally an idealist in philosophy and hence thought truth can be attained only by a deduction from principles known a priori rather than inductively from experience. Critics, however, point out that Kant's universal norms and the middle premises provided by principalism or plurifinalism are so abstract and ambiguous as to give little real guidance in decision. Nor can the use of casuistry remedy this, because a bad judgment made in one case can then give precedence for many more bad judgments, as we so often see in our courts.

The fundamental weakness of duty ethics separated from a grounding in an ends–means ethics is that it makes morality dependent on the will of the lawmaker rather than on the intrinsic character of the act prescribed. Of course, when the lawgiver is God we know that his will is always good and governed by his wisdom. But God's law, whether known through his creation or by revelation, has to be interpreted by humans who frequently err, and human laws are often based on the interests of the lawgiver, not on the interests of those who must obey them. Even when based on goodwill, they can be foolish. Moreover, the history of the probabilist controversy shows that all forms of voluntarism tend to generate unsolvable controversies over whether moral laws are to be applied strictly (rigorism) or leniently (laxism).

The Varieties of Ends–Means Ethics

As the criticism of the dominant duty ethics of principalism in secular bioethics has grown in recent years, more attention is being given to various forms of ends–means ethics. An ends–means methodology in ethics seeks to justify or reject an action, not simply by some accepted code of right and wrong but by determining whether it is an effective or a self-defeating means to the end or goal of true human fulfillment in the community. Some persons choose as their goal in life some kind of illusory self-fulfillment that when it is attained leaves them miserable, such as the man who devotes all his energies to financial success only to discover he is rich, lonely, and afraid of death. Yet even when we have chosen the true goal in life, a happiness that is authentic, we still have the right to choose means that will really achieve it and avoid those that promise to achieve it but will ultimately fail.

Two very different schools of thought whose debates are responsible for many of the hottest controversies in bioethics today use an ends–means ethic. One of these schools, utilitarianism is so popular that some identify all ends–means theories with utilitarianism. Utilitarians believe that the goal of human life is maximum pleasure, or at least a state of affairs that produces more satisfactory consequences than unsatisfactory ones. Similar to utilitarianism but more vague is consequentialism, which does not attempt to provide any specific criterion of what is a positive or negative value but simply says that an act should be judged as good if its positive consequences exceed the negative ones. Both utilitarians and consequentialists attempt to set up norms based on their weighing of positive and negative values in certain kinds of acts, that is, they have a rule type of ethics that provides general norms such as "Thou shalt not kill" as prima facie rules that generally oblige but admit exceptions in some circumstances. To avoid reducing their system to plurifinalism, they contend that the supreme principle of ethics is not merely my maximum satisfaction in life, but "the greatest good for the greatest number." But there are also ethicists who deny any universal ethical rules and therefore hold that every action must be judged in its unique context and advocate a purely act ethics. A pioneer medical ethicist, Joseph Fletcher (1954), argued for a situationism that had only one ethical rule, "Do what is most loving in the circumstances," but he was never able to define what "most loving" means in practice.

The strength of such kinds of duty ethics is their pragmatism, which enables it to be empirically tested by actual results. This makes it very appealing to those who live in the very pragmatic American culture. The weakness of these kinds of duty ethics is that they can be manipulated to justify almost any action because they provide no objective way to measure the good and bad consequences of an action except the pleasure it gives. Yet what seems greatly pleasurable may, like heroin addiction, lead to great pain. Nor is this difficulty removed by including long-term as well as short-term satisfaction, because the long-term satisfactions to be gained are far from predictable or certain. Jeremy Bentham (1748–1832), the English philosopher famous for his defense of this system, believed it possible to establish a "unit of satisfaction" and thus measure satisfaction much as we weigh economic values in units of dollars and cents. But how can we find a common quantitative unit of measurement for the qualitatively very different kinds of "satisfactions" that make up a truly fulfilled life? Can I weigh the price of friendship, success in my work, and good health one against another? Can we sacrifice the life of one innocent person to save the lives of ten others? How in medical ethics can we predict whether the patient's future health will give enough pleasure to outweigh the pain of surgery?

Proportionalism

Proportionalism is another widely influential ethical theory that also claims to be "teleological" and is often criticized as a form of utilitarianism or consequentialism, although its proponents deny this. Proportionalism was developed by Josef Fuchs, Peter Knauer, and Bruno Schüller and defended in the United States by Richard McCormick (1973). Similarly, Bernard Häring (1976), in the moderate voluntarist tradition of St. Alphonsus Ligouri, sought to find pastoral exceptions to what seemed to be too rigid moral norms, such as the condemnation of contraception in all cases by Paul VI in *Humanae vitae*, by invoking the legal principle of epieikeia or "lenient exception." Similarly, his student, Charles E. Curran (1979), proposed a "theory of moral compromise," according to which actions seemingly contrary to classical ethics might in exceptional circumstances become objectively good. This proportionalist methodology reduces all ethical decisions to the single fundamental principle of proportionate reason (or principle of preference): "Do only those acts that have a proportionate reason in their favor." Hence they deny they are utilitarians or consequentialists, because they do not simply weigh the good and bad consequences of an act, but more inclusively weigh all its "values" and "disvalues." Yet in common with utilitarianism and consequentialism, proportionalists reject the traditional view that some kinds of concrete acts can *never* serve as means to true happiness and hence are *intrinsically evil* and are forbidden by absolute (exceptionless) moral norms. They reject such absolute norms because they maintain that it is always possible to imagine unusual circumstances in which what would ordinarily be an evil act can be justified, especially when performed for a good intention. For example, some proportionalists argue that in certain circumstances and with good intention contraception and even abortion are morally good, because they are done with a good intention in order to achieve positive values that outweigh the disvalues of the act.

In the encyclical *Veritatis splendor* (1993), Pope John Paul II rejected proportionalism as contrary to the Catholic tradition (no. 79) and declared that there are some actions that are intrinsically evil, that are morally wrong no matter who performs them and no matter what the circumstances. "If acts are intrinsically evil a good intention or particular circumstances can diminish their evil, but they cannot remove it" (no. 82). Yet some proportionalists still claim that the Pope misunderstood their position (Selling and Jans 1995). They continue to deny the validity of concrete negative, exceptionless moral norms, the essential point that John Paul II insisted on, and allege that their position is based on the teaching of St. Thomas Aquinas. We will discuss this contention further in chapter 2.

After John Paul II's decisive rejection of proportionalism, today there is a growing interest among Catholic theologians in developing an ethics not merely as a method of moral decision but also of character formation, under the name of "virtue ethics." Although plurifinalism recognizes that good moral character is formed by the virtues, it regards virtue theory as secondary in ethics, because it is alleged that it is of little help in providing the middle principles needed for actual decision making (Grisez 1983, 58–61, 192–95). Nevertheless, virtue theory, although it has not as yet greatly influenced bioethics, will surely play an important role in its future development, because professional codes cannot keep pace with the rapid advance of medical technologies. Hence the application of bioethics to actual medical practice is more and more in the hands of professionals who alone are acquainted with the complexities of these new situations. If they lack moral integrity such applications will be seriously at fault. Furthermore, in preventive medicine, as individuals take more and more responsibility for their own health care, their need for virtue in making these decisions will also increase.

The Need for Virtue

The freedom we all have to make good decisions in any particular situation is not the same as the ability to do this consistently and in especially difficult circumstances. For that we need experience and discipline that produce character or "virtue." We form "good" character by acting according to ethical principles or norms based on the needs or goods of the human person, as these are determined objectively, not simply by our own feelings or by the imposed will of a lawmaker. It is difficult to see, however, how a virtue theory can by itself constitute a complete methodology for ethics. Character can be vicious as well as virtuous. Hence the study of the virtues presupposes a methodology that can distinguish between what is virtuous and what is vicious (Porter 1990). The plurifinalists can be criticized for minimizing the role of the virtues in ethical theory, but they are surely correct in saying that virtue theory cannot substitute for criteria of moral discrimination. One cannot help but suspect that the present popularity of virtue theory derives from the desire of some Catholic ethicists to find a substitute for the now condemned proportionalism (Connors and McCormick 1998). They formerly favored proportionalism as a way of relaxing what they consider the overly rigid moral teachings of the Church. Now, by emphasizing "virtue" and "values" instead of decision making, they hope to minimize the obligation of absolute negative norms. A sound virtue theory, however, will deal with how to acquire skills in applying these norms in a consistent and intelligent way that takes fully into account the circumstances of an act without using them as an excuse for fudging the norms, including those that admit of no exceptions. In chapter 2 we will present what we believe to be a sound virtue theory of the ends–means that can be called prudential personalism, because it is grounded in the innate needs of the human person and it judges the morality of concrete human acts by the virtue of prudence.

Liberationism used certain social categories derived from Marxist ethics but claimed a primary grounding in biblical theology rather than philosophy because it took as its historical paradigm the Exodus of the Jews from slavery in Egypt (CDF 1984, 1986; Boff 1987; Gutiérrez 1988; Rowland 1999). It can be considered an ends–means ethics with a strong emphasis on the common social good as an intermediate goal to the ultimate end. What characterizes it, however, is the principle of "the preferential option for the poor and oppressed" that is so often excluded from the common good. Unfortunately this emphasis by its proponents sometimes seems to minimize the fact that this common good consists not just in economic well-being and social freedom but even more in truth. Moreover, it sometimes accepts questionable political and revolutionary means to economic justice. Closely related to this liberationism are Black liberation (Cone 2000) and feminist ethics, which differ from it only in that they are concerned in a special way with "oppressed" African Americans or with women. Feminist bioethics is extensively developed in the literature, although in quite diverse ways, some writers claiming that women's experience has produced attitudes of caring that have been largely neglected, others stressing health problems unique to women, and others preferring to argue that women's welfare is neglected by a male dominated society without stereotyping these interests as peculiarly feminine (Wolf 1996; Donchin and Purdy 1999; Curran, Farley, and McCormick 1996).

The ethical views of analytic philosophers, who during the last half of the twentieth century predominated in British and American universities, but who are now under sharp attack by postmodernists, originated in disillusionment with Kantianism. These thinkers, originally led by Bertrand Russell (1872–1970) and Ludwig Wittgenstein (1889–1951), were initially concerned with clarifying the language of modern science (Smith 1997; Gross 1980). Their disciples at first followed the eighteenth-century thinker, David Hume, in attributing ethical judgments to simple emotional preferences, the utilitarianism already discussed. When it became evident how inadequate this is to solve current practical problems, the analysts sought a better method for ethics. Their principal concern remained the clarification of scientific discourse, but because they accepted Hume's notion of the fallacy of deducing an "ought" from an "is," they did not turn to scientific discourse to provide an anthropology on which to base ethics, as virtue theorists have done. Instead they have sought to clarify the "ordinary language" of moral controversy. Thus they attempt to sort out in ethical discussions the "good reasons" people give for their behavior from the "bad reasons" by which people rationalize bad behavior (see figure 1.1). They generally seek to do this only for particular, concrete points of debate, eschewing any effort to develop a general set of norms. Sometimes,

Figure 1.1   Ethical Systems

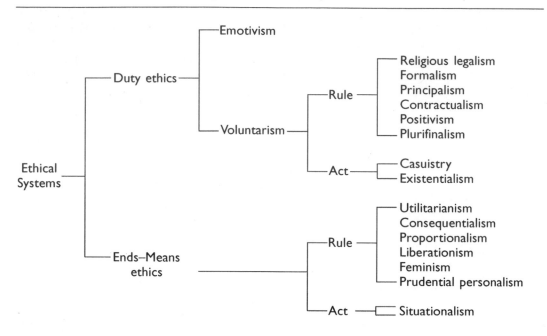

as in the writings of Gertrude Elizabeth Anscombe and her husband Peter Geatch, analytic ethics approaches the thought of St. Thomas Aquinas.

If we now sum up the strengths and weaknesses of ends–means ethics, we can conclude that such an ethics is more fundamental than a duty ethics because it cannot be moral to obey a law that commands one to choose a means contrary to one's true end. In fact it is one's duty to disobey such an intrinsically bad law. Only an ends–means ethics really tells us why an action is morally good or bad. The weakness of an ends–means ethics not also formulated in moral norms, however, is that none of us has such a perfect knowledge of what makes for true happiness that we can figure this out for ourselves in all cases, as Kant would seem to require us to do in order that our decisions be purely autonomous. Thus in actual practice we need moral norms, laws, precepts (duty ethics), and at least enough understanding of the intrinsic goodness of these norms (ends–means ethics) as prescribing realistic means to a true human fulfillment that we can also apply them intelligently to the changing circumstances of life. Thus we must have good reasons to trust those who are our moral mentors, who in turn must rely on the guidance of the only true and all wise mentor, God. Of course this raises a serious problem for any secularist bioethics that claims to be based purely on human reason, unless it also acknowledges that there is a God and that his wisdom is somehow manifest to us in his creation and providence in history.

We have also shown why, among the forms of means-ends ethics, we promote prudential personalism. It relates moral decision directly to basic human needs, as these can be determined objectively, rather than falling into the subjectivity of situationism, or the arbitrary calculation of utilities, consequences, and proportionate values, or the one-sidedness of feminist ethics and liberation ethics. Yet it remains open to the moral insights of all these positions and to the emphasis on character formation of virtue theory.

1.4 FAITH AND REASON IN HEALTH CARE ETHICS

Given the great diversity today in bioethical methodology, with their different strengths and weaknesses, how can such different opinions be resolved or at least be brought into fruitful dialogue? Kevin Wildes, S.J., in *Moral Acquaintances: Methodology in Bioethics* (2000) has addressed this question directly. He contrasts two views: one he calls foundationalism, under which he groups those methods that, although they differ greatly, all adopt some "starting point . . . whatever it may be," which "is the correct starting point for ethical deliberations" on the basis of which an integrated body of principles or rules can be developed. Wildes judges all foundationalist theories inadequate to the current pluralistic situation because it is precisely on basic assumptions that the diverse schools of bioethics diverge. Postmodernist writers such as Jacques Derrida (Johnson and Sheringham 1993) also attack foundationalism because they claim that human thought has no ultimate foundations, as it is a circular process that forever defers any final conclusions. Hence, as an alternative to foundationalism, Wildes describes the proceduralism proposed by the political philosopher John Rawls (1971) that has been applied to bioethics by H. Tristram Engelhardt Jr. (1991). Engelhardt argues that when, in bioethical dilemmas in health care theoretical agreement proves impossible, consensus should be sought only on procedures of dialogue and compromise. Proceduralism has much in common with the "civil discourse" that the philosopher Jürgen Habermas (1984, 1987) has shown to be central to our modern multicultural situation. Wildes, however, prefers to speak of "moral acquaintances" in the sense of helpful interchange between diverse views even when there is little hope of fundamental agreement.

Wildes concludes his analysis by arguing that a bioethicist in a pluralist community has four tasks: (1) to help a particular community of which he or she is an authoritative member to know its tradition and effectively speak out for it in dialogue with a larger community; (2) to be a "translator" facilitating effective dialogue by clearing up semantic differences between the different moral approaches of diverse groups; (3) to be a "geographer of authority and ideas" who studies the factors that lead to different ethical views and their practical implementation in institutional and public policies; and (4) to "analyze institutions, organizations, and organizational ethics." Wildes, therefore, sees secular ethics as primarily a matter of "moral acquaintances" that require only a relatively shallow consensus for dialogue but still look for ways to both widen and deepen this consensus.

The present book is concerned principally with the first of these four tasks that Wildes assigns to the bioethicist, namely, helping a group, in this case Catholics, that has a particular tradition to know their own tradition and to speak out for it effectively in dialogue with other traditions in the pluralistic American culture. In the first part of this chapter we have already made our own comparison of the strengths and weaknesses of the various ethical methodologies, most of them treated also by Wildes, that are today influential in bioethics. We agree with Wildes that foundationalism, as he describes it, is a faulty methodology, but we are convinced that the Catholic ethical tradition is truly foundational in its understanding of human nature in the light not only of faith but also of reason. Consequently it can make a very positive contribution to secular bioethics. As for proceduralism, we accept it if it is taken in the sense that there is an urgent need for a dialogue between all methodologies. This is necessary for the healing professions in our multicultural times, which John Paul II has in brief described as a "culture of death" (1995, no. 4). Catholics are called to work with others to transform this culture into a "culture of life." In the rest of this chapter we must consider what these diverse methodologies in current bioethics can contribute to a Catholic health care ethics founded on Christ the Healer. In chapter 2 we propose such a Christian ethics capable of dialogue with others seeking true health.

Ethics in a Pluralistic Society

Any ethics based on natural moral law, and most especially an ethics of health care, inevitably runs into the accusation that it is really religious morality in disguise. In a culture that is as religiously diverse and highly secularized as ours is today, Catholics, because they have pioneered in bioethics, are especially liable to the accusation that they are trying to impose their religious values on public policy. The word "religion," however, is a very ambiguous term. Experts in comparative religion emphasize that to make such comparisons meaningful "religion" cannot be defined substantively as to content because the so-called world religions differ too much in their doctrines. For example, on the one hand, Buddhism is certainly a great religion, yet it is not clear that Buddhists believe in either God or the eternal life of human persons. On the other hand, such beliefs are essential to Judaism, Christianity, and Islam. Hence, in comparing "religions," it is better to use not a substantive but a functional definition of "religion" as a "worldview and value system." This definition does not exclude but includes the worldviews and value systems of agnostics and atheists, such as secular humanists, who would deny that they have any religion (Baird 1971; Ashley 2000d).

Therefore, in our pluralistic society, if we are to promote ethical dialogue it is necessary that all parties, whatever their worldviews and value systems, talk on equal terms (Habermas 1984, 1987). To assume that secularist views are religiously neutral and objective and hence alone have a right to be heard in the public forum, while other views are subjective, nonrational, and merely "religious," is a fatal barrier to genuine dialogue among worldviews and value systems, a dialogue necessary in any pluralistic society. Some of this misunderstanding about "religion" and "ethics" can be cleared up if among worldviews we distinguish those (1) that claim to be based purely on reason, such as secular humanism; (2) those that claim to be based on mystical insights accessible to all who undertake disciplined meditation, such as Buddhism, Hinduism, and certain New Age systems; and (3) those that claim to be based on divine revelation that must be received on faith, such as Judaism, Christianity, and Islam (Al Khayat 1995). Catholic Christianity is based on revelation but also believes that God has manifested his existence and given us some ethical guidance that is accessible even to those who do not have faith through reason. While Protestant Christians do not deny the importance of ethical reasoning, they tend to hold that human reason has been so darkened by sin that it provides little ethical help (Gustafson 1984). Jews and Muslims also place little emphasis on natural law, relying almost exclusively on revelation.

Our dialogue on bioethics, however, is less often conducted with other views that are recognized as "religious" than it is with secular views. Modern political systems, such as that of the United States, are based on "the separation of church and state." They provide health care for a religiously diverse population. Hence in the public forum we must all, whatever our religious beliefs, use an ethics based solely on reason and neutral to any "faith."

Yet is it really true that the "public philosophy" that dominates our government and our public institutions is simply based on reason? Or is it in fact based on the unacknowledged domination of a special system of values whose complete reasonableness is also debatable? Engelhardt (1991) distinguishes between "secular humanism" and "the secular as a neutral framework." Secular humanism claims not to be a faith, but to be based solely on hardheaded reason, but it is certainly a worldview and value system that places its faith solely in the human potential (Ashley 2000d). Thus it seeks to refute other worldviews or religions that, although they too exalt the human potential, believe its fulfillment is dependent on some spiritual reality that transcends humanity. While we would agree with Engelhardt that we must seek a neutral secularity based on common experience and reason in this dialogue with all worldviews, including that of contemporary secular humanism, we cannot permit secular humanism to go unchallenged in its claim to be "neutral."

Is There a Christian Ethic?

Recently some Catholic ethicists have raised the question "Is there a Christian ethic?" and claim that Christian revelation adds no moral guidance beyond what can be achieved by human reason but only additional motives for observing its norms (Curran and McCormick 1980; Walters 1999, 157–76). They have supported their arguments by quoting St. Thomas Aquinas's statement that the Ten Commandments are simply "natural law." But Aquinas's statement must be read in the context of his other statements that what motivates any free act is a person's ultimate goal in life. Because moral decision has to do with the choice of means to that motivating goal, the character of that goal modifies every decision. We have, Aquinas says (although certain theologians deny it), two ultimate goals, a natural goal of fulfilling the needs of human nature and a supernatural or graced goal of attaining an intimate friendship with God that utterly exceeds our human needs but to which God has freely called us by his grace. There is no conflict between these two goals, as the fulfillment of the natural goal is included in the fulfillment of the goal of grace, not obliterated by it but only subordinated to it. Thus God's forgiving grace heals the weakening of our natural powers that God planted in our human nature so that we can attain our natural goal, but that grace also calls us beyond our natural goal to the infinitely higher goal of eternal life with the Trinity and gives us the power to attain that as our truly ultimate goal.

Thus in Catholic tradition there is an extensively developed natural ethic based on human nature and also a supernatural ethic, traditionally called "moral theology," the former based on reason, the latter on the revealed Gospel (Pinckaers 1995, 2002). These two levels of ethics cover much the same ground but cover it in the light of different principles, namely, our natural and the supernatural goals. Yet the revealed ethics clarifies and supports the rational ethics without, however, denying its autonomy. In pluralistic dialogue, human reason necessarily comes into play, and all parties are forced to make arguments based purely on reason and experience. These, whether they are or are not labeled "natural law" arguments, in fact have to refer to human nature and its needs. For example, in discussing problems in the ethics of health care, arguments concerning human rights inevitably enter the dialogue. These "human rights" are not easy to explain or defend without reference to human nature and human equality, as they are known to reason, that is, to *natural law*, a term adopted by St. Thomas Aquinas from a tradition originating not with Aristotle but with the Stoics. The meaning he gave it, however, is a means–ends ethics based on the empirical observation and critical analysis of those basic human needs that are not merely the products of a particular culture but also are rooted in the human genetic biological and psychological structure as it has evolved and are therefore universal to the human species, as, for example, the human need for a community that fosters and protects human rights.

Catholics, therefore, in dialogue with those of other worldviews and value systems, should have no difficulty restricting this dialogue to arguments that rely on reason and experience without reference to revelation and Christian faith, unless their dialogue partners are ready to go deeper. Yet in their own thinking about these topics Catholics should also look to their faith in the Word of God both to support reason and to provide deeper insights than reason can provide. Thus they should not hesitate to explain the role that doctrines of their faith play in their thinking, while making clear that they do not intend to impose them on others but are perfectly willing to base dialogue on reason and experience accessible to all parties.

Consequently, in this book we attempt always to study each particular issue first in light of an ethics of health care based on reason and the natural law, then afterward to integrate these rational arguments with other deeper insights provided by Christian faith, keeping the two levels of ethics explicitly distinct. In the next chapter we first outline an ethics with a methodology based wholly on reason and the natural moral law, that is, the basic needs of human nature. In the latter part of that chapter we show how this natural law ethics is transformed harmoniously by a Christian ethics in the Catholic tradition. We emphasize that such a Christian ethics not only is open to ecumenical dialogue but obliges us to engage in that dialogue with those of other worldviews and value systems and to seek common ground with them both on the natural law level and, if they are interested, on the level of other valid faith experiences. In what remains of this first chapter, however, we will discuss why, from the point of view of faith and its harmony with reason, openness to the teaching of the Church in moral matters in general, and in bioethics in particular, is so important for Catholics.

How the Church Solves Moral Controversies

As times change, controversies inevitably arise over moral issues. The post–Vatican II debate within the Church on the respective roles of the bishops and of theologians in teaching morality led to the encyclical letter of John Paul II, *Veritatis splendor* (1993), which provides a clear direction for the Church in conscience formation. Pastoral ministry makes a very special contribution to the church's teaching effort (Dulles 1991). This ministry, taken in a broad sense, is not limited to the ordained but is carried on by many men and women whose experience in applying the faith to actual life is essential if the Gospel is to be effectively preached to the poor and to children (Mt 11:5; 18:5–14). For example, religious sisters and brothers probably have contributed more to the active teaching work of the church in the United States than have the ordained clergy (John Paul II 1987).

Nevertheless, a special leadership responsibility falls on the bishops, together with their priests and deacons in local churches, and on the Pope for the whole Church to unify all these different witnessing voices, to express their consensus in clear terms suited to the times, to correct this in the light of the Bible and sacred tradition when necessary and link it to the tradition of the Christian community throughout the world in its historical development. As in the very first years of the Catholic Church's life, St. Paul wrote to Timothy (2 Tm 4:2–4), whom he had appointed in authority over a local church: "Proclaim the word; be persistent whether it is convenient or inconvenient; convince, reprimand, encourage through all patience and teaching. For the time will come when people will not tolerate sound doctrine, but following their own desires and insatiable curiosity, will accumulate teachers and will stop listening to the truth and will be delivered to myths."

Without such unifying leadership, the spiritual riches of faith and insight contributed by the members of the Church would be dissipated, and the community would be divided in its faith and life, as history shows. Thus, whereas the role of theologians is primarily critical and analytical, the role of bishops is primarily pastoral, aimed at unifying the community of faith (Theological Commission 1976). In particular, bishops have the hard task of reconciling partial and extreme views within the Church that might lead to heresy or schism. If they did not exercise this moderating role, the polarization of opinions would so increase in the Church that it would be torn apart or become so diluted as to lose all meaning and vitality. The bishops rightly prefer to do this not by condemnation but by wise emphasis on those principal truths and values that keep a straggling flock moving toward its goal. In moral matters, prudent bishops do not burden the freedom of individual consciences by insistence on secondary issues (1 Cor 10:23–33), because they recognize that the members of the Church are at many different levels of moral development. Rather, such bishops constantly emphasize the primary goals of Christian life.

Sometimes, however, bishops and popes are confronted with dangerous crises in the life of the community when, as leaders and pastors, they have the painful duty of using their authority "to bind and to loose" (Mt 16:19, 18:18), to protect the community from disruption, and to strengthen its public witness. This is why in extreme cases a bishop may have to resort, as did St. Paul (1 Cor 5:1–13), to excommunication or exclusion from Christian life of those who "will not hear the Church" (Mt 18:17), observing, however, all the care for justice, which today is called "due process."

Church teaching, however, has various levels of certitude and finality. Pope John Paul II (1998b), the Congregation for the Doctrine of the Faith (CDF 1990, 1998), and the Code of Canon Law (CIC 1983 [2000], cc. 749–54) have recently distinguished the following levels of teaching:

1. When the magisterium makes an infallible pronouncement and solemnly declares that a teaching is found in revelation, the assent called for is theological faith. This kind of adherence is to be given even to the teaching of the ordinary and universal magisterium when it proposes for belief a teaching of faith as divinely revealed.

2. When the magisterium proposes "in a definitive way" truths concerning faith and morals, which even if not divinely revealed are nevertheless strictly and intimately connected with revelation, these must be firmly accepted and held.

3. When the magisterium, not intending to act "definitively," teaches a doctrine to aid a better understanding of revelation and make explicit its contents, or to recall how some teaching is in conformity with the truths of faith, or finally to guard against ideas that are incompatible with these truths, the response called for is that of "religious submission of will and intellect." This kind of response cannot be simply exterior or disciplinary but must be understood within the logic of faith and under the impulse of obedience to faith.

4. Finally, in order to serve the people of God as well as possible, in particular by warning them of dangerous opinions that could lead to error, the magisterium can intervene in questions under discussion that involve in addition to solid principles certain contingent and conjectural elements. It often only becomes possible with the passage of time to distinguish between what is necessary and what is contingent. While it must be received with reverence, its authority for the most part is based on the reasons given for the particular statement.

Why Four Levels of Teaching?

Why there must be these four levels of teaching, if the Christian community is to fulfill its mission of witnessing to the Gospel, can be explained as follows (Gaillardetz 2003).

First, there are truths that are certainly part of God's word and known to be so because they are (a) clearly stated in the Bible (e.g., the Ten Commandments as stated in Exodus and Deuteronomy and confirmed by Jesus in the Sermon on the Mount in Matthew); (b) clearly stated in the sacred tradition of the Church (e.g., that Exodus, Deuteronomy, and Matthew are the inspired Word of God); (c) or have been solemnly declared to be revealed explicitly or implicitly by God in the Bible and/or sacred tradition by the magisterium. This can be either by the Bishop of Rome witnessing for the whole Church or by an ecumenical council of bishops with the Pope's consent (then it is said to be "extraordinary" teaching), or by all the bishops with the Pope's consent but without a conciliar meeting (this is said to be "ordinary and universal teaching"). Because Christ has promised that the church is infallible in its faith, teaching of this first level is infallible and must be received by all Catholics through an act of the gift of divine faith.

Second, there is a class of truths (whose scope has not yet been precisely defined by the magisterium) (Sullivan 1983) that are not revealed, yet are so intimately connected with revealed truths that to deny them is equivalent to denying what is revealed. For example, scripture and tradition do not determine who is pope or what council is ecumenical, yet if such doubts could not be *definitively* settled, the Church could not teach revealed truth with certitude. Hence such definitive declarations are also infallible, not because revealed but because of their necessary relation to revealed truths. The proper response to such teaching is to hold them to be true with firm conviction not as revealed to faith but as definitively and authoritatively settled by the Church under the Holy Spirit's guidance.

Third, there are truths that the magisterium presents at a given time in her "ordinary" teaching, *not definitively*, but with such consistency and universality that it is clear they must somehow involve principles that are true, although the exact consequences to these principles are still unclear. Hence, to deny them may risk denying the Word of God, but it is not yet certain just what this risk is. Thus it may not yet be clear how to formulate a certain truth in a way consistent with other truths. For example, the Church could not define the Immaculate Conception as a truth of faith until it was clear how to reconcile it with the truth that all are saved from sin by Christ.

Fourth, the ordinary teaching of the Church contains guidance concerning matters that require a prudential judgment on how revealed principles apply to complex and changing situations. For example, Pius XII at a time of crisis urged the Catholics of Italy to vote against the Communist Party, and the bishops of the United States have expressed strong opinions on certain issues that affect political action. Historically, when the Church applied the revealed, unchangeable Biblical teaching against usury to the medieval economy, it had to modify its application when the economic system changed. On such matters Catholics must show obedience to the Church's judgments and for the common influence of Catholic action but may have differing views on what is best to think or do. Some such judgments come into play in bioethics because of the advances in medical practice and the need for Catholic health care to avoid "scandal" by seeming in borderline cases to approve exceptions to absolute moral norms.

Is There a "Right to Dissent"?

After Vatican II there were theologians who claimed that a Catholic has the right to dissent from all teaching of the Pope or bishops that is not an extraordinary, infallible definition. Some went so far as to also claim that the Church has never made any infallible definitions in the area of morals, and hence they were free to teach any opinion they found reasonable, being accountable only to their academic peers. Although it is true that it has been the custom of the magisterium to define as revealed only matters of faith rather than of morals, without doubt the moral norms of the biblical Ten Commandments, the Sermon on the Mount, and the New Testament Epistles are infallible, and the bishops and Pope have the authority from Christ to confirm and interpret these norms by infallible definitions if they choose to do so.

Moreover, as John Paul II has declared, the universal and ordinary teaching of the bishops based on scripture and tradition has already made it clear that some moral teachings, such as the condemnation of abortion and the killing of the innocent, are definitive and infallible (John Paul II 1995, 1998b; CDF 1998). Then Cardinal Joseph Ratzinger has also noted that the Council of Trent solemnly defined the indissolubility of the marriage covenant. In general it can be said that the moral teaching of the Church for the most part is infallible by reason of the fact that the universal ordinary teaching authority of the bishops has confirmed it as the teaching of the Church.

The principal argument for a "right to dissent" in matters of Church teaching is that history shows that the Church has in fact sometimes changed its teaching and been forced to admit serious mistakes in the past, as, for example, in the Galileo case and in some teaching revised in Vatican Council II; for example, the relationship between church and state and the right to freedom of religion (Dulles 1991). This argument can be answered first of all by noting that most of the alleged mistakes pertain to the fourth of the levels of certitude listed earlier that were matters of prudence in which particular popes and bishops can err, yet retain their authority that we must respect. This book is not the place to explain the process of dissent to prudential teaching (CDF 1990), except to note that the Catholic Church's record even in prudential statements is relatively good compared to most major human institutions.

What is more important in replying to these accusations is to understand what is meant by the "development of doctrine" in the church (Nichols 1990). Such historic development is in fact possible because as the whole church meditates on the revealed Gospel given once for all to the church and strives to live by it, certain truths already implicitly present in that revelation become clearer and more explicit by the light of the Holy Spirit as the signs to the presence of these truths in the completed revelation become more evident.

For example, it took a long time for the church to see that the inspired words of St. Paul to Philemon, that he should treat his slave Onesimus "as a most dear brother" (Phlm 16), imply that slavery is always unjust.

Before the final and conclusive sign that a truth is revealed, given by its definition as such by the extraordinary act of pope or council or through its ordinary unanimous teaching by the bishops with the pope's approval, a doctrine remains more or less probable and hence may be in some respect inadequately expressed or even obscured by error (CDF 1990). Thus it is possible, and this is what happened in the Galileo case, famous precisely because such cases have been so rare, that in an effort to defend a certainly revealed truth the teaching authority may imprudently deny some other less certain truth. In that notorious case papal authority, in an effort to defend the infallible doctrine of the inspiration of the Bible, supported a merely probable interpretation of certain biblical passages against the very probable, but at that time by no means certain, theories of Copernican astronomy. It must also be recognized that truths necessary to the consistency of infallible teaching must themselves also be infallibly true. For example, although it is not revealed that Jesus ever laughed, because he was truly human it is infallibly certain that he did so.

Nevertheless, Catholics are obliged to follow all the authoritative (authentic) guidance of the Church not as a matter of divine faith, but out of an obedience based on faith in the Church's authority to guide the consciences of its members, and because the Pope and bishops have such authority is part of the *depositum fidei* and has been infallibly declared to be a revealed truth (CCC 2000, no. 888-892; Cessario 1997; DiNoia 1988). The authoritative teachers in the Church can add nothing to that apostolic revelation or *depositum fidei* (1 Tim 6:20; 2 Tim 1:12, 14), the Greek original for Latin *depositum* is *paratheke*, or "property entrusted to another," but in the course of history the church humanly struggles to understand this revelation more clearly and fully. In this learning and teaching process there are at any given point in history levels of teaching in the church requiring somewhat different responses.

Teaching of Vatican II

This obedient assent to church teaching even when it is not infallible requires not only an obedience of will and action but also the intellectual conformity of Christian discipleship to the church's guidance in life and thought, a guidance superior to that of any merely human authority or expertise. No one, however, is ever obliged to affirm as true what he or she is objectively and prudently *certain* is false. Galileo in 1632 had strong probability that the Earth moved, but as he himself recognized, he did not have certitude about that fact, because the final empirical evidence of the motion of the Earth in its orbit was not obtained by science until 1838 (Wallace 1991)! Hence, if a Catholic were really to discover *with certitude* an important error in Church teaching, he or she is obliged to do what he or she can to inform the teaching authorities of the facts so that they can correct this error, but must do so in a manner that does not cause "scandal," that is, weaken general trust in the Church's teaching authority. In cases where those who are expert in a question have only a strong probability that a revision of teaching is needed, they should continue a learned discussion of the problem but in a manner that respects the superior magisterial authority and does not in any way encourage dissent in practice from the church's norms (CDF 1990).

Those who hold for "right to dissent" also often claim that they are following the teachings of Vatican II or at least "the spirit of" Vatican II. In fact Vatican Council II (1964, no. 25) rejected this so-called "right of dissent." It is true that the teaching authorities of the Church leave many details of our Christian living to our own intelligence and to charitable and fruitful debate within the Church, not only among theologians but also among the whole laity, such as the choice of political parties, ethnic customs, and personal vocations and devotions. Nevertheless, according to Vatican II, all Catholics in the formation of their faith and conscience have the obligation not only to believe on divine faith whatever the magisterium teaches by its infallible "extraordinary" pronouncements but also to accept the guidance of its ordinary teaching. Thus the CDF, in its *Instruction on the ecclesial vocation of the theologian* (1990, nos. 23–24), says:

When the Magisterium proposes "in a definitive way" truths concerning faith and morals, which, even if not divinely revealed, are nevertheless strictly and intimately connected with Revelation, these must be firmly accepted and held. When the Magisterium, not intending to act "definitively," teaches a doctrine to aid a better understanding of Revelation and make explicit its contents, or to recall how some teaching is in conformity with the truths of faith, or finally to guard against ideas that are incompatible with these truths, the response called for is that of the religious submission of will and intellect (Vatican Council II 1964, no. 25; CIC, c. 752). This kind of response cannot be simply exterior or disciplinary but must be understood within the logic of faith and under the impulse of obedience to faith. Finally, in order to serve the People of God as well as possible, in particular by warning them of dangerous opinions that could lead to error, the Magisterium can intervene in questions under discussion that involve, in addition to solid principles, certain contingent and conjectural elements. It often only becomes possible with the passage of time to distinguish what is necessary and what is contingent.

Examples of a moral teaching proposed "in a definitive way" are Pope John Paul's declarations against abortion and euthanasia in *The Gospel of Life* (*Evangelium vitae;* 1995). For examples of a doctrine not yet definitive given "to aid a better understanding," which nevertheless requires "the religious submission of will and intellect," one might cite some detailed items of the CDF's "Instruction on Respect for Human Life" (1987), such as its rejection of artificial insemination by the husband (AIH). Another example of teachings that involve, in addition to solid principles, certain "contingent and conjectural elements," are the remarks of John Paul II on capital punishment (1995, no. 56) in which he says "as a result of steady improvements in the organization of the penal system, such cases [of absolute necessity that require capital punishment to protect the common good] are very rare if not practically nonexistent."

Sensus Fidei

Some may also object to the foregoing analysis that the Church has always taught that the *sensus fidelium* or "opinion of the faithful" also shares in the infallibility of the Church, because certainly the people of God *are* the Church. They then cite the fact that today it is well known that many persons who consider themselves good Catholics not only do not obey some moral teachings of the Church but also seem to be convinced from their own experience and knowledge that these teachings are mistaken. Thus we see the widespread practice of divorce and remarriage, abortion, contraception, premarital sex, and even sodomy by Catholics who claim to act in "good conscience" because they think the Church is wrong and will surely someday come to admit its mistakes as it has in other matters.

This line of argument fails to take into account the fact that historically great sections of the Church have at times claimed to be "good Catholics" while dissenting from Church teaching by defending their rights to be slave owners, racists, sexists, militarists, and anti-Semites! They no doubt thought that their "Christian experience" had confirmed them in these attitudes that in the light of the Gospel are certainly false. Hence much talk about the *sensus fidelium* fails to recognize that, as we have already pointed out, the witness of the Church, though infallibly true to the Gospel, is not always perfect but may be obscured by sin and ignorance. At any given time or place, therefore, the lives, experiences, and religious and moral opinions of the members of the Church, including the clergy, bear imperfect witness to the unchanging faith of the whole church throughout history.

This occasional obscuring of the faith in this or that time or place is one of the reasons that Jesus provided an authoritative teacher in the church to discriminate between the *sensus fidelium,* or human opinions within the church, and the *sensus fidei,* or "sense of the faith" or genuine witness to the Gospel of the perennial church as a whole. To discern the infallible *sensus fidei* on these controversial questions, therefore, we ought not take public opinion polls at face value, but should explore what the Christian community, and especially its most holy and faithful members, seriously believe to have been revealed by God in the scriptures and sacred tradition and confirmed in their efforts to live in obedience to this Word of God.

Note especially that, just as the magisterium has no right to teach its own opinions but only the *depositum fidei*, so all the members of the Church cannot claim as Gospel anything except what has been transmitted to them from this same "deposit of faith" under the living guidance of the magisterium. Within the Church it is the critical task of theologians to help the development of doctrine in the Church by explaining and clarifying magisterial documents and their levels of authority and by suggesting better or more consistent formulations of their teaching.

Theologians must also explore the roots of magisterial teaching in scripture and tradition, as well as apply their principles to solve problems on which the magisterium has not yet pronounced. But the opinions of contemporary theologians are without theological value if they are not based on and consistent with the teachings of today's magisterium. Just as in the natural sciences the final criterion of truth is the empirical evidence, so in theology the final criterion of truth is scripture and tradition as understood in the living tradition of the Church. Consequently, for Catholics, moral conscience must be informed by and conform to the teaching of the Church, not to the opinions of theologians, however numerous, learned, or academically distinguished.

Finally, it must be remembered, in considering the historic examples where Church teaching seems to have changed, that as the CDF (1990, no. 24) stated, "certain contingent and conjectural elements" have been corrected by the passage of time. But these errors in ordinary, noninfallible teaching do not make the authority of the Church untrustworthy.

These chiefly prudential errors have been of several types. Most commonly cited is the rescinding of the former condemnation of taking interest on loans. But in fact usury, that is, charging interest without a just title for doing so, is still condemned by the Church. What has changed is not this principle, but our economic system that now justifies taking interest on other titles than were supplied by the medieval economy. Again the Galileo case is frequently cited, but at most this was a regrettable judicial error in a particular case, not a matter of universal magisterial teaching. Much more serious have been the Church's change of teaching as regards human rights and the relations of church and state, as it has now repudiated its former stance on slavery, the use of judicial torture in cases of conspiracy derived from Roman law, the Inquisition's use of force to defend religious orthodoxy, and the jurisdiction of the church over the state in civil affairs. In these matters the Church has come to see that it had too much conformed to the customs and opinions of secular society from which it has had to free itself to be true to the Gospel.

Human Rights Sensitivity

The Catholic Church is grateful that it has been aided in this greater sensitivity to human rights by the progress in secular government itself in the legal recognition of such rights. Note, however, that this increasing sensitivity to human rights by the Church has not been in the direction of a greater moral permissiveness—which is the common "liberal" demand on the Church—but rather in the direction of greater moral responsibility. Thus the fact that the Church has had to refine some of its moral teaching to support stricter standards of justice, far from showing that it is not to be relied on as a moral guide, demonstrates its growing fidelity to the Gospel and its increasing trustworthiness.

Bioethics has raised new questions to which the Church, in the interest of the dignity of the human person and the value of human life, has found it necessary to make a response. The ordinary teaching of the Church regarding bioethics is to be found in many recent documents, especially in the encyclical *Evangelium vitae* (John Paul II 1995) and the instruction *Donum Vitae* of the CDF (1987). These teachings can be found in practical form in the ERD (2001) of the United States Conference of Catholic Bishops, which have been recently revised, updated, and supplied with fuller theological and pastoral explanations. While Catholic health care professionals may also profitably seek the council of theologians in understanding and applying these directives to particular cases, they should be aware that some claiming theological expertise are not in fact in honest conformity with these magisterial directives. Hence, in doubt, recourse should be had to the bishop of the diocese, who alone has authority to give a final interpretation of the directives. Of course, the bishops too must conform to the teaching of the Holy See. Their responsibilities are not easy.

Finally it can be asked whether prudential personalism, as the Christian tradition has favored it, is the best basis of an ethics of health care today. Is it not too much colored by this Christian advocacy, by ancient and medieval philosophy, and by social biases that are alien to the modern scientific character of medicine and to our pluralistic society, to serve this purpose? But precisely because our society is pluralistic it is necessary for health care professionals to be sure of their own ethical stance and to be able to present it honestly. Moreover, as we have seen, an ethics based on reason and basic human needs is the only common ground among different faiths with which dialogue can begin. The philosophical tradition that most effectively defends such a reasoned approach to morality is one that favors an epistemology that grounds abstract theory in empirical data, as chapter 2 will show is the case with the prudential personalist version of natural law ethics. Moreover, this reliance on an anthropology that can be related to modern scientific findings is also congenial to modern medicine and the life sciences. An ethics of health care grounded in this way is therefore the best practical point of departure both for research and for dialogue with other views.

1.5 CONCLUSION

Bioethics as we know it today is generally based on secular humanism because that worldview and value system dominates modern culture. It is rooted, however, in the Christian tradition of the Catholic Church that originated our system of health care facilities. This basis has tradition attempting to balance faith and reason, as well as the two main types of ethics, duty ethics and ends–means ethics. This tension between the two kinds of ethics has persisted in secular bioethics. Today there is also a multicultural broadening of health care ethics to include the world religions and also special oppressed or neglected social groups. Only an ethics that respects the basic needs common to the entire human species throughout its history, that is, a "natural law" ethics, is adequate to this multicultural situation to which any Catholic health care must today make its special contribution. Thus a Catholic bioethics rests on the foundation to which John Paul II appealed in his encyclical *Fides et ratio* no. 100: "The church remains profoundly convinced that faith and reason 'mutually support each other'; each influences the other, as they offer to each other a purifying critique and a stimulus to pursue the search for deeper understanding."

Chapter Two

ETHICS AND NEEDS
OF THE COMMON PERSON

OVERVIEW

MORALITY IS NOT MERELY A MATTER of obedience to rules but is the free and realistic choice of means to meet human needs in the order of their importance in achieving true personal and communal happiness. It is based, therefore, on a sound understanding of human nature and its needs attained through historical experience and enhanced by the modern life sciences. Jesus Christ has provided us with a historical model of human moral perfection that can strengthen and refine this empirical understanding of the human potential. Consistently good moral behavior, however, cannot be achieved without the development of a sound character, that is, through the development of virtue. Hence virtue theory supplies us with an analysis of what such a virtuous character consists of. Bioethics thus must be more than a set of general principles, but must be grounded in a sound anthropology and virtue theory.

2.1 AN ETHICS BASED ON INNATE HUMAN NEEDS

Ethics concerns the needs and values of human persons. Health is a vital human need; nothing is more human, more personal, and must always be one of the main concerns of any human community. To develop an ethics of human health care, therefore, we must have an accurate notion of what it means to be human and what it means to be a healthy human. As we saw in chapter 1, the most basic form of ethics is of the ends–means type. Therefore we must determine the end or ends for which persons need to strive in order to be healthy in mind and body, and the best means to achieve that goal or goals. Hence we will not follow the a priori, *deductive* procedure of Kantian idealism that is open to the charge of "foundationalism," that is, of being an ethics resting on arbitrary assumptions. Instead we will follow an *empirical, inductive* procedure based on the observation of actual human behavior, pragmatically tested in experience.

An ends–means ethics must be based on those needs that all human persons are born with and it must order and unify the satisfaction of these needs in relation to true human happiness, the fulfillment of the human potential. Human needs are satisfied by human values, but the term *value*, borrowed from economics (Perry 1980), is vague and often connotes a duty ethics rather than an ends–means ethics. The philosophical study of values is called "axiology" (from the Greek *axios*, worthy). A value is what satisfies some need, a negative value frustrates some human need, and a neutral value neither satisfies nor obstructs a human need. A value, therefore, can be something as trivial as a cup of water to satisfy thirst or as sublime as the love of God and neighbor.

As we mentioned in the previous chapter, in the twentieth century British and American ethicists conducted a long and rather tedious debate about the relation between "facts" and "values" (Rachels 1986; Doeser and Kray 1986). Scientists today carefully formulate scientific statements in value-free language, but in ethical and political discussions this is self-defeating, because ethical and political talk not only describes facts, but also asks how these facts can be changed for the better. This long controversy is still not over, but it has led to some points of agreement. First, ethical debate clearly cannot be divorced from all reference to facts; for example, every bioethical debate depends on an accurate knowledge of the medical facts (Thomasma and Kushner 1996). Second, the debaters must give good reasons for their ethical positions in terms of these certified facts (Hare 1991). That is, it is irrelevant in bioethical debate merely to talk about how one *feels* about abortion; there must also be reference to its consequences for those involved. Third, in all ethical discussions people refer to evident human needs (e.g., it is "good" to be able to see and walk, "bad" to be blind and crippled), so that serious ethical issues arise when it is a question of blinding or mutilating a human being. Fourth, ultimately ethical debates return to questions about value *systems*, that is, the religious or philosophical view of the meaning and value of human life as a *whole* and what values have priority in decision making.

There is, however, also much controversy as to whether human behavior is based chiefly on needs that are natural or innate or on those that are freely chosen or cultural. On the one hand, sociobiologists (Pinker 2002) defend the view that evolution has adapted us to our environment by implanting certain needs in the human genome. Thus Paul Lawrence and Nitin Nohria, in their book *Driven: How Human Nature Shapes Our Choices* (2001), argue for four natural human needs that they call "acquire, bond, learn, and defend." Long ago St. Thomas Aquinas, in *Summa Theologiae* (I–II, q. 94, a. 2), argued that we human persons have as our most basic and universal innate needs four goals:

1. Bodily health and security supported by useful certain material possessions;
2. A good family in which to be born and raised and that will ensure the reproduction of our human species;
3. A larger community than our family because this is required to meet all our needs;
4. A true understanding of ourselves and the world we live in so we can (a) make free choices of means to satisfy our other needs, and (b) find "meaning" in life.

Because of the clarity and simplicity of Aquinas's list, we will base our analysis on it. Modern psychology, for example, as in the work of Abraham Maslow (1970), recognizes similar lists of human needs, as well as of rights based on them, as does the United Nations' *Universal Declaration of Human Rights* (1948).

On the other hand, some anthropologists, observing the great diversity of human cultures, deny the existence of a single "human nature." We Americans live in a technological age in a highly artificial environment. We must recover a sense of our difference from robots and even from the rest of nature that has become subject to scientific probing and technological manipulation (ITEST 1975). Indeed, the basic four innate human needs listed by Aquinas can now be adequately satisfied only in a culture that is technologically very advanced. We must, therefore, make political decisions that will ensure that *all* these needs can be satisfied in an integrated and consistent manner. This obviously requires us to set priorities, to formulate our aims and objectives, and to explore the practical steps to be taken to achieve them. We are forced to subordinate and even sacrifice our less important needs to greater ones. The exact mix or proportion will depend on both the culture and the individual. Thus today it is better not to exaggerate the role of either nature or culture but to speak in terms of their interactive relationships. To exaggerate the role of nature in ethics contradicts human freedom, while to exaggerate the role of culture leads to *cultural relativism,* which renders all ethical discussion arbitrary.

How should we rank these human needs in importance? Certainly it seems that sometimes health needs must be subordinated to social needs, as when soldiers risk their lives or bodily integrity to defend their country. From one perspective our needs should be ranked in *descending* order: with the need for health, material goods, and security as the most important, since without a sufficiency of health, material goods, and security we cannot satisfy any of the other needs. Yet from another perspective these four needs should be ranked in *ascending* order, because it is the achievement of knowledge that makes it possible to satisfy the other lesser needs and to find meaning in doing so. It is this second ranking that is most significant for ethics, because when necessary we very reasonably risk our health and property to attain the other three goods. We also realize that we must sometimes sacrifice family happiness to serve our larger community. Finally, the greatest value in community life is our exchange of experience and knowledge, without which there can be no truly personal relationships. Thus when we see in today's culture that so many make material wealth the ultimate goal of their life, or violate the common good of their country to serve their family interests, or seek political power by lying and spreading false propaganda, we see how widespread immorality is and the human misery it spawns.

Health Needs

Just what is human "health" that supports the satisfaction of all our other needs? Etymologically "health" is related to the Anglo-Saxon word from which is derived not only "healing" but also "holiness" and "wholeness." The root of that word denotes "completeness," a whole that has all its parts optimally functioning. Henrik Blum (1983, 93) found no less than eight definitions of "health," each with experience-tested advantages and disadvantages when he synthesized them into a working definition: "Health consists of the capacity of an organism (1) to maintain a balance appropriate to its age and social needs, in which it is reasonably free of gross dissatisfaction, discomfort, disease or disability; and (2) to behave in ways which promote the survival of the species as well as the self-fulfillment or enjoyment of the individual. . . . [H]ealth is the state of being in which an individual does the best with the capacities he has, and acts in ways that maximize his capacities." This definition will suffice for our bioethical purposes, but it should be kept in mind that it is not easy to apply it concretely. A number of difficulties need to be kept in mind.

1. Some think of health simply as the opposite of feeling sick in a *subjective* sense. Yet a person may have HIV or cancer and feel perfectly well, or they may deny that they are chemically addicted or their fears are paranoiac.

2. Some confuse the notion of "normal" with "average." They neglect such well-known facts as that in the U.S. population the "average weight" is not normal but is abnormal obesity.

3. Sociologists such as Eliot Freidson (1971) speak of "the social construction of illness." Some physical and psychological disorders such as a broken leg or smallpox or catatonic schizophrenia are unambiguously, and objectively, "illnesses," but, according to Conrad and Kern (1981), in the United States we tend to assign the term *illness* to more and more phenomena previously given other labels. These social constructions can result in labeling persons as "sick" merely because they do not conform to average behavior in that society. Thus the psychoanalyst Thomas Szasz (1987) argued that drug addiction and alcoholism should be treated not as diseases but as personal preferences and that, if they do any harm, they harm only the addict. We also often use euphemistic names for diseases and disabilities in order not to "stigmatize the victim."

4. Historically in the medical profession the pendulum has constantly swung between two approaches to disease. The *ontological* concept regards diseases as separate entities (devils, contagions, bacteria, genetic defects, neuroses, psychoses). Those who think in this way tend to diagnose diseases in terms of clearly classified and labeled entities and to treat them by seeking specific remedies (e.g., specific drugs, specific surgical procedures). In contrast, the *physiological* concept views disease as a breakdown of the internal harmony of the organic system because of hyperfunctioning or hypofunctioning of some organ or organ system. Such dysfunctions expose an organism to attack by external agents such as bacteria, but the bacteria are not the primary cause of the disease. If the organism were functioning properly, it would resist such bacteria. Some, therefore, resist classifying diseases and emphasize regimen or lifestyle. They use drugs and surgery only secondarily to assist in the adjustment of the individual organism.

5. There are two other opposed tendencies in medical thinking: one *mechanistic*, the other *holistic* (Collinge 1996). Mechanists in medicine emphasize the condition of the parts of the organism; holists pay more attention to the organism as a whole, as one made of interrelated parts whose healthy functions have an ordered interaction. Actually both aspects of an organism need to be kept in mind, but too many physicians still think mechanistically because of three factors: (1) specialization in medicine, which emphasizes the treatment of particular organs or organ systems rather than the whole patient; (2) the increasing use of a multiplicity of drugs, of complex surgery, and of various measuring devices in diagnosis; and (3) the theoretical suc-

cess of molecular biology that explains the whole human organism by listing its ultimate atomic parts.

6. One must also keep in mind that an organism as a system is constantly adjusting by means of feedback to changes in the environment. These minor fluctuations are not diseases; rather, they are health itself. If the system fluctuates beyond a certain range, however, it cannot recover normal health without a major readjustment during a period of sickness in which many normal functions must be minimized while the organism uses all its energies to readjust. Such a disease is an *acute* illness. Or the organism may readjust but only at the cost of a permanent diminishing or suppression of some functions. Then the disease becomes *chronic* or permanent disability results. Finally, an adjustment may be too great for the organism to achieve, and death results. As for *aging*, some scientists still accept the theory of August Weisman (1834–1914) that organisms have been adapted by evolution to die in order to make room for the next generation, but this has not been proved, since life span has relatively minor effects on reproductive rates (Gavrilova and Gavrilova 2001). More probably, aging is the gradual debilitation of a living system that already had some genetic defects and was also during its lifetime exposed to repeated disease and trauma (Gavrilova and Gavrilova 1991, 2001).

7. Many of the foregoing problems have arisen because medical professionals in their scientific training have absorbed a *reductionistic* view of the human person that is closed to the traditional conviction that because we are persons we have a spiritual soul as well as a physical body. They try to reduce the human mind simply to the working of the brain. In fact, modern science has not solved the "mind–body" problem. Conversely, from the time of Plato and again in the seventeenth century with Descartes, a *dualistic* conception of the human person has influenced many to think of the human person as a "mind in a machine" (Wozniak 1995). The problem is still the subject of lively debates among philosophers and between them and biologists (Szubka and Warner 1994; Chalmers 1996).

   Some Catholic theologians have unwittingly accepted dualism by claiming that to take the physical character of an act into account rather than the psychological intention or motivation of the act is "physicalism" or "biologism" (Curran 1984). In fact, in most human actions our psychological intention is directed toward causing some physical change in our physical world and is specified by the change we intend to produce. Thus we cannot judge the morality of those acts without taking into consideration their physical character. Therefore both the physical and psychological aspect of any human act must be considered in any moral judgment. Our spiritual soul and our material body are causally *correlative*, always in mutual interaction. The spiritual soul unifies our body as a living organism, yet our intellects cannot think or make free choices without the information supplied through the bodily senses and the brain. Thus physical health and psychological health are intimately related.

8. The World Health Organization (1958) insisted, "Health is a state of complete physical, mental, and social well-being and not merely the absence of disease or infirmity." Although the health care professions are concerned with health in the narrower sense of optimal functioning at the biological and psychological levels, our thinking about health must always be kept in the context of the integration of all

levels of the person (Pellegrino and Thomasma 1988). Thus, although physicians specialize in dealing with biological or psychological functions, they must never neglect or ignore the social and spiritual needs of their patients if they wish to be truly concerned about health.

For example, to determine whether alcoholism is a sickness without reductionism or arbitrary social construction, we must first define it in behavioral terms and then ask five questions.

a. Is "alcoholism" a biological disease, that is, a change in physiology that puts a strain on biological homeostasis?
b. Is it a psychological disease, that is, a persistent emotional conflict that restricts the victim's capacity for intelligent free choice?
c. Is it a vice, that is, a restriction of free choice in behavior that is inconsistent with the full actualization of the person in community and which leads to antisocial acts?
d. Is it a spiritual disorder, that is, closure to intuition, creativity, and commitment?
e. How are these different levels of dysfunction interrelated? The terms *disease* and *health* are used at each of these levels in very different but analogous ways.

The Unity of the Human Person

In view of the foregoing definition of human health as "optimal human functioning," therefore, we must judge the human need for health as our most *necessary* need but the gaining of truth as the need that most fully realizes the human potential and hence is ethically our *final goal* (or ultimate end), that is, true happiness. This conclusion may, as the plurifinalists (Grisez 1983; Grisez, Boyle, and Finnis 1987) discussed in chapter 1 (section 1.3) argue, seem unconvincing because so many people make the satisfaction of one of the other three needs their supreme value. Moreover, a great many appear to think that *physical pleasure* is true happiness, but as we have seen in the preceding section, Aristotle pointed out that although we certainly all need some physical pleasure for the sake of the recreation that is required for health, we need it not for itself but as a support in seeking one of the four real values. It is only as we learn the truth about ourselves, our community, and the world in which we live that we become free to seek the satisfaction of all our needs in a unified way and thus free to fully enjoy the beauty and wonder of reality. Yet not only highly intelligent or very learned people can be happy, because in a good community the wisdom that some few achieve can be shared with others. Yet only in a community where truth is sought and shared can human happiness rise to a high level.

Although we have many needs, they are all unified in the reality of a human person, and we cannot make good decisions about health needs if we ignore their context in the totality of that person. We have a nature that is constituted by the unity of a material body freely controlled by a spiritual soul. This embodied intelligent *freedom* defines us as human and gives unity and continuity to the human family across time and space. To have this need and capacity for intelligent freedom is to be a *person* (DeKoninck 1945; Ashley 1972, 1985a, 1990, 1998, 2000a, 2000b, 2000c; Adler 1993; Radical Academy 2000). The reason ordinary language does not apply the term *person* to an animal, even a pet, is because although animals sense and feel somewhat as we do, they cannot talk back.

Those who like Peter Singer (1975, 2000) argue that subhuman animals have "rights" in the same sense that humans do because they feel pain misplace the foundation of human rights. Subhuman animals lack the abstract intelligence that makes free choice possible and therefore are not members of the human community who have rights in justice and are obliged to respect the rights of others. It may seem hard to say that one's beloved animal pet is not a member of the same community to which one belongs, but is one's "friend" only in an analogical sense, yet to deny this is to fail to recognize what essentially makes us human. This is not our feelings, but our freedom and the intelligence from which it flows and which subhuman animals that live only by instinct and training completely lack. For that reason subhuman animals do not have rights, but human animals are morally obliged to use animals "humanely," that is, with respect for their God-given natures and without cruelty or waste. Those who become accustomed to abusing animals soon abuse human persons.

Also some ethicists have recently proposed a distinction between being *human* and being a *person* (Engelhardt 1986; Tauer 1985). They define "person" as a self-conscious, free, moral agent; thus infants or victims of senility, although human (i.e., biologically members of the human species), are not, at least in a proper sense, persons. Engelhardt (1977) goes so far as to title one essay "Some Persons Are Humans, Some Humans Are Persons, and the World Is What We Persons Make of It." Does this imply that "moral agents" are free to grant personal status or to deny it to their inferiors—a position that elites have always found very convenient in justifying their neglect or oppression of the powerless? Such a view is very difficult to reconcile with any scientific account of the unity of human nature and does violence to ordinary language. Yet, according to our ordinary use of language, to be a human person does not require that here and now one is functioning as an intelligent, free, moral agent, but one has to have the essential organic structures necessary to develop such capacities and to activate them more or less effectively under favorable and appropriate conditions. Indeed, the very notion of a living being is that, given the proper environment and matter-energy input, it has the innate capacity to develop itself to maturity long before it is able to function in the adult way characteristic of its species, and many living things have periods of dormancy during which their characteristic activities are not apparent.

Humans with Potential

The immature or dormant living thing is not "potentially" a member of a given species. Rather, it is *actually* a member of its species because it is already essentially capable of developing mature and effective behavior characteristic of that species, though the exercise of that behavior remains only potential. Thus an infant human being is already actually and not only potentially a member of the human species years before its behavior can be clearly discriminated from that of other animal species by the exercise of intelligent freedom. Hence we are actually persons, in the sense of having human rights, even when we are not actually, but only potentially, moral agents. Thus the fetus, the infant, the seriously debilitated, the senile, the comatose, and those who are asleep or drugged are still persons (O'Rourke 2006).

As we have already noted in speaking of Platonic dualism, some philosophers identify the human person or self only with the mind and treat the human body as only a sort of garment that is put off at death and reassumed in "reincarnation." In refutation of this idealistic notion of the human person as a "self-conscious mind," recent philosophers (Parfit 1984; Moore 1995) have come to agree with the Bible and St. Thomas Aquinas that bodily identity is necessary to the notion of the human person. For Aquinas, the human soul after death is not a complete human person and that is why God will return it to its body at the Resurrection (*Summa Theologiae* I, q. 76; Suppl. q. 79). Human life involves a development of this unique body–mind in constant interaction with its environment (Ashley 1985a).

Thus human nature is an open system with several functional subsystems. The term *integrity* indicates that in a perfect whole, each part must be fully differentiated and developed. Furthermore, each part must be fitted into the whole and harmonized with it by correct interrelations and interactions with the other parts of the whole. Integrity is lacking when a part is suppressed or unduly inhibited in function, or when, alternatively, one part is hypertrophied due to the injury of other parts. Persons share biological and psychological needs with other animals, whereas human persons share social and spiritual needs only with other human persons. Nevertheless all these needs and their correlative values, whether generically animal or specifically human, are *equally* needs and values of the human person, none of which can be neglected without harming personhood.

At the biological level, the human body is divided into organ systems and these further into organs, each having specific functions (Human Body Adventure 2003). The organ systems are usually enumerated as follows: (1) nervous, (2) endocrine, (3) skeletal and muscular, (4) integumentary (skin), (5) alimentary, (6) respiratory, (7) circulatory, (8) excretory, and (9) reproductive. These systems are interrelated in very complex ways and not in any simple, linear hierarchy. However, the nervous system (with the intimately related endocrine system) is obviously the one that coordinates the others and is the most directly involved in the psychological and higher functions. Greater unification of function occurs at the psychic level of personality. Psychic life, however, is also composite. The organs of the external senses clearly differentiate their functions. Other psychological functions have some type of localization in various parts of the brain, but also involve other centers and the endocrine system as well. Furthermore, as depth psychology has shown, the field of awareness itself is differentiated into an unconscious, a subconscious, a superego, an ego, and so forth.

At the rational and ethical levels, still greater integration and unification of functions into the self-aware, conscious, free, self-controlling subject or person take place. Even at this level, what have been traditionally called the reason and the will (*Summa Theologiae* I–II, q. 1–5) are differentiated as distinct but ultimately correlative functions. Only at the spiritual level do the intellect and will come together in the "still point" (Ashley 1972, 2000c), or top of the mind or heart (in the biblical, metaphorical sense) of the human person, in which peak experiences (Maslow 1970, 1994) and basic decisions, commitments, and fundamental options take place to complete the total integration of the person.

True Human Happiness

What then is true human happiness? The definition of happiness must include the satisfaction of all our basic needs, but it must include them in their proper hierarchy or rank of importance so that the less important are subordinated to the more important. They must be integrated and unified by their relations to each other and especially to the need that is most important, which, we have argued, is knowledge of ourselves, of other persons, and of our environment (*Summa Theologiae* I–II, q. 1–5). Without this knowledge, human life is not human, it is meaningless and empty, as so many people who have made other things their highest value discover too late in life. With this knowledge, an invalid, without a family and living in loneliness, can still have a rich life. Furthermore, because serious thought about ourselves and the world around us ultimately comes up against the question of the Creator and of our death, those who come to the conviction that a personal God is the supreme good, source of all life, wisdom, freedom, and morality, realize that the most important need in our life is to know God and live according to his wisdom and love.

Though the founders of modern science believed in a Creator, scientists today are reluctant to face this question (Jaki 1989; Furton 2003). Yet most people throughout history, including many of the greatest minds, have asked and answered it affirmatively: *There is a God, and death is not the end of human existence.* Those who evade this question or answer it agnostically or atheistically do so either because they think, "Science will explain everything, and we will soon find a cure," or because they are shocked by the immense evil that humans have produced in the world. Yet that God permits us to do evil only shows that he respects the gift of freedom that he gave us.

Thus in this lifelong search for an authentic happiness every person has a biography that consists in the mature actualization of intelligent freedom and the manifestation of a unique personality. This life story passes through many phases of fetal and infant development before the brain can function at higher levels. Getting sick and getting well are both parts of this continuous, struggling process of living development. Thus defining human personhood as "embodied intelligent freedom" presupposes a life process that goes on at many levels of activity, but that is more clearly manifest and definable by its maximum, its high point of integration. Medical ethics must always take into account that the person who needs help in a particular crisis of illness is a being who not merely exists here and now but also has a history and a future, and for all worldviews, except the materialist ones, a future even beyond bodily death. Christians, Orthodox Jews, and Muslims are all convinced that this future will be completed with the reunion of soul and body in the Resurrection, so that the body-person will be fully restored. Hence the great dignity of the human body that Jesus called "the temple of God" (Jn 2:21; cf. 1 Cor 3:16).

Note, however, that "person" and "personality" are not identical; a person *has* a personality that is his or her unique *expression* of personhood. Peter Singer (1975) and the environmentalist Michael W. Fox argue that from an ethical point of view there is no essential distinction between human beings and animals, at least the higher animals. Fox asserts, "One's own selfhood is no less and no more sacred that any other sentient being" (Fox 2001, 33). Yet what makes us human is not that we, like animals, can feel pleasure and pain, as Singer and Fox assume, but that we have intelligence and free will that other animals lack. However, precisely because the essence of human nature is embodied intelligent freedom, each human being transcends the commonalities of this nature and attains a unique biography of personal choices. To be truly human, I must also be truly myself. I must live out my life as being responsible for its ultimate direction. Such is a reasonable interpretation of the paradoxical view of some existentialist philosophers who claim, "Man has no nature, but only a history." Individual differences between one human being and another are not trivial. Even genetically similar monozygotic twins are still able to live personal lives and have distinct biographies. Twins can disagree, can go separate ways. No doubt, if someday science produces human clones, these human beings will still each have their own lives to live and will live them differently.

2.2 JESUS CHRIST, HEALER, AS ETHICAL MODEL

If we are to develop an ethics that is not merely idealistic and a priori but empirically based on actual human behavior, we must base it on historical models of human beings who have realized the full potentialities of mature human nature. Although not everyone will agree on choosing such models, certainly Jesus Christ is among the noblest of historical figures. For Catholic Christians Jesus is a divine person, the Son of God, but he is also truly human, "like us in all things but sin" (Heb 4:15; 2 Cor 5:21). In his earthly life he was, and in his resurrected life is, an existing model of what it is to be truly, fully, and virtuously human. He has won for us also the grace of the Holy Spirit that empowers us to become truly like him.

Moreover, Jesus had special compassion for the sick and the disabled, and because he is the great healer, he is the perfect model for health care professionals. They do not, as he did, perform real miracles, but they use their God-given intelligence to heal by the medical art, as he did by his touch and word. The Catholic Church does not pretend to invent a code of morality but only to transmit the memory of Jesus as handed on from the apostles, recorded in the Bible, and continuously practiced in the life of the community that Jesus himself organized. It is not surprising, therefore, that Catholic health facilities play a major role in health care in the United States and that Catholics pioneered in developing medical ethics.

Although Christian morality is based on the power of God's grace and our call to eternal life in the community of the Trinity, since "grace perfects nature," as St. Thomas Aquinas so often insists, it includes as well as transforms an ethics based on innate human needs as we have analyzed them earlier (*Summa Theologiae* I, q. 1, ad. 8, a. 12; I, q. 62, a. 5; I–II, q. 94, ab. 6). The Christian view of the worth of persons who share with Jesus a human nature is based on the biblical teaching that God creates each person in his own image and likeness, different from lesser creatures in the possession of a spiritual intelligence and free will (Gn 1:26–31). Although God in the order of nature produces the human body through biological evolution and the cooperation of man and woman, the creation of the human soul is a direct act of God (Gn 2:7; 2 Mc 7:22–23) that calls each person into existence in unique relation to God himself (Ps 22:10–11). It may seem strange that God produces a soul for the child born out of wedlock, even though the begetting of that child was a sinful act on the part of the parents. If eventually human clones are artificially reproduced, no doubt God will also create a soul for that cloned human body, although the act of producing a human person in that way is sinful on the part of the technician. Yet the Creator rightly maintains the natural biological forces involved in human reproduction and, so to speak, "does his part," but human beings sin by misusing these natural forces that the Creator has given them to use rightly. We insult God by so misusing his gifts contrary to their true purpose.

Each person is unique and irreplaceable (Mt 10:29–31) to complete the cosmos, and all are called not only to earthly but also to eternal life (1 Tm 2:4). The differences of sex, race, and individual talents or disadvantages in no way detract from this basic equality of all human beings (Rom 2:11; Gal 4:7; Eph 6:9). The Christian foundation for this respect for the person in its integrity is faith in the wisdom of the Creator, who has given persons the gift of human nature, as the Psalmist says (139:13–14):

> Truly you have formed my inmost being;
> you knit me in my mother's womb.
> I give you thanks that I am fearfully, wonderfully
> made; wonderful are your works.

Therefore Christians recall God's own respect for the body of his son, for although he permitted Jesus's death, he inspired the prophets to declare, "Break not one of his bones" (Jn 19:36) and "Nor will you suffer your faithful one to undergo corruption" (Acts 2:27). St. Paul also tells us that our bodies "are temples of the Holy Spirit" (1 Cor 6:19) and that after death they will be resurrected to eternal life (Rom 8:11).

Yet although we are all equally of one human nature with Jesus, God does not give his gifts equally to all, as each person is unique and the good of the community in which all share is enhanced by the complementarity of *different* gifts (1 Cor 12). The extreme inequality between persons we see in our world today, however, is not the work of God but of human sin through which the stronger and less moral oppress the weak and more innocent (Rom 3:9–18). The defects of health that contribute to this inequality are due in part to chance and natural causes, but they are also due to unjust social conditions and the pollution of the environment resulting from human ambition, greed, and neglect. God wills only what is good for us, including good health (Ws 1:12–15), but he gives us as stewards of his creation the responsibility of using natural resources intelligently (Gn 2:15) to overcome disease and preserve health. In his love for his creation, God never permits any evil except as the occasion of a greater good, although if we refuse to be patient with the evil he now permits, we will not enjoy that greater good.

This greater good that is to be fully realized only at the end of history was anticipated by the presence of Jesus among us. He recalled us to our dignity and restored to us the hope for the perfect happiness that God intended for us in our creation. This goal of perfect happiness with God infinitely exceeds the needs of our limited nature and the kind of imperfect happiness that it demands. "Grace perfects nature" so that Jesus in calling us to live with him in the Trinity also enables us to fulfill our natural needs. Our natural happiness is to be included in and transformed by our eternal blessedness. This is why an ethics of reason (of natural law) has autonomy independent of moral theology, yet is also of great service to moral theology. Thus a Christian ethics of health care is based on the historical fact that Jesus Christ worked healing miracles (Mk 1:32–39) to encourage us to use God's gifts for the health care of even the most neglected and powerless members of society (Mt 26:31–46).

Of course non-Catholics, in accordance with their various worldviews and value systems, have much in common with us, and we all need to continue sharing the truths we have in a sympathetic and honest dialogue. Yet such dialogue cannot be really honest unless the proponents of each worldview propose their beliefs and their arguments for their beliefs and expose them candidly to a mutual process of criticism. Others who do not share those views should not take this advocacy of one's own convictions as superior to other views as an offense. That is what honest and charitable dialogue is all about. This applies especially to questions of health care ethics, because in a multicultural society we must all cooperate in preventing illness and caring for those who suffer.

Jesus has showed us the way to the higher goal of eternal life with God and gives to all who will receive it the gift of the *virtue of faith* by which we accept and live by his teachings. It is the most basic of the three supreme Christian virtues of *faith, hope,* and *love* (or charity, Greek *agape,* or *caritas* in Latin). Love is the greatest of the three (Rom 13:13; Outka 1972), because without it the others are lifeless. These three virtues direct the whole of the Christian life to its supreme goal, that is, union with God, and hence are called the "theological" virtues. Christian morality and "spirituality"—a word that today is taken in many very different senses—is simply the flowering of these three virtues. It is these virtues that enable the Christian not merely to perform this or that ethically good act but to form a Christian *character.* A health care professional ought not to be simply a skilled technician but should be of good moral character, a person who can be trusted to act ethically in her or his profession even in unusual and difficult circumstances. Consequently, it is helpful to provide an analysis of character.

2.3 CHARACTER AND THE MAJOR MORAL VIRTUES

Because so many ethicists have overemphasized decision making to the neglect of the *character* required for making good decisions, virtue theory has recently become the "cutting edge" of ethical discussion (Porter 1995a). By a "virtue" we mean a skill to behave in an ethical way *consistently and without excessive internal conflict.* It is by the acquisition of these skills that personal character is formed. Yet a virtue is not a mere habit (in the current English sense of that word). A habit is a learned pattern of behavior that conditions the instinctive behavior of animals, and especially of human animals, because we live more artificially than other animals. For example, we acquire a habit of typing that enables us to perform most of the required actions without much attention except when something unusual occurs. Thus habits are routine behaviors that free us to give attention to more important or unusual problems. But a virtue, although it may be supported by such good habits, is also a capacity to meet new problems, to act flexibly and reasonably. Medical students learning to be surgeons acquire certain physical habits, but if they are to be really good surgeons, they must acquire a skill or virtue that enables them to solve problems that unexpectedly arise in certain cases. Thus successful practice of the medical profession depends not only on theoretical knowledge but also on extensive *clinical experience.*

The opposite of a virtue is a *vice,* a skill in effectively and consistently doing something that is morally evil. It differs from an "addiction," as a vicious person acts freely and intelligently, though from bad motives. Addicted persons, however, act compulsively with diminished freedom. They are so driven by their desire for a certain physical satisfaction that they often act in most unreasonable ways, contrary to what in their more sober moments they really want for themselves and others. Vices enslave the person in wrongdoing because they form habits of perception, feeling, and thought that blind the vicious to the consequences of their evil ways. Hence vices of indulgence in intense pleasures easily result in addiction, but so can vices of extreme aggression, because there can be great pleasure in power and domination.

Figure 2.1   Correlation of Theological and Moral Virtues

Intellect ———————— Prudence	FAITH	
Passions { Pleasure drive ——— Temperance / Aggressive drive——— Fortitude	HOPE	Theological Virtues
Will ————————— Justice	LOVE	

Virtues (Conway 1960; Ashley 1996a) can be (1) theoretical *intellectual* skills, such as learning to think mathematically, or they can be (2) practical *productive* skills, productive of objects that are either (a) *useful,* such as the food raised by a farmer or the healing skills of medical professionals, or (b) *entertaining,* such as the works of fine art or performance in sports. We are free to use such skills in a variety of ways, but we have to decide just whether, how, and for what purpose we are to use them. Alternatively, (3) *ethical* skills, that is, the moral virtues, deal with the satisfaction of our basic needs, and hence we *must* use the moral virtues if we are to be happy, and we *cannot* really want to be unhappy. The four principle natural moral virtues are traditionally called the "cardinal" (from Latin *cardo,* hinge) virtues (Pieper 1966). All four cardinal or chief virtues also have subdivisions and are supported by a number of lesser virtues, which we will not consider here in detail, but which are treated in Benedict Ashley's *Living the Truth in Love* (1996a). Each moral virtue is related to one of the theological virtues (see figure 2.1).

Faith and Prudence

Of these four cardinal virtues, correlated earlier with the Christian theological virtues, only one, traditionally called the cardinal virtue of Prudence, is also an intellectual virtue, namely, a skill in thinking about how to choose the right means to satisfy our basic needs in a unified way (figure 2.1). In English, "prudence" often simply means acting cautiously, but the virtue includes skill not only in being cautious but also in being imaginative, taking reasonable risks, foreseeing possible consequences, and so on. In fact, the virtue of Prudence is the same skill as ethical behavior or good moral judgment, although a distinction needs to be made between someone who has merely studied ethics in an abstract way and someone who has acquired the complete skill so as to be able to actually make good ethical decisions in real life. Studying bioethics is a good way to begin to learn how to make good bioethical decisions, but one needs extensive experience and practice in actual cases in a health care facility to be a prudent bioethicist. That is why some people who have never studied ethics formally are more prudent than some who have only read about it in books.

Christian Prudence, however, is transformed by a vision of a higher goal rather than merely worldly happiness. To recognize who Jesus is and the way he has opened to us, however, we must accept the gift of the theological virtue of Faith that, as we have shown earlier, Jesus offers to all through his church. Faith is a virtue of the human intellect that helps one believe the Word of God although God in his mystery is invisible to us (CCC 2000, no. 26, 142–84, 1814–16, 2087–89). Yet God does not ask anyone to accept this faith blindly or as a "leap in the dark," as it is sometimes wrongly described, because God, who gave us reason, does not ask us to be credulous fools. Jesus has given us signs that demonstrate to our reason that we ought to believe the Word of God on faith just as we have faith in our physicians because of their certification as medical doctors and their good reputations as professionals. To go to a doctor who is not thus certified is to put our bodies in the care of a quack. Thus it would be foolish to believe the Christian, Catholic faith if it was not somehow authenticated.

Though faith has a power that greatly exceeds that of natural human reason, it is also *reasonable*, not because we can see its intrinsic truth but because we can see by extrinsic signs that God has given to show us that he is speaking through these signs, and they oblige us, if we are reasonable, to believe him on his word (CCC 2000, no. 156, 812; Kreeft and Tacelli 1994). These signs were given during Jesus's earthly life by his fulfillment of ancient prophecies and by his many miracles of healing and raising the dead and by his own great miracle of resurrection from the dead. It was unreasonable and prejudiced for the persons who witnessed these signs not to have put faith in his teaching (cf. Lk 10:12–16). Today we cannot be eyewitnesses to these signs as were the holy women and the twelve apostles, yet we can observe the Catholic Church in its witness to these events and see that it too is a miracle of Jesus and is animated by the Holy Spirit he sent upon it, as, in spite of the failings of its members that are common to all human organizations, it strikingly differs from all of them in its universality of membership, its continuity in time under every kind of persecution, and its unity of government and developing faith. Hence the Catholic Church that rests on faith has always been and is today also a major defender of the power of human reason and of natural law morality in the face of the skepticism, cynicism, and moral relativism that dominate modern culture.

Christian Prudence, cultivated by the Catholic theology, is human prudence as it is transformed to guide us not simply to the end of natural happiness but to God in eternal life. It supports natural prudence but goes beyond it, because it makes us thoughtful about whether our own lives will lead us beyond death to eternal life, and it also provokes a concern in us to help others to this same goal. It helps us understand that the world we actually live in has from the beginning of human history been a very troubled world because of sin. The influence of all this sinful history has turned us, our families, and our communities away from seeking God to seeking worldly goods of pleasure, power, and material possessions that can never of themselves bring us happiness but only conflict, disillusionment, addiction, and despair. Our lives and our culture are too much governed not by true faith and transformed Prudence but by "worldly (carnal) prudence," that is, shrewdness and cunning in gaining these false goals at the expense of our neighbors and our own integrity. Jesus Christ worked miracles of healing (Mk 1:32–39) to encourage us to use God's gifts for the health care even of the most neglected and powerless members of society (Mt 26:31–46). Christians must therefore, as Jesus urged, "be as prudent as serpents, yet innocent as doves" (Mt 10:16). Yet, in the ironical parable of the fraudulent servant, Jesus also sadly remarked that the children of this world are more "prudent . . . than are the children of light" (Lk 16:8).

In chapter 1 (section 1.4) we discussed the various degrees of authority, concluding that Christian faith and prudence require that authentic church teaching in all its degrees be the principal guidance of our conscience and should never be disobeyed unless we are objectively *certain* that this teaching is in error, never simply because its teaching seems to us less probable than our own thinking, popular opinion, or the views of theologians, however scholarly. The constant controversies among bioethicists make it perfectly clear that opinion about ethical questions based on reason alone is rarely more than probable.

Even in such a rare case as when one could be certain that church authority was mistaken in its ethical teaching, dissent from it should be expressed in a way that will protect proper respect for church authority (CDF 1990, nos. 24–28). Thus Catholic health care ethicists, while by no means neglecting a rational ethics of natural law, will always measure their professional as well as their personal decisions by the moral teaching of the Catholic Church as summed up in the teachings of Vatican Council II and systematized in *The Catechism of the Catholic Church* (CCC 2000), and in other official documents of the Holy See directly relating to bioethics and most proximately by the U.S. bishops' *Ethical and Religious Directives for Catholic Health Care Services* (ERD 2001).

Love and Justice

Even small children playing games or dividing among them a bag of candy recognize that we ought to be "fair" and not "cheat" or "play favorites." Because two of our basic needs are for good family and social relationships, the human person as a social being greatly needs relational skills. The basic skill for such relationships is the virtue of Justice or Fairness, which makes us concerned not just for our individual good but also for the common good of the family and/or society. Because life is difficult and we need first of all to care for our own needs, it is not easy for us to always remember to think about the needs of others. In an ends–means ethic this does not imply, as Kant's duty ethic claimed, that to act morally we must be altruistically disinterested and think only of what kind of behavior is good for all. In fact, such lack of self-concern is psychologically impossible. We ought and must think first of our own needs. But because we have a need for social relationships for our own happiness, only if the common good is achieved can we satisfy these needs by sharing many good things with others. To think of others, therefore, requires a virtue not in the intelligence such as Faith or Prudence but in the *will*, a consistent determination to respect the rights of others, and this is called the cardinal virtue of Justice, often referred to in the Bible as "righteousness."

Three different kinds or degrees of justice are needed in a community. The first is *exchange* (commutative) justice between individuals, as in buying and selling, or between a physician and his client when the doctor gives medical treatment and the patient pays a fee. This is also the justice that is required by contracts. In chapter 1 we pointed out that some ethicists have tried to reduce all bioethics to contractual obligation (contractualism). The second kind of Justice is *justice to the community*, traditionally called "legal" justice, because we fulfill it in part by obeying the legitimate laws of the community. The third is *distributive* justice of the community to it members, giving to each the share in the common good that they deserve or need, well summed up in the formula "From each according to ability, to each according to need." Because legal justice and distributive justices are reciprocal, the second and third forms of justice are today often joined and called *social justice.*

The Christian point of view on social justice—and which also has support in many other religions and philosophies of life—rejects both collectivism and individualism (whether that individualism be conservative or liberal). Christianity repudiates collectivism because the community should exist to serve persons and not persons to serve a superpersonal totality as in totalitarianism. Christianity also renounces individualism, because Christianity teaches that the highest and most important goods of the person are not private property but are spiritual goods that can be achieved and fully enjoyed only by sharing with others. Because modern states, both collectivistic and individualistic, are oriented to maximizing material goods and economic power rather than maximizing spiritual goods, the struggle between person and community has become chronic.

It is often overlooked that, because our need for family and society and true knowledge ranks higher than our own need for health, security, and possessions, there really is no intrinsic opposition between the individual good and the community good, between private property and social welfare. A distinction must be made between those goods of the human person that are private and those that are shared in common (DeKoninck 1945). They are both personal, but one is private, the other common. Private goods are largely material goods, because if one person uses or consumes something material, others cannot share it. Common goods are chiefly spiritual goods because when these are shared no one loses, but all gain. A teacher does not lose the knowledge that she shares with her students; instead by sharing it she understands it better herself. Thus the church in light of historical experience (Bellah 1986, 1991) rejects both totalitarianism and individualism. It also rejects the Marxist attack on private property and equally rejects the libertarian view that economic justice should be left to an unregulated free market. The kingdom of God begins here on Earth, as we pray in the Our Father, with social justice, as modern popes have constantly preached, and no one will gain heaven that has neglected to work for social justice on Earth. Jesus said, "I was hungry and you never gave me food. . . . Insofar as you neglected to do this to one of the least of these, you neglected to do it to me" (Mt 25:31–46). In the parable of Lazarus and the rich man (Lk 16:19–31), he taught the same lesson.

Consequently a genuine Christian ethic cannot be written from the viewpoint of the status quo, which in a sinful world tends to reflect the materialistic spirit of domination and possessiveness. It must also view the world from the side of the oppressed, whose needs have been ignored and neglected. Thus Jesus pointed to his preaching of the Gospel to the poor as the best sign of the authenticity of his own mission (Mt 11:5). A Christian politics of health care must then be based on this "option for the poor." Christians therefore must join in a common effort with all those who are sincerely concerned about human needs and human rights, including the right to health. This ecumenical search for ethical consensus in regard to needs and rights has its solid legal and political foundations in the United Nations' *Universal Declaration of Human Rights* (1948), signed by most of the countries of the world and supported by all the major religions as well as by humanists. The recent popes have all urged Catholics to support this declaration as a sound basis for social justice. It furnishes for the twenty-first century a basic consensus on the fundamental ethical values on which world peace and community must be based and on which health care for all human beings must be sought.

Yet every individual has the primary responsibility for his or her health, because society cannot compel its members to do many of the things required for health, and hence the work of health care professionals must be conceived as a cooperative service for individuals in their personal search for health. Consequently, to ensure the participation in decision making by all persons whose interests are involved, it is important to observe the three factors of good organization found in the social encyclicals of the popes and adopted in the treaty on which the European Union is founded: (1) solidarity (i.e., to make decisions in view of the fact that we all form part of an interdependent, human community), (2) subsidiarity (i.e., to keep decision making as close as possible to the persons concerned in the vertical organization of society so that all actively participate and cooperate), and (3) functionality (i.e., to divide responsibility for decision making through a division of roles in the horizontal organization of society). At the same time, those who have the highest authority must protect and promote the unity of the community and its common good. The principal official Catholic documents on social justice and other helpful bibliographies can be conveniently accessed on the Internet: www.justpeace.org/docu.htm and www.osjspm.org/cst/doclist.htm.

The Christian point of view is neither idealistic nor altruistic. The words of Jesus were, "Treat others the way you would have them treat you; this sums up the law and the prophets" (Mt 7:12), and "You shall love your neighbor as yourself" (Mt 22:39). According to this teaching we are not asked to love our neighbor and *not* love ourselves, but to love our neighbor as ourselves. In other words, if we really love ourselves, not selfishly, but intelligently, we will realize that we cannot be happy in isolation, because we were created as *social* beings. The New Testament also teaches, "Faith without works," however, "is dead" (Jas 2:17). The Sermon on the Mount makes clear that the "works" in question are not the external rituals on which the Pharisees placed so much emphasis, but on "faith working through love" (Gal 5:6) of God and neighbor. The teachings of Jesus in the New Testament, though they also speak of Justice or "righteousness," go further and emphasize that the greatest commandment is the "love of God and neighbor," or in other terms the Golden Rule, "Do unto others what you want them to do to you." While the virtue of Justice respects others' rights, the virtue of Love goes beyond this to help even those who do not deserve help but nevertheless need it (Wadell 1992; Jackson 2002). Jesus illustrated this "extra" effort of love in the parable of the Good Samaritan, who recognized that right in the wounded stranger and "was moved with pity at the sight. He approached him and dressed his wounds, pouring on oil and wine" (Lk 11:33b–34) and then took him to an inn, promising the innkeeper to pay for any extra things the wounded man might need. At the same time, Love degenerates into sentimentality unless it is also assisted by the virtue of Justice, that is, the consistent will to respect the rights of others (John Paul II 1991).

The term *love* in this New Testament context is in Greek *agape*, not the word "eros" for sexual love, and it does not mean simply sentimental attraction. That is why it used to be translated "charity" (from the Latin *caritas*) but in present English "charity" has the connotation only of doing good to another, while, as St. Thomas Aquinas says, New Testament love is the love of true friendship that not only seeks another's benefit but also wants to share life with the other (*Summa Theologiae* I–II, q. 65, a. 5e). Jesus loved even his wicked enemies not only because he wished to do them good but also because he hoped to convert them so that they might enter with him into the eternal life of God where all are intimate friends. Few of us when we give "charity" to homeless persons really want to live with them as intimate friends! Therefore in any Christian ethics the fundamental truth is that there is a Triune God and that "God is love" (Jn 4:8). God loves us not because he has first needed our love but because his love for us has made us lovable and able to love him and our neighbor in return. As St. John of the Cross said, "In the end, what counts is love."

Hope, Temperance, Fortitude

After discussing the norms of faith and prudence and love and justice, what theologians call the *eschatological* aspect of ethics can be better understood. Eschatology is the study of what has been revealed about the final coming of Jesus Christ in the fully realized kingdom of God. Communities of persons are not structures of static relations but are dynamic—loving, growing, developing, and evolving. This is why we have opted for a goal-directed, means–ends ethics. Furthermore, human goals are not always clearly envisioned in advance. The kingdom of God, on which Jesus centered his preaching, is a goal so mysterious that he could express it only in terms of parables. Recently, Christian theologians have developed theologies of hope and theologies of liberation to bring out that the Gospel is not merely a declaration that heaven is better than Earth, but a call to transform the Earth as we journey heavenward. Thus we are finding areas of agreement with the claim of secularism and Marxism that to be human is to work for the future. This sense of hope is the source of all healing, so that to be a health care professional is to affirm constantly the possibility of turning suffering into a victory over disease and death.

Christian theology though, as previously indicated, has freed itself from Platonic dualism; however, it recognizes a certain measure of truth in a body–soul dualism reconcilable with the deeper unity of the human person. The human person is a unified complex subject prey to internal conflicts, so that any person's integration and self-individuation can be achieved only by a sane *asceticism,* or impulse control. Such ascetic discipline, however, does not imply that the human body in its biological functions is evil or of little value, but rather that it shares in the spiritual dignity of the total person and yet needs to be integrated with the whole (Van Kaam 1985). Thus the body cannot be suppressed or ruthlessly sacrificed to higher values or even trivialized as of no moral significance. Catholic ethics have sought a middle way between the dualistic extremes of asceticism and antinomianism and to respect the intrinsic teleology of bodily structures and basic biological functions. This takes on symbolic value in the Church's liturgical cycle where an ascetic Lent prepares us for a joyful Easter.

Morality is not, as some writers seem to think, only a matter of our relations with others. The first responsibility of our human freedom is that each person must seek his or her own true happiness and form his or her own good character, because without a good character with its virtues we cannot move consistently and efficiently toward true happiness. Yet human intellect and free will cannot operate except with the use of the instruments of the human body: our senses and affective drives that we share with other animals. These drives to satisfy the needs of the body are not as such conscious, but they cause changes in our bodies that we then sense as "feelings" or "emotions." The sight of food starts the digestive juices flowing and the stomach contracting. We then sense this change in our bodies and speak of it as a feeling or emotion of hunger. Emotions as such are ethically neutral, neither good nor bad, and take on positive moral value only when controlled by reason, or negative moral value when opposed to reason. Controlled emotions that support and facilitate realistic decisions of our reason are morally good, but those that obstruct realistic, prudent decision and lead us into destructive acts are morally bad because they lead to unhappiness.

Therefore, because Christians hope for a kingdom that has not yet been realized on Earth and that will last forever, they are willing to undergo a more rigorous discipline (asceticism) of their natural biological drives for pleasure and the avoidance of pain, and of their fears and aggressive tendencies, than might seem reasonable if their only goal were temporal happiness. Hence Christian hope is assisted by the two cardinal virtues of Temperance, or moderation in regard to the pleasures of food, drink, sex, and recreation, and Fortitude, or courage in the endurance of suffering and risk taking to attain goals. The first of these virtues by which one can control these basic biological drives, Temperance, is the skillful control of our desires for physical pleasure or the avoidance of physical pain. The alcoholic cannot make prudent judgments about his life because his addiction has restricted his freedom to think realistically about practical decisions and sometimes has even destroyed that freedom altogether. While some of our politicians have shown remarkable prudence, their uncontrolled sexual appetites have led them to do utterly foolish and self-destructive things.

But besides the pleasure drives that we share with animals, we also share with them aggressive drives that enable us to endure the pain of a struggle to attain our goals or to wait patiently until the danger can be attacked or is over. Such aggressive drives are necessary if we are to meet the difficulties and dangers of living, but they, like the pleasure drives, can get out of control and become self-destructive. The skill or virtue in controlling these aggressive drives is called Fortitude. It supports Temperance, because it takes great courage to overcome the addictions to which we can so easily succumb.

These two virtues of Temperance and Fortitude are not primarily intellectual because what they control is our drives or emotions, and these are primarily bodily functions. Yet Temperance and Fortitude exert their control by conforming the body and its drives to what the virtue of Prudence tells us is reasonable and realistic. Thus someone with Fortitude does not merely control anger but also gets emotionally angry in a reasonable way appropriate to the real situation to be faced. A temperate person may like a drink but is not inclined to drink more than what is reasonable and finds excessive drinking distasteful. Thus as adolescents grow up they find their physical drives to be very violent and rebellious ("raging hormones"), but if by practice they gradually learn self-control, they acquire those virtues that will help them satisfy their basic needs in realistic, efficient ways without such struggles for self-control. Accordingly, Aristotle distinguished "continence," or what today we call control by "will power," from a true virtue, because persons with true virtue no longer need to exercise "will power" to control their emotions, since their emotions obey their reason easily, as a trained horse knows what its master wants it to do without being whipped.

Christian Sexuality

Genuine Christian teaching on sexuality is clear enough in the scriptures and was given a rich and accurate expression by Vatican II and the encyclicals of Paul VI, *Humanae vitae* (1968), and of John Paul II, *Familiaris consortio* (1981), based on that council. Genesis 1:3 teaches that God created persons as male and female and blessed their sexuality as a great and good gift. Jesus confirmed this teaching, and perfected it by affirming that men must be as faithful in marriage as women (Mk 10:2–21; 1 Cor 7:10). Nevertheless, Jesus also taught that although sexuality is a great gift, its use in marriage is only a relative value, which can be freely sacrificed for the sake of higher values. Thus, for the Christian, the celibate or single life, with its freedom from domestic cares, so as to be free for the service of others, can be even more personally maturing and fulfilling than married life. St. Paul (1 Cor 7:25–35) also emphasizes the value of the single life in view of the "shortness of the time" (i.e., the time to achieve holiness and complete one's mission in life), but also teaches that marriage is a sacrament in that the love of husband and wife is a symbol that teaches us the love of Christ for his people (Eph 5:22–23). Thus in the church the married and the single complement each other. The married give celibates an example of fruitful love. The celibates remind the married of the peace of the still more loving life to come.

In the Jewish and Christian view, based on the first chapters of Genesis, human sexuality is always seen in relation to the *family*, which is the basic community into which we are born and educated and on which the larger community is built. Hence sexuality is not merely a private matter, although it involves the most intimate of relationships; it concerns the common good of society and requires public support as the basic social institution. The Church's moral teaching on sex, therefore, can be understood primarily as support for the family, and it opposes certain kinds of sexual behavior not because Catholicism is antisex, but because centuries of experience show that such behaviors undermine the family institution and deprive children of their right to a secure home life.

As for suffering and death, Christian faith understands these in two different ways. On the one hand, death is evil because it is the result of sin. On the other hand, it is a liberating and grace-filled experience, if the proper motivation is present. These two views are not contradictory; rather they are complementary. Suffering and death, joined to the suffering and death of Jesus, the Lord of life, represent not dissolution but growth, not punishment but fulfillment, not sadness but joy. God allows suffering and death to enable us to live with Christ now and forever. The principle, supremely exemplified in the Cross, is rooted in the basic human need to preserve life, because people suffer only in order to achieve a renewed, purified, and enriched life.

Jesus taught us not only to believe in God and to love Him and our neighbor but that such love would not be possible if we did not have firm hope of attaining friendship with God and our neighbor forever. In the worldview of the secularism dominating our culture, many place their hopes in the myth of constant technological progress. Yet this progress has failed to solve some of our worst problems and has produced many of them. Hence we need a virtue of Hope that rests not on human power but on our faith in God whom we know loves us and would never permit any evil to happen to us that he cannot ultimately use for our greater good.

It might seem strange to relate this virtue of Hope to the virtues of Fortitude and Temperance that we need to control our physical drives for power and for pleasure. Yet the weakness of people in the face of the difficulties of life and the temptations to self-destructive pleasures arise from the fact that these people have lost hope in true happiness and have come to substitute cowardice and indulgence as the only kind of life they can trust to give them some kind of satisfaction. In health care also, *prevention* of disease requires the promotion of considerable discipline in diet, exercise, simplicity of life, and so forth that make us healthy but whose practice can also develop these virtues. Every physician knows that a patient who hopes to get well is more likely to do so than one who gives up. Christian hope supports these lesser forms of hope but extends to hope even in the face of fatal illness and death. Yet as bodily pleasure should be sought only as the fruit of the satisfaction of some basic need of the total human person, so suffering and even bodily death when endured with courage can and should be used to promote personal growth in both private and communal living.

2.4 PRUDENT DECISION MAKING

We have explained that Prudence is the intellectual virtue that, while it presupposes the other three cardinal virtues in the will and the biological drives, and requires elevation by Christian faith, enables us to make good moral decisions. Thus it is the completion of ethics, and health care ethics is the virtue of Prudence applied to decisions about how to meet health needs. Because decisions about human health needs are so complex, we need to ask, "What is the prudent way to form our consciences so as to make moral decisions in general and in particular about health care?" The term *conscience* refers to our judgment of what is right and wrong to do, both as to general norms but also as regards actual concrete situations. Traditionally it is said that "conscience is the voice of God," but this is true only if our decisions are prudent, that is, made reasonably in relation to human needs properly ranked and unified.

Thus we must understand and keep in mind the true needs of our human nature and their relative importance. Then we must get the best information available to us as to the possible means to that goal in the concrete circumstances of our lives. Our conscientious judgment must rest on the reliable information we have gathered in a realistic way and not on prejudice or unreasoned feeling, impulse, or addiction. We need to come to a definite and consistent moral judgment, and not just drift or conform to what others are doing. Yet it is not enough just to make good moral judgments; we must also decide to act on them and carry them through. Once we have acted we should not waste time on second-guessing or neurotic guilt, but we should also not make excuses or rationalize our mistakes or our failures to follow our best moral judgment. We should admit our mistakes honestly, confess our failures to follow what we knew to be right, learn from our failures, and try to correct the damage we may have caused. The honesty and humility of this responsibility for our own free acts is the best guarantee of future improvement.

In classical ethics the supreme goal of human life was called "the ultimate end." Commitment to this goal involves the whole person and may be made implicitly in action rather than by some explicit verbalized decision. Consequently some authors today, in order to avoid the implication that it is always explicit and coldly rational, prefer to term it the "fundamental option" (Poddimatam 1986; McInerny 1987). John Paul II, in *Veritatis splendor* (1993), insists that our life commitment, whether it is called our "ultimate end" or our "fundamental option," must be a free and conscious human act that can be changed only by a free and conscious human act. Unfortunately, this new terminology has given rise to the erroneous opinion of some that it is possible to remain committed to God and neighbor by a subconscious fundamental option while at a conscious level committing objectively serious sins. This theory is supposed to explain why some Christians who seem sincerely committed to God nevertheless habitually commit what are traditionally objectively mortal sins, for example, drunkenness or masturbation.

Objective and Subjective Morality

The fundamental option theory overlooks the way classical theology quite adequately accounted for this phenomenon by distinguishing between the *objective* sinfulness of an act and the *subjective* guilt of the agent. It is essential, however, to distinguish between the *objective morality* of an act, that is, whether it is really helpful or harmful, and the *subjective morality* of conscience, that is, whether it appears to the agent helpful or harmful (Ashley 1996a). We are often mistaken about the objective morality of acts that subjectively appear good to us but are in fact quite harmful.

Thus persons struggling to overcome addictive sins of weakness, while remaining committed to God, may repeatedly fall into objectively wrong acts, but are not fully culpable because of lack of freedom and full deliberation (John Paul II 1995, no. 18). We can make such mistakes either because we act under extreme emotion or so quickly that our judgment is blinded or because we lack the needed information to make a realistic judgment. In the latter case this ignorance may be due to our own failure to seek that information so that we are still morally responsible for our bad judgment. But we may also be blinded by "invincible ignorance," that is, ignorance for which we are not responsible, and hence we are not morally guilty for our mistaken action. Yet we and perhaps others will still suffer the harmful consequences. A physician is not committing murder when he mistakenly kills a patient, even though treating his ailment according to the best information available at the time; nevertheless the patient dies.

Also some current authors do not clearly explain the difference between what the Catholic tradition has always called "mortal" and "venial" sin. This difference is not just one of degree but of our *relationship* to God and neighbor. When we perform an act that we know is objectively harmful yet not seriously so, or when subjectively we act without full freedom, deliberation, and consent, our action weakens but does not destroy our relation of commitment to God, to neighbor, and to the integral fulfillment of our own human nature. In contrast, when we knowingly, freely, and with full consent perform an action that seriously harms our neighbor, ourselves, or our relation to God, that is a *mortal* sin and turns us aside from our true goals in life. We then no longer share in the divine life that God gave us in baptism.

It is also a serious mistake to think, as some have done, that we can commit a mortal sin only by sinning seriously against faith, hope, or love of God, because "If any one says: 'My love is fixed on God,' and hates his brother, he is a liar" (1 Jn 4:20). In biblical language, to "hate" someone is to be willing to do them serious harm. Just as a divorce is usually the result of a long series of lesser quarrels, we ordinarily fall into mortal sin only as the conclusion of a long series of more and more harmful and deliberate sins that have prepared its way. Thus health care professionals who think themselves to be good Catholics or respectable citizens, but who knowingly and deliberately seriously neglect or misuse professional skill or status so that others are harmed or the professional's own development as a person is seriously impaired, commit mortal sins that must be forgiven in the sacrament of reconciliation and, insofar as possible, repaired.

In making a moral decision one must first consider the action one might perform as it relates as a means to the true goal of life happiness, as the satisfaction of the four basic needs in the order of their importance. Thus one must (1) *intend* to act only in such a way as to what one knows to be true happiness and (2) *intend* to perform an act that one knows to be a realistic means to further one's intention of true happiness. This is to intend a *moral object*, that is, some act to be performed as an appropriate means to that goal. Thus we must distinguish between a merely *physical object* of an act and that object as a moral object. For example, an act of sexual intercourse with one's wife or a prostitute is the same act physically but is morally different, as the former act strengthens one's marriage and family, while the latter weakens it.

Thus in every deliberate human act there are always at least two intentions, the intention of the end and the intention of the means, because we cannot intend a means as such without intending the end. For an ends–means ethics, therefore, the *essential* determination of the morality of a decision is whether its moral object is good because it is a fitting means to the true end of life or evil because it blocks one's pursuit of true happiness. If it is an act that is contradictory to this goal it is a "mortal" or serious sin, as for example, is clearly the case for an act of intercourse that will cause AIDS infection. But if the act is simply inconsistent with the intention of the goal because it weakens one's drive toward it, the sin is said to be "venial." For example, a husband's impatience with his wife would be venial because it only slightly weakens their relationship, whereas his act of adultery with a prostitute weakens their relationship critically and makes divorce likely. In either case, however, whether an act contradicts or merely weakens our striving for the true goal of life, the fact that the act cannot by its essential character serve as a means to the true ultimate end of life makes it morally bad. The act can be said, therefore, to be *intrinsically evil*, whether mortally or venially so, because by its essential character it diverts one's search for true happiness and leads toward unhappiness.

Yet the fact that the moral object is the essential determinant of morality does not necessarily make it the sole determinant of morality, because it is possible that these first two kinds of intention are qualified by (3) one or more *accidental circumstances*, for example, *by whom, when, where, how,* and so on the act is performed. These circumstances can increase the goodness of a good act or lessen it, or they can increase or even lessen the evil of a bad act, but they *cannot make an intrinsically bad act good* (John Paul II 1993, no. 80). For example, the circumstance that a doctor treats a patient even if the patient cannot pay increases the goodness of his healing act, while if he overcharged the patient it would lessen the good of that healing act, but would not make it essentially a bad act. Alternatively, if a doctor performs an abortion in circumstances that might lead to an infection, his evil act is made worse, while if he performs it with special care to avoid complications, this lessens the evil of the act, but it remains essentially evil (Mullady 1986).

Note, however, that one kind of circumstance is a *circumstantial intention*, for example, when a physician performs a legitimate operation with a good essential intention of the moral object, namely, the healing of the patient, but in addition to this essential intention has the accidental circumstantial intention of making money. Thus, in every human act there are at least two kinds of intention: (1) the intention of the ultimate end; (2) the intention of the means, namely, the moral object that essentially determines its morality; and there may also be (3) one or more circumstantial intentions that accidentally modify its morality. Indeed many of our acts are performed with mixed intentions, that is, an essential intention of the object and other circumstantial intentions.

2.5 MORAL NORMS ESPECIALLY RELEVANT TO HEALTH CARE

We have argued in the previous chapter that any ethics should be based on human needs knowable to us from experience in an inductive, empirical way and should thus be fundamentally an ends–means ethics. We can, however, concede to those who defend a duty ethics made up of an ethical code or set of moral norms that, once specialists have worked out, as we have attempted to do, an empirical ends–means ethics, it is useful to formulate on the basis of its conclusions a set of norms to guide persons in their prudent decisions in particular cases. Without such a set of norms it is very difficult for any individual to work out the foundations of the whole of ethics every time he or she makes a decision.

These moral norms, however, must not be understood in the way that principlists understand them. One cannot simply deduce moral judgments from the principles we are about to formulate as if they were "middle principles" in a mathematically deductive system. Instead, ethical norms are only general guides to prudent reflection on concrete moral questions. Even when a norm declares that some type of action is intrinsically evil so as to exclude it from further deliberation, this still leaves it open to prudence to determine whether in fact a particular act under judgment actually involves the intrinsic evil that the norm absolutely forbids. Thus one can formulate the true norm that "Lying is intrinsically evil, because it violates our need for membership in a community of mutual trust," but this still leaves it open to prudence to determine whether a certain communicative act is in fact a lie.

To formulate all of ethics in a series of norms is an impossible task. The Ten Commandments are valid and universal norms, but even they are not exhaustive. In this book we are concerned only about those norms that commonly arise in the discussion of health care ethics. Sometimes, however, even after much reflection we find ourselves faced by what seems a moral dilemma. Here ethical theory can help, because over the centuries ethicists have worked out important norms for prudent reflection when we are faced with ethical dilemmas. These concern decisions that have some evil effects: cooperation with wrongdoers, obtaining informed consent, and respecting confidentiality.

Double Effect

The first type of moral dilemma arises in situations where the moral object intended is good and thus has ethically beneficial results, but it is foreseen that it may also have some physically harmful effects. Such an action should still be performed if the following conditions, usually called the "principle of double effect" (PDE; Mangan 1949; Marquis 1991; Cataldo 1995), are met:

1. The directly intended object of the act must not be intrinsically contradictory to the true ultimate goal of human life.
2. The intention of the agent must be to achieve the beneficial effects and as far as possible to avoid the harmful effects (i.e., the agent must only indirectly intend the harm).
3. The foreseen beneficial effects must be at least equal to the foreseen harmful effects.
4. The beneficial effects must follow from the action at least as immediately as do the harmful effects (otherwise the harmful effects are the real means chosen to effect the good end).

Sometimes a fifth condition, "There must be a grave reason for permitting the evil effect" is added, but this is already covered by the third condition.

Because it is not possible to avoid all harmful side effects and at the same time to fulfill our obligations to do the good from which these harmful effects also result, we need a principle to guide us in such dilemmas. For example, to save someone's life, a physician may perform an amputation. Although the disablement caused by the surgery is foreseen, it is not what is desired or chosen as such and would be avoided were it possible to heal the person in a better way. Thus it is not a moral effect, but only a physical effect, because morality always pertains to *free* choices (nor is it "pre-moral" as proportionalists claim, as it is the physical effect of a moral decision). In this case the effect that is freely (directly) chosen is *morally* good, while the other effect is *physically* harmful, but of itself neither moral nor immoral because it is not freely chosen (it is only indirectly "chosen").

Moreover, John Connery, S.J. (1981) has shown that only the first of the four previously listed conditions is really essential. The other three merely suggest prudential tests by which one can better determine if the first condition is actually being fulfilled. Consequently, all that the third condition demands is not the precise, determinative weighing of values on which the entire methodology of proportionalism depends, but merely that an action, already determined to be intrinsically moral (first condition), is not vitiated by circumstances that produce obviously greater evils than the good intended. The second and fourth conditions are required for the same reason, to ensure the agent directly intends only the intrinsically good effect.

A common bioethical example of the application of this principle is an operation to remove the cancerous uterus of a pregnant woman that will also kill her unborn child. The physician rightly decides that this operation is ethical because

a. his direct intention is to save the woman's life (the first condition);
b. he would save the child's life if he could (second condition);
c. the moral value of the mother's life equals that of the child's life (the third condition); and
d. it is the removal of the cancer not the child's death that is the means to save the woman's life (fourth condition).

Legitimate Cooperation

A second type of moral dilemma frequently arises when to fulfill our responsibilities we have to seek the cooperation of others. We often foresee that this may involve us somehow in conduct on their part that we believe to be objectively wrong, although we realize that those with whom we cooperate may not in their own consciences perceive it as evil. When possible, we should inform them of the evil and try to dissuade them, but often we know that this will have no effect and may even make them more obstinate in their evil intention or result in injury to ourselves such as losing a needed job. Must we therefore refuse to cooperate with them? This question can be answered in terms of what is called the "principle of legitimate cooperation" (Haas 2003; O'Rourke 2003).

It follows that people must be careful not to cooperate in or promote the evil actions of others. However, it sometimes happens that a person may perform an action that is morally good, which will be used by another person to further his or her evil purpose. What is the moral responsibility of a person performing the good action? Must he or she avoid all cooperation with the person doing evil? Traditional moralists considering this problem offer distinctions that help answer this question (Merkelbach 1949; Prummer 1958).

First of all they distinguish between formal and material cooperation. Formal cooperation occurs when one assents to the evil intention of the person mainly responsible for performing the evil action. Formal cooperation may occur if one advises, encourages, or counsels the person principally responsible for the evil action, even though one does not take part physically in the action. Of course, if one is in agreement with an evil action and also contributes physically to the action then it is clearly a case of formal cooperation. Alternatively, one may be opposed to the evil action being performed insofar as the intention to do evil is concerned. This would occur if the person who merely cooperates in the evil action does so due to another motive. If one becomes involved in an evil action without having the same intention of the evildoer, then one cooperates not formally but materially.

In order to understand material cooperation as considered in the more traditional manner, another distinction is needed. The manner in which one is involved in the evil action becomes significant. Does the cooperator participate in the evil act by doing something necessary for the actual performance of the evil act, or does the act of the cooperator precede or follow the evil act (see following example)? If one's action contributes to the active performance of the evil action so much so that the evil action could not be performed without the help of the cooperator, then this is known as immediate material cooperation. This method of cooperation involves the cooperator acting in conjunction with the person primarily responsible for the evil action. If the act in question is intrinsically evil, then immediate material cooperation is always prohibited. If one's cooperation is not needed to perform the evil action, but only assists in the performance of the action, then this is known as mediate material cooperation. This type of material cooperation may be justified if there is a serious reason for it because the action on the part of the cooperator is fundamentally good. A serious reason is required to justify mediate material cooperation, because one should avoid cooperation in evil if at all possible. Clearly, allowing mediate material cooperation in the evil act of another is an application of the principle of double effect, though this has recently been denied (Keenan and Kaveny 1995).

Some theologians use a different nomenclature than that indicated earlier (Aertnys and Damen 1947). They identify immediate material cooperation with implicit formal cooperation. Thus Bernard Häring (1963) distinguishes two kinds of cooperation, formal and material. But instead of describing two different forms of material cooperation, he describes two kinds of formal cooperation. Implicit formal cooperation indicates that a person who cooperates intimately in performing an evil act *should know* the evil he is helping to perform. We do not concur with this nomenclature because it involves an interpretation of another person's subjective state of mind. While we do not concur with the use of this distinction, we recognize it as legitimate. However, we would prefer to keep the analysis in the objective order. For this reason, we will continue to use the distinction of immediate and mediate material cooperation, but caution that when applying this principle of cooperation to practical cases, it is important not to confuse the two methods of nomenclature.

An example may clarify the difference between formal and material cooperation and the two kinds of material cooperation. If a person is associated with an abortion clinic and approves or encourages the practice of abortion, this person cooperates formally in the evil action, whether or not he is physically involved in the abortion procedure. If one does not approve of the procedure, having another intention besides abortion, for example, simply to make a living or to keep one's job, then the degree of involvement in the evil act must be discerned. If one is a nurse physically involved in the abortion process, for example, using a suction pump to remove the fetus from the mother's womb, then one is involved in immediate material cooperation even though he may declare vigorously that he is not in favor of abortion but is "only protecting his job." (Häring and others would call this formal cooperation of an implicit nature). On the other hand, the nurse who cares for a woman after an abortion is not intrinsically involved in the evil act of abortion and cooperates in a mediate material manner. She may continue her work in the abortion clinic if there is a justifying reason, for example, if she cannot find other employment as a nurse.

In a case of mediate material cooperation one must also consider the element of scandal because it is sinful to lead a third party to sin or think less of the teaching of the Church, even though one may not be committing a sin by reason of one's personal action. Thus she would still have to avoid scandal, that is, avoid bringing the teaching of the Church into disrespect by seeming to condone the abortions. This might be accomplished by expressing her opposition to abortion whenever possible.

The difficulty that arises in efforts of Catholic health care facilities to enter into cooperative agreements with non-Catholic facilities will be taken up in chapter 3. It is important to note the following statement of the United States Conference of Catholic Bishops in the ERD (2001):

> This new edition of the *Ethical and Religious Directives* omits the appendix concerning cooperation, which was contained in the 1995 edition. Experience has shown that the brief articulation of the principles of cooperation that was presented there did not sufficiently forestall certain possible misinterpretations and in practice gave rise to problems in concrete applications of the principles. Reliable theological experts should be consulted in interpreting and applying the principles governing cooperation, with the proviso that, as a rule, Catholic partners should avoid entering into partnerships that would involve them in cooperation with the wrongdoing of other providers.

This problem had been caused by divergent interpretations of an appendix to these directives in which the definition of legitimate cooperation seemed to permit cooperation with intrinsically wrong medical procedures "under duress" (Ashley and O'Rourke 1997, 197). While it is true that the difficulties arising from "duress" (external pressures) must be taken into consideration in estimating the possible negative effects of noncooperation, such duress can never justify formal or immediate material cooperation with intrinsically wrong acts. Footnote 44 in the 2001 ERD to Directive 70 quotes a 1975 reply by the Congregation for the Doctrine of the Faith to a question about "cooperation" that states, "Any cooperation institutionally approved or tolerated in actions which are in themselves, that is, by their nature and condition, directed to a contraceptive end . . . is absolutely forbidden. For the official approbation of direct sterilization and, *a fortiori*, its management and execution in accord with hospital regulations is a matter which, in the objective order, is by its very nature (or intrinsically) evil." This controversy shows how important it is to apply the principle of legitimate cooperation in a way that preserves its essential condition, that no intrinsically evil moral act can ever be justified.

Free and Informed Consent

In a principalist ethical methodology, among the issues of justice and the protection of human rights of special relevance for health care ethics, much stress is put on the principle of *autonomy* and the right of *free and informed consent* derived from it. Principalists argue that all decisions about medical treatment, and even about whether a pregnant woman will bring her child to term or whether some sufferer may choose suicide, pertain to the right to free control over one's own body. Though a prudential personalist ethics also holds that because everyone has primary responsibility for her or his own health, no physical or psychological therapy may be administered to him or her without his or her free and informed consent, or, if he or she is incompetent, the proxy consent of his or her legitimate guardian. Yet personalist ethics rejects the view that persons or their proxies have a right to consent to procedures that are intrinsically unethical, such as abortion or suicide. No one has a right to do what is intrinsically evil, though sometimes it is necessary to permit someone to do evil, as when a parent permits a child to do what the parent has forbidden in order to let the child learn responsibility.

This right and obligation of consent to any treatment is an essential feature of the physician-patient relationship. Responsible consent to therapy must be *informed:* the essential elements of informed consent are:

1. Information. The essential information that should be provided for the patient concerns the purpose of the procedure, anticipated risks and benefits, alternative procedures, and hoped-for results. Information should never be withheld for the purpose of obtaining consent, and truthful answers should be given to patients who have a right to such information.
2. Comprehension. Comprehension of the necessary information is a complex requirement. Because information varies so greatly, the material must be adapted to the subject's capabilities. Health care professionals cannot be excused for failing to make sure that the subject has comprehended the information, especially if the risks are serious. If the patient cannot comprehend, then some third party, usually a family member but sometimes a person appointed by the court, should act in the patient's best interest.
3. Freedom. Freedom implies that the person understands the situation clearly and that no coercion or undue influence is exercised by the health care professional. Freedom does not imply that the patient will be free from all pressure or persuasion in a given circumstance. For example, a person with an inflamed appendix is limited insofar as freedom of choice is concerned. (Reardon 1994; ACHAN 2003)

The question of "advance directives," "living wills," "powers of attorney," and so on by which someone states the kind of medical care they wish to receive if they become incompetent will be further discussed in chapter 6.

If the patient is not competent to make a decision for herself, then another person, usually called a proxy or a surrogate, is called upon to make a decision. In "proxy consent," the legitimate guardian should always act not for the guardian's interests but for the patient's benefit and should respect the patient's known or probable wishes, provided these are ethical and reasonable. If professionals have good reason to think a guardian is not acting in this responsible way, they must make serious efforts to protect patients' rights, by legal action if necessary. Thus the *principle of autonomy* used by many moralists (Beauchamp and Childress 2001) is neither an a priori assumption nor a merely formal principle, as it gets concrete content from the understanding of the nature of the human person as a free, responsible, *social* being. It does not, therefore, favor an individualistic autonomy by which someone becomes "a law unto himself," but supports the mutual, communal responsibility we have for each other.

Confidentiality

To fulfill their obligations to serve patients, health care professionals have the responsibility to strive to establish and preserve mutual trust at both the emotional and rational levels.

They should also share whatever information they possess that is legitimately needed by others in order to have an informed conscience, and they must refrain from lying or giving misinformation. Finally, they must keep secret information about the patient that is not legitimately needed by others and that if revealed might harm the patient or others or destroy trust (Roberts 1997; Eisenberg 2003; Kenny 1997). For more than two thousand years physicians taking the Hippocratic oath have sworn, "Whatever, in connection with my professional service, I see or hear, in my patients' life, which ought not to be spoken of abroad, I will not divulge, since all such should be kept secret."

There are now federal regulations in regard to confidentiality in health care that must be observed by all health care professionals (Annas 2002). If they are not truthful to patients, there cannot be free and informed consent. Hence good communication is needed between professional and patient, which is impossible without (a) trust, (b) contact among people who have the needed information, (c) clear formulation and expression of this information, and (d) continuous feedback by which failures in communication can be corrected. Modern communication theory has shown that this work of communicating depends above all on good emotional relationships among the parties, as emotional conflict is a powerful barrier to communication and brings into play all sorts of uncontrollable, unconscious factors.

Professionals are sometimes asked about confidential matters in such a way that even to refuse to give some answer will betray that confidence. For example, a psychiatrist may be asked whether a certain person, who wants no one to know he is seeing a psychiatrist, has visited him. May the professional lie in order to preserve confidentiality? Catholic tradition holds that lying is intrinsically wrong because even venial lies break down social trust and habituate the liar to coping with difficulties by lying and thus eventually lead him to begin lying about very serious maters. Priests, of course, often have this problem regarding confessional secrets. Yet we must remember that human communication is always in a *context* that must be taken into consideration in interpreting the meaning of a statement. For example, the same statement said in one social context is a joke, but in a serious situation it is perjury or calumny. Reasonable persons know that they have no right to inquire of professionals about their clients. Hence in that context whatever evasive answer the professional gives is not a lie, even if he or she says, "No," because the questioner who has no right to the information will understand that the answer he has been given is simply a polite way of saying, "It is none of your business. I can't answer such questions." Traditionally such evasive answers to improper questions were called "mental reservations."

The duty to tell the patient the truth does not, of course, relieve one from the responsibility to do so in a sensitive, compassionate, and tactful manner and in the proper circumstances. Moreover, professional secrecy has some limits. Although a Catholic priest is absolutely bound by the secrecy of the confessional, the medical professional may in some rare situations reveal confidential matters, namely, when the patient is a minor, is considering suicide, is involved in a serious crime or serious injustice to a third party, or is seriously incompetent or when child abuse is involved.

The virtue of Justice and its related virtues give us the consistent will to respect the rights of others whether in individual or communal relationships, and in particular to respect their autonomy in their decisions about their own persons and their right to privacy and confidentiality within ethical limits. Social justice requires that the members of a community promote the common good and requires that the leaders distribute the common good fairly to the members. The members of the community should participate in its decisions at the level of their own competency, and the leadership should promote cooperative action. In health care this means that government needs to have some supervision over health care institutions to ensure that they perform their functions justly but should insist that the institutions also accept due responsibility for their services.

2.6 CONCLUSION

The natural goal of human life, true happiness, is integral satisfaction of basic human needs for physical health, security, and moderate material possessions; formation in a good family and the passing on of life; friendship in a community cooperating for the common good; and an understanding of the world, other human persons, and a personal God. Such happiness can be achieved only if one's personal, family, and community life are guided by realistic, prudent decisions that respect the rights of others and are not hampered but facilitated by moderation in one's drives for pleasure and courage in difficulties. Such decisions require us to develop skills or virtues. Catholic Christians believe that Jesus perfectly possessed such virtue and gave us both a model and the power of the Holy Spirit in the teachings and sacraments of a community, the Catholic Church, that will ultimately not only restore humanity to happiness but lead them beyond mere human happiness to a share in the eternal happiness of God, Father, Son, and Holy Spirit. Christ heals and perfects the character of human persons by faith that clarifies prudence, love that extends justice, and hope that makes moderation and courage easy. The Catholic health care mission is one of the ministries of this church and is directed to physical healing as a component of this true Christian happiness extended to all humanity by love, inspired by hope, and guided by faith.

Part II

Clinical Issues

Chapter Three

SEXUALITY AND REPRODUCTION

OVERVIEW

BECAUSE SEXUALITY IS SUCH AN IMPORTANT part of human character and plays an integral role in moral behavior, the topics of sexuality and human reproduction give rise to many ethical issues. Before considering these issues we will study two fundamental concepts: First, what is the meaning of human sexuality? How does it affect our health and social relationships, and does it influence one's perspective in regard to bioethics? Second, when does human life begin? These considerations will influence the answers to specific questions concerning human conception and the prevention of human conception. Hence, after considering these two pivotal topics, we consider questions of natural family planning, artificial reproduction, surrogate motherhood, cloning, contraception, sterilization, abortion, ectopic pregnancy, care of anencephalic infants, and treatment of rape victims. To pursue all these topics in an orderly manner, we divide our considerations into four parts: (1) The Meaning of Human Sexuality, (2) When Does Human Life Begin? (3) Ethical Issues in Reproduction, and (4) Pastoral Approach to Ethical Problems Arising from Sexuality.

3.1 THE MEANING OF HUMAN SEXUALITY

The biological determination of sexuality depends on the presence or absence of the Y chromosome in the one-cell zygote, which in the beginning constitutes the human person. When present, the Y chromosome produces testicular determinant Y (TDY) as early as the eight-cell stage of development, and the person begins to move toward maleness;

otherwise, all zygotes develop as females. All embryos originally have undifferentiated gonads and two sets of sexual ducts, the Wolffian and Mullerian, but at seven weeks the male gonads differentiate and begin to produce hormones that destroy the Mullerian ducts and cause the development of the male genitalia. Otherwise, the Wolffian ducts are absorbed and the gonads and the Mullerian ducts develop into the female sexual system. At the same time, the differing hormonal balance in the two sexes causes certain differences in the male and female brains, in particular, preparing the female brain to regulate the menstrual cycle. It seems that neurological differences also result in behavioral differences in the two sexes (Roberts 2000).

All these biological determinations are at work before birth. After birth, it is probable, but not yet proved, that there are *biophysical* events at the unconscious level, similar to the imprinting demonstrated in animals, that also promote sexual differentiation, such as the way the mother cares differently for a female than for a male child. Finally, at the unconscious *environmental* level, the person learns his or her own *gender identity* and assumes a *gender role* in society (http://csd.georgetown.edu). In this long and complicated process something can go wrong at each stage, with the result that in the human population a whole spectrum of conditions exists between the normal masculine and feminine conditions, both physical and psychological (Sultan et al. 2002b). "Normal" here means a condition determined by that sexual teleology designed by God to culminate in successful heterosexual marriage.

Yet *sexuality* in modern conversation is an ambiguous term, used with two different connotations. In the first meaning of the term, sexuality connotes the ability to relate to other persons in a loving manner and to unite with other persons in friendship and community. In this sense of the term, every human being is a sexual person. Our capacity for affection, communication, and sympathy is rooted in physical and psychic sexuality. Human persons are embodied spirits, and hence sexuality in this broad sense grounds human relationships. In accord with nature, persons are born from sexual relations of their parents and achieve their fulfillment through relations with other persons, even if they remain celibate. Through their sexuality, God calls men and women to either marriage or the single state. John Paul II expressed this concept in the following manner (1981, no. 2): "God inscribed in the humanity of man and woman the vocation and thus the capacity and responsibility of love and human union. Love is therefore the fundamental and innate vocation of every human being. Christian revelation recognizes two specific ways of realizing the vocation to love: marriage and virginity (the single state)."

In a second sense, the term *sexuality* is used to refer to actions that are genital, that seek orgasmic satisfaction, and that from their nature lead to the generation of human beings (Ashley 1985b). All persons are sexual in the first sense of the term, but many are not sexual in the second sense of the term. Those who choose a celibate life do not exercise sexuality in this sense of the term, and it is sexuality in this sense that underlies or is involved in most of the ethical issues considered in this chapter. Moreover, in Christian tradition, the exercise of sexuality in this sense is confined to married persons.

The Goals of Sexuality

Overall, human sexuality is a complex of many values that are generally recognized in every culture and ethical theory (Blankenhorn and Browning 2004). Yet the interrelationship of these values is often a subject of disagreement. The generally recognized values of marital sexual activity can be reduced to five major categories. As we consider these five major values, it will be clear that some of them are dependent not only upon genital acts but also upon acts of sexuality in the first sense of the term:

1. Sexual activity is a search for sensual pleasure and satisfaction releasing physical and psychic tensions.
2. More profoundly and personally, sexual activity is a search for the completion of the human person through an intimate and personal union of love, expressed in and through the mutual gift of the lovers' bodies. It is thus the mutual complementing of the male and female so that each achieves an integral humanity.
3. More broadly, sexual activity is a social necessity for the procreation and education of children in a stable family so as to sustain the human community and guarantee its future beyond the death of individual members.
4. Still more broadly, our sexuality opens us, married or single, to all the human relationships of friendship, sympathy, compassion, cooperation, and reconciliation that constitute the network of a peaceful and productive society.
5. Symbolically, genital sexual activity is a sacramental mystery, somehow revealing the cosmic order and our human destiny because it stands for the creative love of God for his creatures and their loving response to him.

Because of this cosmic symbolism, these values are celebrated as sacred gifts in all the great religions and philosophies of life and are protected and developed in every viable human culture. The five values of human sexuality, all of them not limited to genital activity, are affirmed in the natural law (Lawler, Boyle, and May 1985). The Catholic Church, often influenced by the culture or philosophy of the times, has emphasized various aspects of these values at different times in history. When agricultural production required more human labor than it does today, the Church emphasized the need for large families. In contemporary times, in order to respond to our culture's great concern for the subjective factors in human development and the resources that must be devoted to the rearing and education of children, the Church looks at human sexuality from a more personalist perspective, without however, neglecting traditional aspects (Doms 1939; Von Hildebrand 1984).

Modern evolutionary sociobiologists also support this view, although they are now debating whether the primary function of human sexuality is to guarantee the survival of the species by passing on genes (Dawkins 1990) or by promising social solidarity (Eldredge 2004). The Church's position is that the procreative (selfish gene) and unitive (solidarity) goals are inseparable because the committed union of the parents produces the family in which the child is socialized.

Therefore, through the thought of the Second Vatican Council and the writings of Pope Paul VI (1968) and Pope John Paul II (1981), the Church has proposed a new formulation for the value of marriage that better balances its social and personal meanings. The earlier language, contained in the Code of Canon Law (CIC) issued in 1917, spoke of the value of procreation as the "primary end of marriage" (CIC c. 1013, 1), has been clarified by Paul VI's teaching in the encyclical *Humanae vitae* (1968), which declared the basic principle of the theology of sexuality is "the inseparability of the unitive and procreative meaning of marriage." Hence, in the Revised Code of Canon Law (1983), marriage is no longer referred to as a contract but more specifically as a "covenant of the whole of life" (c. 1055), thus confirming the language of the Second Vatican Council (1965, no. 40).

This new formulation has caused confusion in the minds of some theologians who seem to think that the Church has now designated love between the spouses as the primary end of marriage and procreation as merely an optional consequence (Kosnick et al. 1977). However, the real aim of the new formula is not to rank the unitive and procreative values of marriage or to subordinate one to the other but to make clear that they are inseparably connected so that one value cannot define the marital relationship in isolation from the other. This is the major difference between humanists and Christians insofar as human sexuality is concerned. Of the five values of human sexuality enumerated earlier, sexual pleasure cannot be isolated from the unitive or love value of the genital expression of sex as humanists often maintain (Lebacqz 1999). The decline of the family in modern culture provides strong evidence that the secular humanist attitude tends to depersonalize sexual activity, counteracts the possibility of true intimacy, and treats sexual partners as mere objects who can be abandoned when, for one reason or another, they are no longer the source of pleasure.

The fourth or symbolic value and the fifth or relational value are achieved only if the genital act is an act of committed love. Genesis 1–3 teaches that God created us male and female and blessed our sexuality as his great and good gift. Jesus confirmed this teaching and perfected it and demanded that men be as faithful as women (Mk 10:2–12; Mt 19:3–12, 1 Cor 7:10). He also emphasized the dignity and value of the child as a fully human person (Mt 19:13–15).

Childless Couples: Fulfillment

What, then, is the meaning of sexuality for married people who have no children because they are infertile? "Spouses to whom God has not granted children can nevertheless have a conjugal life full of meaning, in human and Christian terms. Their marriage can radiate a fruitfulness of charity, of hospitality, and of sacrifice" (CCC 2000, 1654). Childless couples may love each other no less, but through no fault of their own they cannot enjoy the full generative expression of their love. Yet they can still exercise generativity by extending their love and service to others in need (Browning 1973).

Adopting children, for example, is one way for infertile couples to fulfill their generativity. Hence the bond that holds a man and woman together is not just a bond of self-interest and need, but above all, a bond of self-giving love, yet it also is a special kind of love, specified by human sexuality.

Therefore single persons too can express their generativity by concern for children's welfare or for social justice, and they often do this more effectively than some parents. Jesus taught that although married sexuality is a great gift, its use is only a relative value and can be freely surrendered for "the sake of the Kingdom" (Mt 19:12). Thus the Christian single life, with its freedom from domestic cares, can be of service to others and can be personally maturing and fulfilling. St. Paul (1 Cor 7:25–35; Eph 5:22) praised the holiness of married love as symbolic of Christ's love for the church, yet gave preference to the freedom enjoyed by celibates who devote all their energies to the service of God and human community. Like Jesus, St. Paul and other Christians have chosen the single life to devote themselves in the name of God to the service of others. Hence the Catholic Church has maintained the institutions of sacramental marriage and consecrated virginity or celibacy as complementary to one another. Jesus said, "At the resurrection they will neither marry nor be given in marriage" (Mt 22:30), indicating that after death, the married state will be transcended, although the bonds of love that marriage fostered will endure forever. Through our human sexuality lived as Christians, whether married or single, we prepare through our loving human relationships to enter into that everlasting community, God's kingdom, with Father, Son, and Holy Spirit.

Disordered Inclinations

The Catholic Church teaches that forms of sexual attraction and behavior that do not conform to the natural goals of sex are "disordered," that is, unable to meet these goals. Consequently, as the Congregation for the Doctrine of the Faith (CDF) has stated (1986), "Although the particular inclination of the homosexual person is not a sin, it is a more or less strong tendency toward an intrinsic moral evil; and thus the inclination itself must be seen as an objective disorder." The term *objective* abstracts from the question of actual personal guilt.

In sharp contrast to this traditional view that homosexuality is a "disorder," in 1973 the members of the American Psychiatric Association (APA) removed homosexuality and bisexuality from its *Diagnostic and Statistical Manual of Mental Disorders* by a vote 58 percent to 42 percent and has recently (APA Fact Sheet 2002) reaffirmed this position. The chief argument for this action was that homosexuals and bisexuals, unlike persons with gender identity disorders, can allegedly be well adjusted and comfortable with their orientation, or would be if it were not for the unjust social stigma attributed to their sexual preferences. Moreover, the majority of the APA believes that psychiatry has been ineffective in changing sexual orientation. Thus the only way psychotherapists can help such persons is to remove the social stigma attached to their orientation by recognizing it as a harmless variant of gender identity. Those psychotherapists who dissent from this action of the APA question it on several grounds: (1) Is it true that the discomfort of homosexuals with their condition is only due to cultural homophobia? (2) Is it true that homosexuals cannot be successfully helped to become heterosexuals? And if it is true now, (3) is it not possible to discover remedies for their condition? (Bayer 1987; Satinover 1996; Lamberg 1998).

A study done by the National Opinion Research Center of the University of Chicago (Smith 2003) shows that only about 2 to 3 percent of sexually active men and 1 to 2 percent of sexually active women are currently engaging in same-gender sex of which a considerable portion are bisexual. Because of the professional attitude of systematic denial manifested by the *Diagnostic Manual* and vigorously supported by those who seek political and social approval of homosexual and bisexual lifestyles, including gay marriage, research on the causes of homosexuality has been very biased. At present, however, the evidence for its genetic etiology remains weak (Whitehead and Whitehead 1999). A 2002 fact sheet of the APA reads:

> No one knows what causes heterosexuality, homosexuality, or bisexuality. Homosexuality was once thought to be the result of troubled family dynamics or faulty psychological development.

Those assumptions are now understood to have been based on misinformation and prejudice. Currently there is a renewed interest in searching for biological etiologies for homosexuality. However, to date there are no replicated scientific studies supporting any specific biological etiology for homosexuality. Similarly, no specific psychosocial or family dynamic cause for homosexuality has been identified, including histories of childhood sexual abuse. Sexual abuse does not appear to be more prevalent in children who grow up to identify as gay, lesbian, or bisexual, than in children who identify as heterosexual.

Even if it is eventually proven that homosexuality is genetic in origin, this defect, like other genetic defects, would not excuse aberrant behavior, but would call for continuing efforts to find a remedy. It remains probable that homosexuality has multiple causes of which the principal are a dysfunctional family and early masturbatory or homosexual experiences. Thus the popular stereotype of genetically gay and lesbian persons is a social construct developed in recent times that greatly distorts the historical, biological, psychological, and social facts (Catholic Medical Association 2004). The Church urges health professionals to treat homosexuals with respect and compassion and to encourage them to get help from psychiatrists and psychologists who regard this condition as a disorder that may be remediable. It strongly encourages objective scientific research to gain greater certainty about its etiology and possible methods of treatment. When it is found that it is a disability that makes successful marriage a grave risk, marriage should not be encouraged, because the Church recognizes this as legitimate grounds for annulment. If this is the case, such persons must be counseled to remain chastely celibate (CCC 2000, 2357–59). The Catholic ministry called "Courage" (see www.catholic-pages.com/dir/homosexuality.asp), founded by Fr. John Harvey, O.S.F.S., provides support groups based on the Church's view, whereas those groups called "New Ways Ministry" (Zenit 1999; Courage 1999) and "Dignity" (Helmeniak 2005) have not.

Sexuality and Bioethics

The effects of sexual difference on a man or woman's physiology permeate all of the body's systems, impacting the way his or her body functions, ages, and manifests ailments and disease (Wisemann and Pardue 2001; http://csd.georgetown.edu). Symptoms present differently and diseases progress differently. Proper diagnoses and treatment of both everyday and serious conditions follow from sexual differentiation. Women tend to live four or five years longer than men, but in addition, sexuality affects blood pressure, cardiovascular function, and kidney diseases. Of special concern to women are questions of violence, pregnancy, infertility, birth control, breast cancer, and gynecology (Ruzek, Olesen, and Clarke 1997; Annandale and Hunt 2000). Clearly, medicine has been slow to recognize the differences that are due to sexual differentiation; for example, women were excluded from most pharmaceutical research until the 1990s. To date, the exact causes for the differences in men and women's health are not known. But significant differences between men and women in diagnosis and therapy do indicate serious ethical obligations. First of all, the tendency to neglect the difference between men's and women's health needs must be resisted. With the increased number of women in medical schools perhaps this oversight will be eliminated. Moreover, any implication that women are inferior to men insofar as health care is concerned must be overcome. Pope John Paul II was especially outspoken in this regard, stressing biblical teaching and philosophical anthropology to teach that all human persons, male and female, have basic human rights and that men and women should look upon one another as equal and complementary individuals (CDF 2004). Men are completed by their natural relations to women just as the same social complementarity is true of women with respect to men. It is true that because of original sin men have often both unjustly dominated women and prevented them from using their full complement of gifts, but Jesus offered a true model of masculinity that recognized the dignity and equality of women.

Finally, to correct the oversight in regard to sexuality in ethical health care, bioethics, especially as practiced and developed in the United States, must take seriously the experience of women. There have been several works by women that have pointed out the serious shortcomings of bioethics theory as developed in the United States (Iglesias 1987; Tong 1997; Holmes and Purdy 1992; Donchin and Purdy 1999). These authors stress the importance of recognizing the perspectives and interests of women of different racial, cultural, educational, and socioeconomic class and admit that sometimes feminism has been solely the voice of white, highly educated professional women who have not understood their sisters' circumstances and concerns. Susan Wolf, a leading writer on the topic of feminist bioethics, sums up the situation in this way (1996, 5):

> The answer [for the neglect of feminist perspective] is to be found in the deep structure of bioethics—in its early embrace of a liberal individualism largely inattentive to social context, in its emphasis on deduction from ethical principles rather than induction from concrete cases, in its tendency to view ethical problems either dyadically as problems between individuals, or nationally as problems for the entire society, but rarely at an intermediate level attentive to more significant groups, and in the failure of bioethics to be sufficiently self-critical by examining whom the field serves and how.

3.2 WHEN DOES HUMAN LIFE BEGIN?

To treat this bitterly controversial question (Warnock 1984), on which an objective answer to so many bioethical questions depends, we consider (a) semantic issues (Daly 1987; Brennan 1995; Irving 1993, 1994a, 1994b; Hui 2002; Perry 2005), (b) biological issues, and (c) philosophical and theological issues.

Semantic Issues

Some writers argue that although a human embryo may be considered a "human being," it is not yet a "human person" (Grobstein 1983, 1988; McCormick 1990, 1991a, 1991b). Often they think that to be a "person" is to be "conscious." Thus Peter Singer (2000) argues that because animals are conscious of pain, they are persons with rights, and this implies that the embryo is not a person. Michael Tooley (1974, 1983) and Dean Stretton (2002, 2003) argue that the "value" or dignity of the person is an accidental not a substantial property; hence one can admit the unborn is a person yet deny that they have the moral value of a conscious adult person. However, as we showed in chapters 1 and 2, the classical meaning of "person" is not simply a conscious being, but one with intelligence, the power of abstract thought, which animals lack, although they are conscious of concrete objects and capable of feelings. A sleeping person or one in a coma is still a person, and so is an embryo if it can reasonably be identified as substantially the same organism that develops itself into an adult person (O'Rourke 2006).

Yet to avoid this plain fact some now redefine "conception" to mean no longer fertilization of the ovum but instead the implantation of the embryo or, as some say, the "pre-embryo," a term deplored by other embryologists, in the uterus (Lockwood 1988; Hare 1988; O'Rahilly and Muller 1994; Kischer 2005). Some claim that the "pre-embryo" is only "potentially" human because it is only "gradually" developing into a human person (Bedate and Cefalo 1989; Morowitz and Trefil 1992). If, conversely, we ask embryologists whether with the completion of the fertilization of a human ovum we have a new "organism" that will self-develop into a member of the genus and species *Homo sapiens*, we get an unequivocal affirmative answer, based on modern genetics and embryology, as we shall see (Kischer 1996).

The ovum and the sperm that fertilized it were originally part of the bodies of the parental female and male organisms. Each possessed only half the genome necessary to form a complete organism and when separated as parts from the parent organisms acted in an instrumental manner and then ceased to exist. Thus they were not self-maintaining organisms as is the one-celled zygote formed by their fusion. But once the fertilization of the ovum by the sperm is complete, a new, unified, self-sustaining organism begins to develop itself toward human maturity (Kischer 1992, 1993, 1994; Suarez 1990; De Marco 2000; Tacelli 2005).

As for those who hold that this question can only be settled by social consensus rather than fact (Engelhardt 1977) or that the pregnant woman alone should decide the matter, because her rights exceed those of the intrusive child (Thomson 1971; Boonin 2002), we must insist with Francis J. Beckwith (2004) and others that such views, if consistently applied, would destroy the grounds for defending human equality and human rights. Nevertheless others illogically attribute human rights to the mother but not to the unborn human organism, without seriously inquiring whether the unborn is truly human (Fletcher 1972; Baehr 1990; Claire 1995; Dombrowski and Deltere 2000). Even the Supreme Court in its *Roe v. Wade* decision (1973) made no effort to face the scientific data.

Biological Issues

Because the question is so controversial, *Roe v. Wade* should at least have inquired as to the state of the question in scientific biology. Yet Justice Blackmun confidently wrote (1973, IX B), "We need not resolve the difficult question of when life begins. When those trained in the respective disciplines of medicine, philosophy, and theology are unable to arrive at any consensus, the judiciary, at this point in the development of man's knowledge, is not in a position to speculate as to the answer."

Among writers who have taken this biological question more seriously, Clifford Grobstein (1988) argued for a distinction between genetic and developmental individuation and claimed that, although the zygote is genetically individuated, its developmental individuation only takes place gradually. He questioned its genetic individuation on the grounds that the development of the embryo is determined not only by the nuclear genes but by maternal cytoplasmic deoxyribonucleic acid (DNA) and perhaps also by influences from the mother after implantation. This view, however, disregards the fact that the normal development of the human organism is a unified process of self-development (Moore

1988; Lejeune 1989; Marquis 1995, 1998a, 1998b; Larsen, Sherman, Potter, and Scott 2001; Gilbert 2003; Moore and Persaud 2003). Thus from the very beginning that process must be guided principally by the genetic information present in the zygote. Of course, the development of the child also requires the appropriate environment provided by the mother, yet all known information in embryology show that the organism is not formed by its maternal host, but develops from within itself, implants itself in her womb, and triggers her body to expel it at the proper time.

Others argue more strongly that the fact that identical twins can form up to implantation proves that no organism destined to reach maturity exists before that time (Ford 1988, although he opposes abortion, 2002). They claim that the unicell fertilized ovum (zygote) after the first cell division ceases to be a unified organism and before the time of implantation becomes only a loose collection of cells. This claim is disproved by the fact that even at the first cell division the two cells are not isolated but are still a unified organism that is differentiating its parts under the direction of the human genes. Although each of the cells of this organism is "totipotential," and if separated from the total organism is able itself to begin to develop as a second individual, as long as it remains in the organism it plays a special role, at least by reason of its position, because in animal organisms the future head-tail axis already begins to be established and cell division follows a specific pattern determined by the human genome.

The causes of identical twinning in humans are still not perfectly understood and may occur at any time after the first cell division of the embryo, or the formation of the inner cell mass in the blastocyst and its implantation in the uterus (President's Council on Bioethics [PCB] 2004a, 171; Wikipedia 2005; National Organization of Mothers of Twins Clubs 2005). It is most probable, however, that twin B arises from a separation of one or more cells from the original organism, namely, twin A, that continues in existence, just as in artificial cloning one must first create a human embryo and then separate some cells from it to produce its clone. It may be that twinning is due to a genetic defect in the embryo, as its occurrence is somewhat disadvantageous for both a woman and her offspring (Kirk et al. 2001); or it may be due simply to some accident to the embryo at a stage in which its cells are not as firmly interconnected as they will later be. Because at this very early stage of human development the parts of the organism are not well differentiated, all the cells are "totipotential" and thus any one or a small group of cells separated from the original embryo will become its clone, having the same genes.

Philosophical and Theological Issues

Although biology is able to settle the question of the time of the origin of the individual living animal organism, a further set of questions is raised when we consider the unique character of the human organism as capable not only of sense consciousness but also of human self-consciousness and abstract thought (Warnock 1984, 1987; Arkes 1990; Fisher 1991a, 1991b; Beckwith 1993; Lee 1996; Moreland 1995; Moreland and Rae 2000; Buratovich 2003). In chapters 1 and 2 we presented a view of human persons that shows they have abstract thought and free will, which are powers that transcend the capabilities of any physical system, even the most complex one that we know of, the human brain, and can be explained only by admitting that the human mind is spiritual in nature. Hence it follows also that the soul or organizing principle of the human person that gives life to the body is itself spiritual, and not merely the organizing principle of the body. Yet because of the unity of the human person this spiritual soul requires the body, its senses, and its brain as the instruments by which it gathers information about itself and its environment. On the other hand, because it is spiritual it cannot be formed out of matter as the work of any finite power but must be directly created by God to complete the human body supplied by biological forces and ultimately by evolution, which God uses as his instruments (CCC 2000, 362–68).

Biologists today are very uncomfortable with this spiritual dimension of the human person, yet they are aware that the "mind–body problem," as it is called, remains controversial among scientists (Bole 1992). We will not enter here into this mind–body controversy except to point out that while it is not simply a religious question, but one that science itself cannot avoid, Catholic faith and the long tradition of Catholic study of this question on the basis of the facts of human behavior reject a merely materialistic account of the human being because it renders the facts of human abstract thought and freedom inexplicable (Braine 1992). Any bioethics that assumes a merely material biological explanation of the human organism would eliminate intelligent and free moral decisions and thus would be based on a self-contradiction.

Delayed Hominization

Some Catholic writers still defend what they call the "delayed hominization" theory of St. Thomas Aquinas based on the embryology of Aristotle, historically the first important writer on the subject, who significantly influenced the Church's views in the past (Donceel 1970; Wallace 1989; Shannon and Wolter 1990). This view was based on the previously mentioned sound biological principle that the life of an organism depends first of all on the directive functioning of some main part, but it erred in applying this principle to the scanty embryological data available to ancient doctors (Ashley 1992; Ashley and Moraczewski 2001; Taylor 1982; Austriaco 2002, 2004; Suits 2005; Sullivan 1995). Aristotle thought that the embryo is formed from the homogeneous menstrual blood of the mother by the action of the semen that remained, he thought, in the womb for at least forty days. This matter was not sufficiently prepared to receive a human soul, but was first formed into a "pre-fetus" having only vegetative functions, and then finally into an animal body with a heart when at last it became truly human. Given the facts that we now know, however, this sound principle leads to the conclusion that hominization is completed with the fertilization of the ovum (Johnson 1995, but cf. Porter 1995b, 2002).

As shown in chapter 2, the fact of human intelligence cannot be explained simply as a function of the human body or its brain, although it necessarily uses the brain to form abstract ideas. It is essentially a spiritual function. Consequently, the conception of a human being is not completed simply by the formation of the brain under genetic guidance. Because material processes cannot produce a spiritual entity, human conception must be completed by God's direct creation of the spiritual human soul that uses the brain to unify and guide the body in its human activities. God is the first cause of the biological process we have described, and he completes this process at human conception by creating a unique human soul appropriate to that particular body. This fact is established philosophically but is reinforced by the doctrine of faith according to which at the end of history God will again reunite human souls with the identical, but glorified, body they had in this life. Some theologians have asked whether the large number of fertilized ova that never develop to term casts doubt on their ensoulment (Rahner 1972). Would God ensoul so many persons that can never perform a human act so as to be saved? Yet facts make this doubt inconclusive: Many of these failed cells were probably so defective as to be incapable of ensoulment (PCB 2004a, 163), and countless late abortions and infanticides deprive ensouled children before they ever perform a human act.

Largely because of the former influence of this delayed hominization theory on the thought of the Catholic Church, the Church has never officially based its position against direct abortion on the claim that the human soul is created at conception (Connery 1977). *The Declaration on Procured Abortion* (CDF 1974)—while affirming that from the time of conception direct abortion is always a grave sin because the generation of a human person, however God has designed it, is of immense value—appended note 19 saying, "This declaration leaves aside the question of the moment when the spiritual soul is infused." The advances in embryology, however, have made the Church more confident that the theories of delayed hominization are scientifically obsolete, so that a more recent *Instruction on Respect for Human Life* (1987) states:

> Certainly, no experimental datum can be in itself sufficient to bring us to the recognition of a spiritual soul. Nevertheless, the conclusions of science regarding the human embryo provide a valuable indication for discerning by the use of reason a personal presence at the moment of first appearance of human life. . . . Thus the fruit of human generation from the first moment of its existence, that is, from the first moment the zygote has formed, demands unconditional respect, that is morally due to the human being in his bodily and spiritual totality.

Thus, as embryological research advances, the evidence that life begins at fertilization becomes overwhelming. The medical profession therefore needs to work toward a consensus on this issue of who is a person with human rights on the basis of what is best known, namely in biology and psychology, just as they have for a definition of human death. The definition of what it is to be a human person with human rights must not contradict biological facts or depend simply upon pragmatic considerations. To do so is to become open to racism and all kinds of discrimination (Cunningham and Forsythe 1992).

3.3 ETHICAL ISSUES IN REPRODUCTION

There are several ethical issues that are connected with human reproduction. Before considering them singly, however, we examine the method that the Church sanctions for the limitation of birth and reproduction.

Natural Family Planning

In recent years, the Church has emphasized that in order to be truly human, married couples must consider the intelligent planning of parenthood so as to provide for the proper care and education of their children (John Paul II 1981, 1983). Catholics therefore cannot be indifferent to the growth of population and the ethical problems that it causes (World Council of Churches 1994). They cannot solve such problems by blind trust in

God's providence because God gave us our intelligence to use in perfecting creation. Many recent papal documents address these issues (CCC 2000, 2370; Catholic Pages Directory 2004), as do also Orthodox Christians and some Protestant churches. In general, the Church proposes natural family planning (NFP) as a means of limiting the number of children when there are reasonable and serious reasons for such limitation (J. Smith 1991, 1993; Shivanandan 1997; Arevale and Jennings 2002; NaPro Technology 2005). At the same time, it points out the great value of the family and encourages couples that are able to give adequate care to large families to engage in this great contribution to society. For today in many countries, including the United States, the population is aging (United States Population Pyramids 2005).

Moreover, children in larger families receive many benefits from being raised with siblings (Diamond 1996; Plomp 2000). Hence the words of John Paul II (1998d, c. 680) must be kept in mind: "The use of the 'infertile periods' for conjugal union can be an abuse if the couple, for unworthy reasons, seek to avoid having children, thus lowering the number of births in their family below the morally correct level. This morally correct level must be established by taking into account not only the good of one[']s own family, and even the state of health and the means of the couple themselves, but also the good of the society to which they belong, of the church, and even of the whole of humankind." Some critics of Church teaching have maintained that this approval of family limitation, even if qualified, is not consistent with the teaching on the natural inseparability of the unitive and procreative aspects of the conjugal act. For example, James Arraj (1989) argues that use of NFP is just as unnatural as the use of contraception, because both kinds of sex deliberately separate the natural procreative purpose of the marital act from its unitive purpose. As John Paul II has repeatedly explained in the collection *The Theology of the Body* (1997, 393–403), it is writers like Arraj, not *Humanae vitae* that equivocate on the term *natural*. What is unnatural about contraception is that it deliberately destroys the natural fertility of certain marital acts. NFP, conversely, makes use only of naturally infertile acts. The facts that this restriction of marital relations to the woman's infertile period is deliberate and that NFP is in that sense "artificial" does not make it "artificial" in the sense of violating nature, as contraception does. When art is abused and violates nature, it is unethical, but when "Art perfects nature," it is an ethical use of human intelligence and freedom (Ashley 1992).

Two modern and well-tested methods of determining the time of ovulation and the periods of fertility and infertility are the symptom-thermal method and the ovulation method, often called the Billings method after the physicians who developed it (Kippley and Kippley 1996; Klaus 1995; Hays 2001; Weschler 2001; Natural Family Planning Site 2004). In addition to these methods, Dr. Thomas Hilgers, working at the Pope Paul VI Institute for the Study of Human Reproduction in Omaha, Nebraska, has designed NaPro Education Technology, sometimes called the Creighton method program (Hilgers 1995; Hilgers and Stanford 1998), which is based on new research and combines various methods both to control and to promote fertility.

Scientific studies conducted under the auspices of the World Health Organization (WHO 1981) show that the *method effectiveness* of NFP is approaching 98 percent, as good as or better than any other method of family limitation, except that achieved by surgical sterilization (WHO 1981; Hilgers 1995; Kippley 2004). The *user effectiveness*, of course, depends on the motivation of the users, but studies made in Austria, Canada, Colombia, France, Germany, Mauritius, and the United States have demonstrated a user effectiveness ranging from 85 to 99 percent, which means that this rate is "equal to or higher than the user effectiveness of any other non-permanent method of birth control except the Pill" (Kippley 2004) and, of course, surgical sterilization. Proponents of NFP also point out the following:

1. Such methods place responsibility on both partners, not merely on the woman, as do most methods of family limitation.
2. Many women who use NFP report an enhanced sense of personal dignity resulting from an awareness of their own bodies and their natural rhythms.
3. Abstinence from intercourse can help a couple to have confidence in the strength of their love and express it in other ways besides orgasm.

Periodic abstinence removes something of the sexual routine and enhances the experience when it is actually decided upon (Billings 2003). The degree of abstinence it requires is not significantly greater than that couples often accept today as a matter of course for reasons of occupations, travel, and health. Moreover, couples practicing NFP report that overall they engage in marital intercourse more often than couples using artificial methods to prevent conception.

Contraception

Contraception is the performance of sexual intercourse with the deliberate intention of rendering infertile an act that could be fertile. The most common form of contraception practiced today is the hormonal pill (the pill) taken orally to prevent ovulation and thus deliberately render the sexual union of the couple infertile. Other forms of contraception, such as an intrauterine device (IUD), condoms, and contraceptive jellies, are also used to prevent conception. These latter mentioned devices are often ineffective. Moreover, the IUD sometimes causes permanent sterility (Barnhill 1989).

The practice of contraception has become so common today that many Catholics practice it and do not understand why the Church has always (Catholic Answers 2004) judged it to be sinful (Hoyt 1969). These Catholics think that the Church's condemnation of contraception is some arbitrary rule made up by conservative clergy. In fact, however, contraception, like abortion, has been present since the very beginning of Christianity and was opposed by Christians as a feature of a decadent paganism that had no regard for human dignity. The question for Pope Paul VI in regard to family limitation in the 1960s was not whether contraception was wrong, but whether the pill was a contraceptive. Though the ancient practice of contraception was less effective than modern methods, it was very common and if not successful, often led, as it still does today, to abortion (Grisez 1964; Noonan 1965; John Paul II 1995, no. 13).

Ethically considered, contraception is intrinsically wrong, not because of any arbitrary rule of the Catholic Church, but because it destroys the true meaning of sexual love and in the long run leads to serious personal and social evils. While married couples practicing it may deny its harmfulness to their relationship, what has happened in our society to marriage proves the contrary. Throughout history contraception was condemned not only by the Catholic Church but also by all the other Christian churches, because they understood that it was contrary to the Creator's design for human sexuality and that it was a violation that would be harmful to the human family and social welfare (Armstrong 2005; Klimon 2004). Its acceptance by some Protestant churches in the last century, often under the influence of eugenics-minded Margaret Sanger (Arias 2004), has proved to be disastrous, as it is a principle factor in the so-called sexual revolution that, in the name of freedom, has in fact enslaved persons to depersonalize sex (Smith 1988). In our culture, sexual abuse, rape, the treatment of women and children as sex objects, teenage sexual activism, divorce and its harmful effects on children, and injustice to women have become common. In this disintegrating milieu the Church's wisdom in preserving the true meaning of human sexuality for the sake of human happiness has become very clear.

Pope Paul VI, in the encyclical *Humanae vitae* (*On Human Life*; 1968, no. 12), argued chiefly on the basis of the natural law when he wrote, "The church's teaching on Contraception, 'often set forth by the magisterium, is founded upon the inseparable connection, willed by God and unable to be broken by human beings on their own initiative, between the two meanings of the conjugal act, the unitive meaning and the procreative meaning.'"

Pope John Paul II gave more attention to the biblical foundation of this teaching than did *Humanae vitae*, which insisted on its natural law basis (Grabowski 1996) but was careful to show that faith and reason give mutual support to its truth. In *On the Human Family* (*Familiaris consortio*; 1981b, no. 33) he wrote, "When couples, by means of recourse to contraception, separate the two meanings that God the Creator has inscribed in the being of man and woman and in the dynamism of their sexual communion, they act as 'arbiters' of the divine plan and they 'manipulate' and degrade human sexuality and themselves and their married partners by altering its value of 'total' self-giving."

Various conferences of Catholic bishops throughout the world have attested to the truth of this teaching, while at the same time recognizing pastorally, just as Paul VI and John Paul II did, the difficulties that married couples may have in following this teaching of the Church. We discuss these difficulties more when we consider the pastoral aspects of this teaching.

In past editions of *Health Care Ethics* we devoted considerable space to discussing the theological arguments proposed against the teaching of the Church concerning contraception, especially those arguments proposed in opposition to the encyclical of Pope Paul VI, *Humanae vitae*. In recent years, most critics have not mentioned these theological arguments, perhaps because of the affirmation this teaching has received from Pope John Paul II and the *Catechism of the Catholic Church* (CCC 2000, no. 2370) after consultation with the entire episcopate. Instead, those in opposition to the teaching focus on three other objections:

1. The fact that the papal commission instituted by Pope John XXIII and continued by Paul VI produced a majority report that approved contraception in some situations, the implication being that the Pope should have accepted the majority report and approved contraceptive practices because the magisterium of the church should follow what the majority of Catholics believe to be acceptable (McClory 1995). These reports were never officially published (Fehring 2005).
2. The fact that many Catholics practice contraception, or at least do not consider it sinful, proves that the *sensus fidelium* is contrary to the teaching of the Church in this matter (Hartman 1998).
3. Paul VI was afraid that if he changed the traditional doctrine he would weaken papal authority (Wills 2000).

The Papal Commission

The commission that Pope John XXIII formed to study population problems as well as acceptable methods of birth control met once in 1963 and twice in 1964. As Vatican Council II was concluding, Pope Paul VI enlarged it to fifty-eight members, including married couples, laywomen, as well as theologians and bishops. The last document issued by the council, *The Church in the Modern World* (*Gaudium et spes*) contained a very important section titled "Fostering the Nobility of Marriage" (1965, nos. 47–52), which discusses marriage from the personalist point of view. The "duty of responsible parenthood" was affirmed, but the determination of licit and illicit forms of regulating birth was reserved to Pope Paul VI. After the close of the council a fifth and final meeting of the commission was held, again enlarged to include sixteen bishops as an executive committee, in Rome in the spring of 1966. The commission was only consultative but did make a report to Paul VI approved by a majority of members, proposing that he might use his authority to approve at least some form of contraception for married couples. A minority number of members opposed this report and issued a parallel report to the Pope.

One highly influential theologian on the commission who favored the majority report was Rev. Josef Fuchs, S.J., a professor of the Gregorian University in Rome and a leading proponent of proportionalism in ethics, which holds, as explained in chapter 1 (section 1.3), that a human act cannot be judged by its moral object alone, thus denying that there are human actions that are intrinsically evil. This moral theory was later clearly rejected by Pope John Paul II, in the encyclical *The Splendor of Truth* (*Veritatis splendor* 1993, 68–70). Pope Paul VI seems to have hesitated over not whether contraception was intrinsically evil but perhaps whether anti-ovulants (Marks 2004) were contraceptive.

After two more years of study and consultation, Pope Paul issued *Humanae vitae,* which removed any doubt that hormonal anti-ovulants are contraceptive. He explains why he did not accept the opinion of the majority report of the commission when he writes (1968, no. 6) that he had been forced to make a personal judgment on the matter "because certain approaches and criteria for a solution to this question had emerged which were at variance with the moral doctrine on marriage constantly taught by the magisterium of the church"; this was not a new teaching on the part of Paul VI but rather an affirmation of the consistent condemnation of contraception in keeping with statements from several previous popes.

Insofar as invoking arguments under the guise of *sensus fidelium* is concerned, it is clear that this principle does not depend on popular opinion (Gaillardetz 2003). Rather, it is precisely the witness to the revelation contained in the gospel and teaching of the Church. A more apt term for this principle is *sensus fidei*. Hence, to ask, as the media often does, "What percentage of Catholics think that contraception is wrong?" does not touch on the *sensus fidelium*. The question would have to be posed to Catholics who strive to live by their faith, and the question would have to be thus phrased: "What has been transmitted to you through the Christian community of all times as God's Word revealed in Jesus Christ about contraception?" Thus, the *sensus fidei*, or "faith intuition" of Catholics, is their corporate witness as members of the Church to the faith transmitted to them through the Church that they have grown to understand and accept in their prayers and Christian living through the enlightenment of the Holy Spirit.

Does the acclaimed "new insight into human sexuality" that those who approve of contraception maintain to support their opinion have its source in the Gospel and reverence for the Creator, or is its source the influence of today's secularized culture that presents technology as the answer to every human problem? If the rise in the practice of contraception by Catholics had resulted in an increase in the stability of marriage, there might be more reason to think it is in conformity with the Gospel, but the divorce rate among U.S. Catholics has risen to about 25 percent compared to about 35 percent for the general population (Barna Research Group 2004; Hoopes 2004). In fact, Fr. Lestapsis, S.J., one of the members who wrote the minority report of the papal commission, had predicted just such consequences if the Church approved contraception (Cremins 2005).

The history of the church shows that only gradually do Christians see the moral truth of the Gospel; for example, it took centuries for the teaching on human equality to lead members of the Church to realize that slavery, racism, and sexism are incompatible with human dignity. Therefore the fact that, in our century, contraception, which throughout the history of the Church was considered wrong, has now under the pressure of modern economy and the sexual revolution become acceptable to many Christians is no proof that the teaching of the Church in regard to contraception is wrong (Smith 1988, 1993; Santamaria 1988). It has been encouraged also by the proportionalism and "right of dissent" views adopted by some prominent Catholic theologians of the post–Vatican II period that often got more media exposure than the positive explanations of the reasons for the Church's teaching.

As for the third argument cited earlier that Paul VI was afraid to weaken papal authority, it can be granted that this is always a consideration for the successor of St. Peter, and an entirely legitimate one in this case, where the weight of tradition was so great against any change in Church teaching. Yet Paul VI must have known how perilous for his influence this extremely unpopular decision would be.

Surgical Sterilization

Because contraceptive techniques are not 100 percent effective and have medical side effects or hinder full sexual pleasure, many men and women resort to surgical sterilization. Surgical sterilization results from a surgical procedure by which the sexual organs of a person are altered so that fertilization will not result when the act of sexual intercourse is performed. If infertility is the result of a surgical procedure to counteract some pathology in the body, for example, a hysterectomy, it is called an indirect sterilization and can be ethically justified.

Direct sterilization is a more permanent form of contraception. It is more radical than the pill but has the same effect, namely, deliberately to separate the unitive and procreative ends of the marital act. The highly technological culture of the United States is insensitive to deep human needs that are unconscious and often suppressed by cultural influences. Simply because most sterilized persons claim to experience only a feeling of relief and sexual freedom as a result of their surgery is not necessarily a reliable indication of its deeper consequences.

A special problem arises when persons are sterilized against their will. This is done sometimes because a person of low IQ or other disability is thought incompetent to control her or his own sexuality, or as punishment for a sex offense, or as in India and China, in an attempt by government to reduce the birth rate (Ramsay 2000; Reilly 1991; American Association on Mental Retardation 2004). Church teaching opposes the use of involuntary sterilization for these purposes. John Paul II, in the encyclical *On the Human Family*

(*Familiaris consortio;* 1981, 35), stated, "It is a grave offense against human dignity and justice for governments or public authorities to attempt to limit the freedom of couples in deciding about children. Consequently, any coercion applied by such authorities in favor of contraception, or still worse of sterilization and procured abortion must be altogether condemned and forcefully rejected."

Involuntary sterilization has often been practiced on the basis of eugenics theories, for example on Native Americans (England 1993). It is clearly a violation of the principle of informed consent and respect for personal dignity. The U.S. federal government has now become much more reluctant to fund enforced sterilization (Johansen 2000). Nonetheless, there clearly can be considerable pressure exercised for the sterilization of even mildly retarded persons and the poor in public institutions (England 1993).

Sterilization and Catholic Hospitals

Elective surgical sterilization of men (vasectomy) is often performed in an outpatient clinic. Elective surgical sterilization of women (tubal ligation) is more often performed in an acute care hospital, especially if the tubal ligation is performed after a Cesarean section delivery. Because the Catholic Church sponsors many acute care hospitals, performing sterilizations in Catholic hospitals has often been a point of contention. First, the distinction between a direct and an indirect sterilization has not always been clearly defined. Second, given the popular acceptance of surgical sterilization as a means of family limitation, many representatives of Catholic health care facilities have urged a policy of toleration in regard to people and physicians who wish to practice this procedure in apparent good faith. The teaching authority of the Church has stood firm, however, in maintaining that unless there is an existing pathology that needs to be corrected, surgical sterilizations are intrinsically evil and may not be performed in Catholic hospitals, nor in non-Catholic hospitals under the management of a Catholic sponsor (CDF 1975). Thus the *Ethical and Religious Directives for Catholic Health Care Services* (ERD) 2001 state: "Direct sterilization of either men or women, whether permanent or temporary, is not permitted in Catholic health care institutions. Procedures that induce sterility are permitted when their direct effect is the cure or alleviation of a present and serious pathology and a simpler treatment is not available." Moreover, in response to the plea that Catholic health care facilities could perform surgical sterilizations if duress were involved (Keenan and Kopfensteiner 1995), the ERD state: "Catholic health care organizations are not permitted to engage in immediate material cooperation in actions that are intrinsically immoral, such as abortion, euthanasia, assisted suicide and direct sterilization" (D. 70). This statement, in addition to the elimination of the explanation of immediate material cooperation contained in the appendix of the ERD approved in 1994, speaks to the difficulties we pointed out in the fourth edition of *Health Care Ethics* (Ashley and O'Rourke 1997, 197). Would immediate material cooperation in providing direct sterilizations ever be possible for a Catholic hospital?

The declining birth rate in the United States has led to a strong movement for hospitals to consolidate obstetrical departments so that a single center located in one of the hospitals can afford the highest quality care. Would a Catholic hospital be allowed to cooperate with a community hospital if the direct sterilizations were performed under the auspices of the community hospital? It seems that this form of cooperation would be mediate and legitimate if the medical personnel and operating rooms were not under the administration of the Catholic hospital, and if the Catholic hospital made it clear that it did not approve of such procedures and took steps to correct any scandal that might arise. Moreover, the Catholic hospital should not profit from these procedures (Haas and Cataldo 2002; O'Rourke 2002). If Catholic hospitals do not cooperate in such joint ventures they would be accused of wasting health care resources and frustrating an effort to provide quality health care for local communities.

Abortion

Technically, the term *abortion* includes *spontaneous* (miscarriage) and deliberately *procured* (or induced) terminations of pregnancy with resulting death of the human being at any stage of its development. Usually the term *abortion* is used in regard to the latter event. A *direct* abortion is one that is induced with the immediate purpose of destroying the human fetus at any stage after conception. An *indirect* abortion is one in which the direct moral object of the action (the immediate and intrinsic purpose of the procedure) is medical therapy for the mother, but in which the death of the fetus is a side effect that cannot be avoided; for example, removal of a pathological tube containing a fertilized ovum in ectopic pregnancy or removal of a cancerous gravid uterus. Such indirect abortions are justified by the principle of double effect because (a) the act itself is directly aimed at treating a pathology in the mother and hence ethical, (b) the mother and physician would save the child if this were possible, (c) the death of the child is not a means to treat the mother, but only an unwanted side effect of the procedure, and (d) the proportionate reason for allowing the death of the infant is saving the mother's life.

It is not necessary here to review the long-standing public debate over "pro-life" and "pro-choice" (Glendon 1987; Dworkin 1993; Lee 2004; Engelhardt 1995) because the main issues, the definition of personhood and its beginning, have been treated earlier in the chapter (section 3.2). An extensive bibliography on the subject can be found in Johnston (2003), DeHullu (1989), Irving (1991, 2002), and Ladd and Bowman (1999). It should be especially noted, however, that the failure of the medical profession to seek a scientifically objective and ethically responsible position on this question has seriously undermined the profession (Pellegrino 1989, 1991, 1992).

The prohibition of direct abortion has always been consistent with church teaching. Jesus preached the good news of God's love for the "little ones," the outcasts rejected by secular and religious authorities including powerless little children whom he declared should be given special respect in the kingdom of God (Mk 9–33). The sacredness of human life is so fundamental to the teaching of Jesus and the moral exhortation of the New Testament that abortion is not even mentioned in the New Testament. The *Didache* (translation, *Didache* 1991), however, a catechetical instruction for baptism contemporary with the later books of the New Testament, shows that early Christians were forbidden to have abortions. In the times following the early church, abortion and infanticide were widespread in Greek and Roman culture, but the church continued to condemn the practices. The church continued the condemnation of these practices up until modern times (Noonan 1970; Grisez 1970, 1989, 1993; Schwartz and Tacelli 1989; Schwartz 1990; Fisher 2005). The Second Vatican Council, for example, condemned abortion and infanticide as "unspeakable crimes" (1965, no.51). In 1995, John Paul II, in the encyclical *Gospel of Life*, declared unequivocally that abortion and euthanasia could not be reconciled with the

Church's constant teaching (62): "Therefore by the authority which Christ conferred upon Peter and his successors, in communion with the bishops—who on various occasions have condemned abortion and who, in the aforementioned consultation albeit dispersed through the world, have shown unanimous agreement concerning this doctrine—I declare that direct abortion, that is abortion willed as an end or a means, always constitutes a grave moral disorder since it is the deliberate killing of an innocent human being."

This statement has been declared an ordinary infallible teaching of the church (CDF 1998); hence acceptance of this teaching is required of all Catholics. If they are true to their beliefs in the advocacy of the helpless, Catholics need to work for practical legislation defining the subject of human rights, or at least for positive efforts to reduce the number of abortions. Undoubtedly the task of Catholics as a community should first and last be educational rather than merely political. Jesus taught us to trust in the power of truth, love, and forgiveness rather than in the power of law or law enforcement. Political action cannot be neglected, but it must be supported by a transformative educational effort. In the United States, some bishops have reminded Catholic politicians and legislators that they have a serious responsibility to oppose abortion whenever possible. Many politicians and legislators, conversely, maintain that they must obey the Constitution and the laws of the land if they are elected to office. Often these Catholic legislators will defend their reluctance to oppose abortion by declaring abortion to be "a private matter," or a matter of conscience (McCarrick 2004). However, the conscience of Catholics should be formed in accord with the teaching of the Church, not in opposition to it.

Certainly, it is not enough for a Catholic legislator to say, "I personally disapprove of abortion, but I do not believe in imposing my private views upon the public"; this would be equivalent to a person saying, "I personally abhor racism, but I do not wish to impose my private views on others." In the struggle to create a just society and to promote the rights of every person, there will be legitimate difference in regard to what is politically possible and what is realistically obtainable, but the right to life should be promoted as a fundamental cornerstone of a just society. Thus the continued efforts of some to claim that Catholics can be true to the faith and yet pro-choice are groundless (Kissling 2005; MacCrae 2005).

Note that the Catholic position regarding abortion does not depend on the conviction contained in the earlier part of this chapter, that human personhood begins at fertilization, but rather on the proposition stated in *The Declaration on Procured Abortion* (CDF 1974): "From a moral point of view, it is certain that even if a doubt existed whether the fruit of conception is already a human person it is an objectively grave sin to dare to risk murder."

Abortions are sometimes performed at the behest of parents who are unsatisfied with the results of prenatal screening, usually in the form of amniocentesis. Thus while prenatal screening is not in itself unethical, it may dispose for an unethical attack upon a fetus. We shall consider this topic when discussing genetic screening and counseling in chapter 4.

Disputed Cases: Ectopic Pregnancy and Anencephaly

Because the manner in which ectopic pregnancies are removed, and the manner in which an infant might be treated after anencephaly has been diagnosed, may result in direct abortions, over the years the ethical treatment of ectopic pregnancies and anencephalic infants has been disputed (May 1994; Moraczewski 1996).

Ectopic Pregnancy.   An ectopic pregnancy usually occurs when a fertilized ovum embeds itself in the wall of the fallopian tube (though it may occur in other locations) instead of passing through the tube and embedding itself in the wall of the uterus, as normally happens. This results in a pathological condition in the fallopian tube, an abnormal infiltration of the fallopian tube by the placental villus of the conceptus, which could lead to death or a serious morbidity for the woman if the fallopian tube should rupture. (Luciano, Roy, and Solima, 2001) The ERD states that in treating a woman with an ectopic pregnancy, "no intervention is morally licit which constitutes a direct abortion." (2001, D. 48) But physicians and theologians do not always agree on which procedures used to treat the pathology would be direct abortions and which would be indirect abortions. All seem to agree that it would be licit to remove the portion of the fallopian tube that is pathological (salpingectomy) even though the fertilized ovum would also be removed, by reason of the principle of double effect. But there is some dispute with regard to performing a linear salpingostomy (merely splitting the tube and removing the fertilized ovum), which allows the tube to heal and perhaps be useful for future pregnancies.

In contemporary medicine, methotrexate is often used to treat the pathology caused by the abnormal location of the fertilized ovum. While it would be wrong to detach a fertilized ovum from its normal site of implantation, to detach it from an abnormal site that constitutes a serious pathological condition in the woman's body would seem to be licit. Hence, the direct intrinsic intention (*finis operas*) of the surgical or pharmaceutical act (salpingectomy or methotrexate) seems to be to protect the health of the mother, and the death of conceptus is not intended. For this reason, it is our opinion that salpingostomy and the use of methotrexate do not result in direct abortion and therefore are in accord with Directive 48.

Anencephaly.   Anencephaly is a birth defect that inhibits the development in utero of the brain. There is no therapy by which to correct this anomaly and the baby will usually die shortly after birth. Would it constitute an abortion to deliver infants with anencephaly, or some other severe genetic anomaly, before viability? Some moralists have maintained that early delivery before viability would be licit because it may help the mother avoid psychological suffering (Bole 1992; Drane 1992). Furthermore, some have maintained that anencephalic infants could be considered as organ donors even though they would die shortly after an early delivery (Holzgreve 1987). Delivery before viability seems to be a direct abortion because the moral object of the act is to end the pregnancy, and the child dies as an inevitable result. Even if the motive (*finis operantis*) for early delivery is consolation for the mother, the moral object of the act (*finis operis*) still seems to involve a direct abortion. Some ethicists have maintained that delivery could be induced after twenty-six weeks, which they equate with viability. However, these opinions seem to use the term *viability* in an equivocal manner. Viability is not a general characteristic that all infants acquire at the same time. Moreover, no aggressive care, such as an incubator, will be utilized in the care of an anencephalic infant delivered early, while it would be given to a normal infant for whom early delivery is considered a medical necessity (Directive 49). Hence speaking about "viability" for the anencephalic infant at twenty-six weeks seems to be a misnomer. It seems the moral object of early delivery for an anencephalic or a genetically deprived infant is to hasten or cause the death of the infant. Moreover, early delivery of seriously impaired infants does not seem to relieve psychological suffering on the part of the mother (Iles and Gath 1993). Thus it is our opinion that anencephalic infants and genetically deprived infants should be allowed to go to term, be baptized, and be allowed to die in their parents' arms (O'Rourke 1996b). This opinion is in accord with norms published by the National Conference of Catholic Bishops (NCCB 1996).

Treatment of Victims of Sexual Assault

Rape is one of the more common social crimes (Graham 2005). Because many rape victims hesitate to expose themselves to shame and notoriety, and because false charges of rape are possible, it is difficult to ascertain with any degree of accuracy the number of rapes committed in the United States each year. When crimes of violence are tabulated, however, the percentage of rapes increases each year. There is evidence that rape is motivated by hostile impulses—a desire to assert the aggressive power of the rapist and to humiliate the victim—more than a desire for sexual pleasure (Lifshitz 1999). Furthermore, many rapists force the victim to engage in perverse sexual acts. To perform even natural sexual acts, outside or even within marriage, against the will of the partner is contrary to the meaning of sexuality as an expression of mutual love. In *Lust and Personal Dignity* Pope John Paul II (1980) pointed out the sinfulness of the husband who even in thought considers the wife a mere sexual object, without regard for her free personhood. Such behavior is wife abuse, which is at last being exposed to public concern.

A victim of rape should be given the most sensitive and charitable care possible. Such victims often complain justifiably that the police and medical personnel treat them as though they were responsible for provoking the attack, thus compounding the grave injustice from which the woman has suffered. Many cities now have formed rape treatment task forces, not only to help educate police and medical personnel concerning humane treatment of rape victims but also to prevent the crime by alerting the public to the signs of impending attack and to the measures that might ward it off (Sparks 1988). After the police, the responsibility for care of the victim of rape generally falls on the health care profession, although the clergy and especially the family of the victim have important roles as well. Hospital procedures developed by such task forces are designed to accomplish four things:

1. To offer the psychological support and counseling that the woman needs to work through the trauma of the attack and its aftermath. Often this will require follow-up treatment with a counselor or psychologist.
2. To provide medical care for injuries or abrasions that might have occurred.
3. To gather evidence to be used if the rapist is apprehended and prosecuted. This usually consists of a rather extensive examination of the vagina, pelvic area, and clothing.
4. To provide treatment to prevent possible venereal disease and pregnancy.

This last point, preventing pregnancy, raises special ethical problems. Because more probably the woman is in an infertile portion of her cycle and because the trauma of rape has an anti-ovulatory effect (Mahkorn and Dolan 1981), the chances of conception after rape statistically are very low. Becoming pregnant is naturally a very serious concern to the victim, however, and she deserves all the help that medical professionals can give her, provided that help is ethical. Of course, in many cases, it will be possible to ascertain that conception is not at all likely, for example, if the woman is postmenopausal, taking contraceptive drugs, or an examination of cervical mucus shows she is not in a fertile phase. If pregnancy is a possibility, because the victim is in no way responsible for the possible pregnancy, she has the right to avoid it if this is ethically possible (Pemico 1993). A woman who has consented to intercourse takes responsibility as a free person to use the sexual act in keeping with its intrinsic significance of love and procreation. The arguments of *Humanae vitae* against contraception are based on this responsibility. The rape victim, however, has no such responsibility because she has not consented to the sexual act. Thus she has assumed no responsibility to give proper meaning to the sexual act that has been unjustly forced on her.

Therefore most Catholic moralists today admit that a woman who is in real danger of rape may, before the attack and if the danger is real, take a drug to prevent conception or even insert a diaphragm (Bayer 1985). After the rape, through her own action or that of a medical person, she may do what is possible to render the sperm inoperative, to prevent it from joining the ovum, or to delay the production of ova.

Preventing Conception

From the discussion of abortion earlier in this chapter, however, it follows that once the woman has conceived, she cannot take any action that would abort or destroy a fertilized ovum directly or request others to do so, nor may they cooperate with her in doing so. Although she has the right to protect herself from the effects of the aggression, she does not have the right to do so at the expense of the life of a fetus that is in no way an aggressor. There is no proportion between the fetus's right to life and her right to be free of the injury done to her, overwhelming as this is. A woman does not restore her personal dignity and integrity by destroying the life of another person.

Problems arise, however, when methods to prevent conception are proposed that not only prevent conception but also may be abortifacient. As already noted, even though a woman is protecting her rights, it is wrong for her to do so at the expense of the rights of a child already in existence. On the other hand, when honest *doubt* exists as to whether conception has in fact taken place, the probability should favor the certain rights of the woman. Once it becomes certain or highly probable that conception has occurred, however, she must then recognize the rights of the developing embryo to life and avoid any serious risk of abortion.

Formerly, when discussing licit methods of attacking the sperm before conception, Catholic moralists recommended (with some limitations as to time) dilation and curettage (D & C), vaginal douche, or intrauterine douche (O'Donnell 1957). Today, from both the medical and moral points of view, none of these methods seem to be acceptable. The vaginal douche may be used for cleansing and sanitizing purposes to prevent venereal disease but is unlikely to prevent conception. Conception takes place ordinarily in one of the fallopian tubes, not in the vagina or uterus, and studies show that the sperm enters the tubes five to thirty minutes after intercourse (Settlage, Motoshima, and Tredway 1973). Thus the vaginal spermicidal douche might attack some of the sperm remaining in the vagina but would be ineffective for most of them. The intrauterine douche is considered too dangerous because the fluid it introduces could flow through the fallopian tubes into the peritoneal cavity and perhaps cause serious infection. Competent gynecologists do not employ this procedure today.

The theologians who formerly allowed D & C realized that the scraping of the womb made it impossible for an already implanted zygote to survive or for a fertilized ovum to be implanted. They argued, however, that the principal purpose of this action was to eliminate the sperm, and if this was done soon enough after the attack, the principle of double effect could be used (Healy 1956). Given the new evidence of the motility of the sperm, it is no longer reasonable to say that D & C is a specific remedy to remove the sperm when the effective sperm is probably already out of the uterus. While the above few paragraphs may seem to be ancient history, they are included to demonstrate that ethical conclusions may change given new scientific information, though by no means always in the direction of pragmatic leniency.

Another example of changing ethical norms has occurred in the prescribed treatment for rape victims. Prior to recent scientific studies, it seemed that the antifertility drugs that could prevent ovulation would prevent the implantation of a fertilized ovum. Thus, if conception had already occurred in the fallopian tube, the effect of the antifertility drug was thought to be abortifacient. "But recent scientific literature concerning two F.D.A. approved medications for emergency contraception (rape treatment) Preven and Plan B, raise doubts about the effect of these medications" (Hamel and Panicola 2003). While the studies do admit of histologic changes in the endometrium, there is no conclusive evidence that the changes inhibit implantation (Menart 2005). Moreover, they suggest that emergency contraceptive medications act primarily by inhibiting ovulation or disrupting fertilization and mainly employ prefertilization mechanisms in their contraceptive effectiveness (Croxatto 2005).

All commentators on this issue do not agree with the previously described method of treatment (McMahon 2003). They prefer the "Peoria Protocol" (Shea 2004), which was predicated upon the supposition that antifertility drugs would seriously impede implantation and thus required testing to ensure that ovulation either had taken place or was not taking place at the time of therapy for rape. The Committee on Doctrine and Pastoral Practices of the NCCB considered the two methods of treatment and "concluded in part that rape treatment protocols that only provide pregnancy testing prior to administering post coital anti-ovulatory drugs do not violate Directive 36 of the ERD" (Cataldo 2004). Hence it is safe to say that the pregnancy protocol (Hamel and Panicola 2002) may be followed in Catholic hospitals.

In conclusion, the responsibilities of Catholic health care facilities when caring for rape victims are summarized in the following manner:

1. Catholic health care facilities should prepare and carefully observe a protocol for the treatment of rape victims in which the first concern is respect for the dignity of the woman, regardless of her character or socioeconomic condition (Gregorek 1988). This should consist of both medical and counseling help, including the offer of pastoral counseling, to reduce the harm she has unjustly suffered and should shield her as much as possible from embarrassment.
2. The protocol should provide for the collecting of adequate and accurate information for the police so that the aggressor can be brought to trial and conviction.
3. The protocol should also include medical tests to determine if the woman is pregnant. If the tests are positive, nothing should be done that would cause harm to the embryo.

4. If it is determined that the woman is not pregnant and not using contraceptive medications or devices, antifertility drugs may be administered. Although there is very remote risk that implantation might be affected, the risk is not substantial (Cataldo and Moraczewski 2001). If physicians or rape victims wish to avoid even this small risk to a potential third party and thus would not wish to administer or receive antifertility hormones, their consciences should be respected by the Catholic health care facility.

5. Facilities should be aware that, depending on state laws, they may be liable to legal suit if they fail to provide a rape victim with the opportunity to avoid pregnancy. Consequently, if a Catholic facility believes in conscience that it is unable to provide treatment that can be established as adequate in the local courts, it should make sure that victims can be promptly referred to their own physicians for whatever antipregnancy treatment they themselves choose.

Artificial Human Reproduction

Artificial reproduction, often referred to as ART (assisted reproductive technology), is any process by which human sperm fertilizes a human ovum in a manner other than sexual intercourse. While there are many different methods of bringing about conception outside of human intercourse (PCB 2004b, 26), today the more common methods are in vitro fertilization (IVF) and artificial insemination by husband (AIH) or donor (AID).

The process of IVF involves collecting sperm and ova from the couple who will generate the child, starting the process of human generation in a Petri dish and then transferring two or three (or more) fertilized ova to the womb of the woman who will bring the child to birth. This process is performed in private clinics and is very expensive, especially if success is not obtained in the first attempt. Live births resulting from this form of artificial generation occur about 25 percent of the time (PCB 2004b). Excess embryos resulting from this process are often destroyed or frozen with the possibility of thawing and reanimating them should the initial process fail (Edwards and Beard 1997; Seyfer 2003). In artificial insemination, whether AIH or AID, sperm is introduced into the woman's vagina artificially. In AIH, the sperm is obtained from the husband, usually by means of masturbation. In AID, the sperm is obtained from a donor, also usually by means of masturbation. It has been argued that self-stimulation by a man to obtain a semen sample, as opposed to the same for seeking genital satisfaction, is not masturbation; however, this argument seems mistaken. Genital acts are essentially interpersonal, and obtaining semen in this manner is a solitary orgasm and ejaculation. Judging from the number of scientific and popular articles written about these two forms of artificial reproduction in the last twenty-five years, many thousands of children have been conceived in this manner, but it is difficult to obtain accurate statistics. Serious birth defects often result in infants generated by ART (Hansen et al. 2002; Stromberg et al. 2002).

While the Church has often spoken against the assisted generation of children outside of the marital act (Pius XII 1956; CDF 1987), artificial reproduction is not wrong because it is artificial but because of the particular set of techniques used to separate the procreative from the unitive purpose of the marital act, just as contraception separates its unitive teleology from its procreative purpose. "The desire for a child is a good intention, but the good intention is not sufficient reason for making a positive moral evaluation of *in vitro* fertilization between spouses" (CDF 1987). The most complete explanation of Church teaching is contained in the *Instruction on Respect for Human Life*, issued by the CDF, in 1987. The teaching of the Church, as written in this document, is summarized as follows:

1. Human procreation must take place in marriage. The procreation of a new person, whereby the man and the woman collaborate with the power of the Creator, must be the fruit and the sign of the mutual self-giving, love, and fidelity of the spouses.
2. Using the sperm or ovum of a third party is not acceptable because it constitutes a violation of the reciprocal commitment of the spouses. Moreover, this form of generation violates the rights of the child to a filial relationship to its parents.
3. Generation of the new person should occur only through an act of intercourse performed between the husband and wife, in an act that is per se suitable for the generation of children, to which marriage is ordered by its very nature.
4. The fertilization of the new human person must not occur as the result of a technical process that substitutes for the marital act because it separates the procreative and unity aspects of marriage.

Unfortunately, in our opinion, Directive 39 of the ERD concerning assisted reproduction is not stated as precisely as the *Instruction on Respect for Human Life*. That directive reads, "Those techniques of assisted conception that respect the unitive and procreative meanings of sexual intercourse and do not involve the destruction of human embryos or their deliberate generation in such numbers that it is clearly envisaged that all cannot implant and some of them are simply being used to maximize the chance of others, implant may be used as therapy for infertility." Thus the directive seems to imply that an assisted technique of reproduction that would cause fertilization inside the body of the woman is acceptable. The *Instruction on Respect for Human Life* (CDF 1987) clearly maintains that even generation inside the human body is immoral if it separates the unitive and procreative aspects of marriage; for example, AIH would not be an acceptable method of generation, as the *Instruction* states. Moreover, the way that this directive is stated gives the impression that assisted methods of conception that are acceptable do exist. In reality, none have been developed. Some Catholic physicians and theologians have advocated the gamete intrafallopian transfer (GIFT) method of reproduction as ethical if masturbation is not employed to obtain semen (Sparks 1997; Cataldo 1996). But it seems that even if fertilization occurs within the body of the woman, as it does in GIFT, fertilization that is not the direct result of the marital act but rather is the result of a technician's manipulation does not meet the norms of the Church's teaching. Hence the right of the child so conceived is not respected, because this natural bond consists not merely in the fact that the couple supply a sperm and an ovum but also in the fact that they themselves generate the child through the act of love that binds them together and hence their child. The ultimate social result of the spread of such practices, therefore, can only be a weakening of the family institution that for this and other reasons is in rapid decline. In all such questions, the rights of the child are more fundamental than the desire of the couple, as noble as it is, to procreate, because the proper goal of the parents' desire is the good of the child, not their own generativity.

Surrogate Motherhood

Surrogate motherhood occurs when a woman conceives or carries a child for a married couple, the conception involving the gamete of one or more third parties. The conception may have occurred through natural intercourse or through some form of artificial reproduction, the fertilized ovum later being implanted in the surrogate mother's womb. Resort to this technique by infertile couples seems to be increasing (www.surrogacy.com/index.html). The surrogate mother usually makes a promise or signs a contract assuring that she will give the baby to the couple who has paid her to bring the child to term. The courts of the United States do not always honor a surrogate motherhood contract, thus allowing the surrogate mother to rescind her agreement if she so desires during the pregnancy (Incandela 2005; Freeman 1999). One philosopher commenting on the ethics of surrogate motherhood maintained that it calls upon a woman to be everything a mother should not be. In regard to surrogate motherhood the Church states: "Surrogate motherhood represents an objective failure to meet the obligations of maternal love, of conjugal fidelity, and of responsible motherhood; it offends the dignity and the right of the child to be conceived, to be carried in the womb, to be brought into the world and to be brought up by his or her own parents; it sets up to the detriment of families a division between the physical, psychological and moral elements which constitute those families" (CDF 1987).

3.4 PASTORAL APPROACH TO ETHICAL PROBLEMS ARISING FROM SEXUALITY

Difficult moral questions often arise in the life of Catholics, and other persons interested in living a good life, as a result of the Church's teaching on sexuality. Medical professionals as well as theologians and ethicists may often be called upon to act as counselors for people who face difficult ethical decisions. History shows that a "morality gap" between Church teaching and the moral understanding of many Catholics is by no means unusual. Indeed, like the gap between medical knowledge and human health habits, it has always in various degrees prevailed and is immensely difficult to overcome. To cite one notorious example, representatives of the Church—bishops and priests—were reluctant to preach about racism or question racist attitudes and practices. They justified this reluctance on the grounds that given the racist milieu they might drive people out of the Church without actually improving their attitudes or conduct. This pastoral policy was intended to be compassionate in regard to the subjective dispositions of white individuals, but in contrast, objectively it perpetuated a grave social injustice that disregarded the equal dignity of black people.

Objective and Subjective Morality

The Church has no desire to condemn people who abuse or contradict the natural good of human sexuality or reproduction; rather, it recommends patience, sympathy, and time to help people realize the injury they inflict upon themselves and others by contradicting the values of virtuous human sexuality. Typical of the Church's attitude is the statement of Pope John Paul II (1995, 18) on the morality of abortions: "Decisions that go against life arise from difficult or even tragic situations of profound suffering, loneliness, a total lack of economic prospects, depression, and anxiety about the future. Such circumstances can mitigate even to a notable degree, subjective responsibility and the consequent culpability of those who make choices which are in themselves evil."

Thus, even in matters as serious as abortion, the Church recognizes the difference between objective and subjective morality. In the history of Church teaching, the distinction between objective and subjective morality has always been recognized. Thus the objective teachings of morality must be combined with a person's subjective capability of observing the teaching. This truth was expressed once again in a document from the CDF (1989, no. 3):

> Christian moral tradition has always maintained the distinction—not the separation much less the contra-position—between the objective order and subjective guilt. For this reason, it becomes a matter of judging subjective moral behavior within the norm that prohibits the intrinsic disorder. It is perfectly legitimate to give due consideration to actions of the individuals not only to their intention and motivation but also to the various circumstances of their lives and above all to the causes that might impair their consciences and free will. This subjective situation, which can never change into "order" what is intrinsically "disorder" can have some bearing on the responsibility of the individual behavior.

This distinction between objective morality (i.e., what is helpful or harmful to the human person by reason of the moral object) and subjective culpability (i.e., a person's own understanding and responsibility for good or ill) is fundamental to counseling and pastoral care, which seeks to help people overcome the gap that often exists between ethical truth and moral awareness. The acceptance of ethical truth and the development of moral sensitivity are gradual processes. Helping people to fulfill the norms of morality is not accomplished through condemnation but through patience and compassion. We are historical beings. In all things, moral behavior included, we make progress only by invoking and practicing "patience, sympathy, and time" (John Paul II 1981, 34). Hence the distinction between objective and subjective morality does not mean that people have the right to form their own consciences without referring to Church teaching. Rather it implies that Church teaching in some instances will be difficult to follow because of the many situations in contemporary society that impinge upon moral decision making and behavior. We live in an unhealthy society that emphasizes individuality over community and pursuit of pleasure in place of justice and personal virtue. Jesus calls us to be in the world, but not of the world.

3.5 CONCLUSION

Though often used as synonyms, "sexuality" and "gender" have distinct meanings. Sexuality has two different meanings. Every person, in one sense of the term, is a sexual being. Gender refers to a person's self-representation as male or female as determined by environment and experience (http://csd.georgetown.edu). The beginning of human life is also a significant factor in the study of bioethics. Catholic tradition with regard to the generation and birth of children is based on the firm conviction, drawn from sacred scripture and human reason, that the family is the God-given entity for co-creation and flourishing of human life. The acts of love and unity proper to married people are the only human acts worthy of bringing new life into the world. The family is not only the proper source of life but also the proper setting for educating the young in virtue.

Closely allied with the teaching of the Church in regard to family and reproduction is its teaching on the sanctity of each person. Thus the teaching about abortion is of great importance for contemporary society. Unfortunately, contemporary society is blind to the sanctity of life—especially for the weak and debilitated—and the meaning of the family as the only proper context for reproduction. In a word, the teaching of the Church in regard to reproduction and sexuality is countercultural. The task of Catholics is not only to live the teaching of the Church but also to explain and defend it using the science and language of contemporary society.

Chapter Four

RECONSTRUCTING AND MODIFYING THE HUMAN BODY: ETHICAL PERSPECTIVES

OVERVIEW

IN RECENT YEARS, MEDICAL TECHNOLOGY HAS moved from the mere capability of repairing the human body to new capabilities of remodeling the body through surgical reconstruction, and even perhaps by genetic intervention, which will alter not only individuals but also all their descendants. In addition to the possibility of enhancing human function through biotechnology, surgical procedures that modify the appearance of the human body have become commonplace. Some of these new capabilities are already practical, others still futuristic. This chapter deals in some detail with certain current methods associated with modifying the human body but also touches on the futuristic ones for purposes of illustration.

After discussing briefly the theological norms guiding the development of the human body, this chapter then considers the potential of changing the human body through genetic intervention and the need to counsel and screen those who have genetic anomalies. Next we consider the methods of reconstructing the human body through surgical procedures: organ transplantation, reconstruction and transsexual surgery, and finally, ethical norms for research on human subjects, a form of manipulating and improving the function of the human body, are formulated.

4.1 MODIFYING THE HUMAN BODY

A basic axiom of medicine has always been the Greek dictum "Art perfects nature," which implies that human persons can be healed (or patched up) and helped to develop to maturity, but they cannot be essentially remade. Today, however, the situation has changed. By means of surgery and genetic manipulation, the body can be reshaped or modified significantly. Can we change human function without endangering our natural capacities? We must face the following questions: Is it right for persons to become their own creators? Can and should human nature be remade? Can genetic engineering hasten the processes of evolution? Might the technology of the future greatly reduce the complexities of the digestive system, which so often becomes diseased? Can human beings be fed in some simpler way, perhaps by a more effective intravenous method? Might all human beings be sterilized and reproduce artificially? Some answer this question by saying, "If we can, we must," and call this the "technological imperative" (Francoeur 1972; Friedmann 2000). Jonas (1979, 1984), however, cautions against the tendency to accept scientific progress as an unquestioned benefit (Peterson 2001). There is no doubt that medicine and science will not pause (Elliot 2003); in a realistic sense, "the future is now." But we must temper the present and the future developments with ethical principles. Though many seem to agree with this thought, there is a reluctance to control scientific research because of a desire to conquer disease and illness. In other words, many believe that the end often justifies the means.

The first steps toward remaking the human body have already been taken (Shapiro et al. 1986). Three levels of physical remaking seem possible:

1. Surgical procedures which modify the human phenotype (the actual body as opposed to inherited characteristics) in an effort to make the body more physically attractive or function more effectively, for example, procedures that replace existing organs with transplants or artificial organs.

2. Embryological development might be influenced by drugs or surgery (Brownlee 2002) so as to mold the development of the phenotype (the actual body) while not changing the genotype (inherited characteristics). Thus the phenotypic sex of a child could be determined at will despite the genotype by altering the course of development very early in embryonic life (American Society for Reproductive Medicine 1999). There are even possibilities of expanding the human senses so as to extend our senses of sight or hearing beyond their present ranges or enhance their power to resolve colors or pitches (Adelman 2000).

3. Ultimately genetic engineering might be employed to produce any gene combination in the fertilized ovum, thus creating human beings by "recipe" (Nevin 1999). Already the development of the technique of "recombinant DNA" (deoxyribonucleic acid) has made it possible to produce new species of bacteria with useful (and perhaps dangerous) combinations of genetic traits. Related to this is the production of clones from the somatic cells of a parent or artificial reproduction of multiple individuals all having the same genetic composition (Revel 2000).

The basic ethical issue here is seen by some theologians to be how great the extent of human dominion over nature is (Cole-Turner 2000). This is a classical way of posing the issue, but it is perhaps too much influenced by the Greek image of God as a jealous monarch who becomes angry when Prometheus infringes on his prerogatives. Others would see such attempts to improve on human beings as an insult to the work of the Creator, whose masterpiece is humankind, or at least as a fatal temptation to pride (Ellul 1980; Keenan 1999).

Today, however, in considering radical human development, two theological points must be stressed. First, God is a generous creator, who in creating human beings also gave them intelligence to share in his creative power. Consequently, God does not want human beings to leave fallow the talents he has given them, but encourages them to improve on the universe he has made. Second, such improvement is possible because Christian theology can assimilate the scientific view of an evolutionary universe in which the human race has been created through a still continuing evolutionary process, if God is acknowledged as the ultimate cause of that process (John Paul II 1995). Thus God has called us to join with him in bringing the universe to its completion, and in doing this, he has not made us merely workers to execute his orders or to add trifling original touches on our own. Rather, God has made us his genuine co-workers and encourages us to exercise real creativity (Ashley 1995, 2005).

Granted such a theology, however, it is not so clear that the remaking of the human body on new lines is really the appropriate focus for our creativity. Remolding the environment and creating human culture takes time enough and perhaps is a more productive way to proceed (Jones 2000). Someday genetic disease may also be eliminated and even human health advanced eugenically. Yet before technology attempts to produce Superman, it needs to heed the paradox proposed by MacIntyre (1979), who first imagines what types of human beings he would like to produce. They would have the ability to live with uncertainty, to keep rooted in the particularity of everyday life, to form nonmanipulative relations with others, to find their fulfillment in their work, to accept death, to keep hopeful, and to be willing to die for their freedom. He then concludes, "The project of designing our descendants would, if successful, result in descendants that would reject that project" (Reiss 1999).

Cooperation in Creation

It is important to remember, however, that human creativity depends on a human brain. Any alteration that would injure the brain and thus a person's very creativity would indeed be disastrous mutilation, especially if this were to be transmitted genetically, thus further polluting the gene pool with defects that might be hidden and incalculable.

It is generally admitted that knowledge of this wonderful brain is still in its beginnings (ITEST 1975; Edleman 1995; Rosenfield 1995; Penrose 1995; Naam 1995). The complexity of the brain is beyond any other system imaginable, and this complexity is reduced to a relatively small organ capable of self-development from the embryo and of self-maintenance, but only minimally of self-restoration. The human brain may be near the limit of complexity and integration possible in organic, living systems (Ashley 1995). If this is the case, any radical improvement may be illusory, whereas even slight alterations may be very damaging. Thus, to say the least, radical attempts to alter the structure of the human brain must be viewed with the utmost caution, because the risk of producing persons of lowered intelligence is very high.

This is certainly not so true of other organ systems, and it is possible to imagine that someday in other environments it might become necessary, for example, to replace the human lungs with other ways of obtaining oxygen. In principle it would seem that such changes would be ethical if they gave support to human intelligence by helping the life of the brain and if they did not suppress any of the fundamental human functions that integrate the human personality. Thus alterations that would make it impossible for persons to directly sense the external world at least as effectively as they now do with five senses would be contrary to human well-being, as would alterations that would make it impossible for persons to experience the basic emotions, as emotional life is closely related to human intelligence and creativity. Again, alterations that would make human beings sexless and incapable of parenthood would also be antihuman. The power to procreate through intercourse and to form families for holistic development of children and parents are functions that pertain to the very essence of being human. Hence the following conclusions can be drawn:

1. The use of surgery and genetic manipulation to improve human bodies is ethically good, provided that they take full account of such risks and are not carried away by a false ambition to work technical miracles without regard to their real meaning for human living. In particular, Christians should be concerned that such innovations do not weaken the fundamental relations within the family or the sense of the child as a unique gift of God.
2. Genetic engineering and less radical transformations of the present normal human body would be permissible if this improves rather than mutilates the basic human functions, especially as they relate to supporting human intelligence and creativity. Transformation would be forbidden, however, (a) if human intelligence and creativity are endangered and (b) if the fundamental functions that constitute human integrity are suppressed. Experimental efforts of this radical type must be undertaken with great caution and only on the basis of existing knowledge, not with high risks to the subjects or to the gene pool. In this regard we need not draw a firm line between somatic cell genetic intervention and germ-line cell intervention. Surely somatic cell intervention is more problem free, but if germ-line cell intervention could be perfected, it could ethically be utilized if the goals of such intervention were in accord with the norms already mentioned.
3. Natural law should not be conceived of as a fixed pattern of human life to which human beings are forever confined. Rather, the Creator has made human beings free and intelligent, and it is precisely this intelligent freedom that is human nature and the foundation of natural moral law. Human intelligence, however, is not disembodied; it depends on a brain and a body that have a specific structure and purpose. In caring for their total health, persons have not only the right but the obligation to understand their psychological and biological structure and to improve themselves even in ways that may seem novel to past generations. Such improvement is good stewardship of the share in divine creativity with which God has endowed humankind, provided it perfects and not destroys what he has given us already.

4.2 GENETIC INTERVENTION

The most ambitious scientific project, as extensive in its implications as the Manhattan Project that made possible the release of atomic and nuclear energy, is the Human Genome Project (Human Gene Project 2005). Utilizing the resources and skills of the scientific community throughout the world, the Human Genome Project sought to identify the activity of human genes and locate the place of genes on the human chromosome (Dietrich 2001).

Eventually this knowledge, it is hoped, will be used to modify the effect of deteriorative genes and to introduce into the human genotype genes that will improve the structure and behavior of human persons (Stock 2002). To date, astounding progress has been made in regard to identifying the location and activity of human genes (Human Gene Project 2005). Efforts to modify the activity of the human genotype by eliminating from or introducing genes into the human genotype have not been as successful. "As late as the early 70s serious scientists talked more optimistically about humankind's new opportunity to take the reins of its own evolution, than about the predicted confluence of genetic engineering and reproductive technologies. But as scientists have learned how difficult it is to engineer precise genetic change—even to treat individuals with genetic diseases caused by a simple one gene mutation—explicit talk about improving the species has largely faded" (PCB 2003, 31). However, indicators of some future success in manipulating genetic activity should not be discounted (Kolata 1995).

Children by Design

The issue of the parents' need and right to have children or even to "order" the sort of child they want is also at the base of many new problems that loom on the horizon concerning genetic engineering, or—to use an expression with less pejorative connotations— "genetic intervention" (PCB 2004, 93ff). This is the effort to repair genetic defects at their genotypic source in the genes and chromosomes rather than in their phenotypic effects and, further, to control and produce at will new combinations of genetic traits in offspring (Simpson and Carson 2002).

One of the simplest forms of such engineering would be to determine at will the sex of the fetus by selecting sperm that do or do not have the Y chromosome, which determines maleness, and then using selected sperm for artificial insemination or IVF and implantation (Robertson 2002). Most of the techniques used at present involve IVF, which is contrary to the teaching of the Catholic Church (CDF 1987). Even if a technique could be invented that would promote or suppress the production of one or the other type of sperm in the male parent without interfering with the normal process of sexual intercourse, the social and ecological consequences of such intervention could be counterproductive.

The theory of evolution by the selection of the fittest suggests also that this has led to the development of the process of sexual differentiation by a genetic mechanism of the sort we find in the human species in order to ensure an approximate 50/50 distribution of the sexes. The present ratio at birth is 105 boys to 100 girls (PCB 2004a, 59). Some additional mechanism not fully understood even produces a slightly higher number of male zygotes to offset the higher mortality of males. The practice of sex selection, either by means of abortion after sex determination in the womb or by means of preimplantation genetic diagnosis (PGD) following IVF, which involves abortion of unwanted fetuses before implantation, is widespread in many countries around the world and is becoming more frequent in the United States. The sex ratio of boys to girls in India is 117, in China 117, in Cuba 118, and the Caucasus nations as high as 120 to every 100 girls (PCB 2004a, 60). Such ratios portend grave difficulties in the future, especially insofar as the rights and dignity of women are concerned.

Ethically speaking, is this free choice of a boy or a girl an advantage to the *child*? After all, parents should not let their subjective preferences operate at the expense of their children in this matter, just as it is unethical for them to insist that the child be a doctor or a lawyer if this is not truly in the best interests of the child. On the one hand, it might be argued that it is somewhat advantageous for a boy to have a sister, and vice versa, rather than a sibling of his or her own sex, but it would be difficult to prove that such an advantage, if it exists, is of major significance. On the other hand, Christian teaching shows that it is highly significant to children that they be accepted by their parents as a divine gift to be loved for what they uniquely are and not merely because they conform to the parents' hopes or expectations. At present, society is becoming more aware of the immense injustice and harm done to women by cultural patterns and structures that constantly say to a girl, "You should have been a boy." Sex selection by the parents either will reinforce this male preference pattern or, if parents can be reeducated to equal preference, will still say to the individual child, "You are loved because you conform to your parents' preferences." This seems an injustice to the child and further reinforces the cultural message that children exist primarily to fulfill the needs of the parents rather than for their own sake. This implication is already built into many cultural structures, and people have an ethical responsibility to fight against it. The health care profession should discourage such attitudes, not promote techniques to further them.

Complex Forms of Intervention

The same consideration applies to more complex forms of genetic intervention. Although some progress has already been made in genetic recombination at the level of simple organisms, the possibility of using such methods to correct genetic defects or to create new genetic structures in human zygotes or embryos is still remote (Fitzgerald 2002).

One type of possible intervention is the transplantation of nonhuman animal cells, tissues, or organs into the human body or, conversely, human cells, tissues, or organs into an animal either to improve the recipient somehow or for research purposes. An organism made up of such a mixture of animal and human cells is called a "chimera" (from the mythological creature that was a goat-lion-serpent). Another type of intervention would be the formation of a hybrid by combining animal and human genes in the reproductive process. The essential point to remember is that, as argued in chapter 3 (section 3.2) vertebrate animal organisms are most precisely specified by their behavioral or functional abilities, and these are ultimately determined by what kind of brain their genome is able to produce. Therefore the specific distinction between human persons and lower animals must be determined by what kind of brain the chimera will have, whether animal or human. The same holds for a human-animal hybrid. This biological principle is not altered by the philosophical and religious view that the animal soul pertains to the material order, while the human soul pertains to the spiritual order and can owe its origin not to biological processes but only to direct creation by God. This is the case, because, as we argued in chapter 3 (section 3.2), in the natural order the Creator has established, he supplies a spiritual soul to any body that is genetically prepared to constitute a human body and, when it fully develops itself, a human brain.

For genetic interventions whose purpose is therapeutic, the only ethical issue is the proportion of probable benefit to risk. The greatest risk in the formation of an animal–human chimera would be if this would injure a person's brain, or produce a chimera that, against human dignity, had a human brain in an animal body. The same would hold for an animal–human hybrid that proved fertile, which would be even worse because it would produce a race of defective human persons. Nevertheless, as long as the result was an organism with a human brain, even a defective human brain, the victims would be true persons with all human rights.

What if the purpose of the genetic intervention is not therapy for an existing fetus but the production of superior human beings, not through chimerization or hybridization involving organisms of different species, but through germ-line therapy using only human genes (Silver 1997)? Two methods have been proposed. One is to replicate many genetically identical individuals by cloning. In such a process, nuclei from the somatic cells of a "superior" individual would be transplanted into a denucleated ovum, which would then develop into an identical twin of the donor. This would require IVF and implantation into a foster mother's womb (PCB 2002, 6–10). Another method is to recombine genes in the nucleus of a zygote, for example, by using viruses that have the capability of incorporating a section of a chromosome derived from one nucleus and fixing it in a chromosome of another (transduction). Theoretically it may become possible to synthesize chemically new genes that have never existed in the gene pool or to produce them by artificial, controlled mutation. Thus it might also be possible to produce a human being according to "recipe," with the height, complexion, physiological traits, and mental abilities desired. Although this is still remote (Fukuyama 2002), we would not rule it out ethically merely on the grounds that it would be usurpation of God's creative power, because God wishes to share this creative power with human persons if we use it well. But there is simply no guarantee that a child born after such genetic manipulation would grow up with the desired traits. "The interplay of nature and nurture (genes and environment) in human development is too complex and too little understood to make such results predictable" (PCB 2003, 43).

Moreover, grave ethical difficulties arise over whether society has either the knowledge or the virtue to take the responsibility for creating these superior members of the race (Callahan 1981; Kass 2003). Attempts to define *superior* eugenically are so ambiguous as to be arbitrary (PCB 2003, 102). Because human beings are evolutionary and historical beings, *superior* does not mean a being superior in one age and culture, but rather a being with capabilities of meeting the challenges of new and unpredictable situations. Genetic variation assists this flexibility, whereas the production of many identical human beings or those favoring certain supposedly superior types amounts to a restriction on this genetic variability. At most, a eugenic policy would have to be content with introducing into the gene pool some new, apparently valuable traits or increasing somewhat the percentage of their presence. Furthermore, all the difficulties already mentioned about the way in which such techniques tend to separate the child from its relations to parents and family must again be faced. The following conclusions can be drawn regarding these issues:

1. It is more feasible, technically and ethically, to improve the human condition by improving the environment and development of the individual, that is, the *phenotype*, than by modifying genetic endowment, that is, the *genotype* (Jones 2000). Priority in research and investment of medical resources should be given to the former effort. Genetic research is extremely important, however, to understand the interactions of genotype and phenotype.

2. Current proposed methods of genetic reconstruction of human beings involve IVF and other procedures that are ethically objectionable because they separate reproduction from its parental context and involve the production of human beings, some of whom will be defective because of experimental failure and who probably will be destroyed. This contravenes the basic principles of ethical experimentation with human subjects (Ramsey 1970; Hollander 2000).

3. Proposals to improve the human race by sex selection, cloning, or genetic reconstruction are ethically unacceptable in the present state of knowledge. Unless limited to very modest interventions, they would restrict the genetic variability important to human survival, and they would separate reproduction from its parental context.

4. If the foregoing problems can be overcome, it will be ethically desirable to develop and use genetic methods for therapy of genetic defects in existing embryos, keeping in view the risk-benefit proportion (Davis 2001).

Ecology and New Life Forms

In addition to discussion about efforts to manipulate human genes, much dialogue has focused recently on the possible effects on the ecological balance and the possible medical and commercial uses of experiments with and large-scale production of new life forms by the technique of recombinant DNA. This involves the modification of the genetic code of existing life-forms by introducing into their chromosomes fragments derived from the chromosomes of other life-forms, thus producing organisms with combinations of genetic and inheritable traits never before found in nature. For example, it is possible to produce food plants that can directly utilize atmosphere nitrogen and thus eliminate the use of fertilizers, or to produce rather inexpensively the heretofore extremely scarce interferon, a natural substance believed to have many important medical uses, including cancer therapy. The U.S. Supreme Court, in *Diamond v. Chakrabarty,* held that a live, man-made microorganism might be patented, thus opening the way to its commercial development (Ehrman et al. 1980).

Those who favored patenting such biological inventions argue that this will promote research, as it has for drugs. The analogy, however, also suggests the possibility of serious abuses for profit. The same basic ethical principles that govern any form of research apply here (section 4.6), with the additional precautions that what is involved is the total environment, not merely individual human subjects, and that possible widespread epidemics could result if something goes wrong. The greatest worry, but one that should not be exaggerated, is whether some new life-form, against which there is no existent immunity in the human, animal, or plant ecosystem, may multiply beyond bounds, as has so often occurred when alien species are introduced into an ecosystem already in balance (Carson 1994).

4.3 GENETIC SCREENING AND COUNSELING

The medical specialty of diagnosing inherited or genetic defects and their treatment is well established in the United States, as is also the genetic screening of parents in order to counsel them in case a child may be genetically defective (Bennett 2001).

Three basic discoveries have made it possible sometimes to predict inherited traits of a child before birth (Beurton, Falk, and Rheinberger 2000): (1) Gregor Mendel's theory of the laws of the combinations of units of inheritance, (2) the fact that these units are located in the chromosomes of the nucleus of every cell, and (3) how to map the genetic code consisting in variations in a fundamental substance, DNA, out of which the genes are composed. Techniques of diagnosing these defects at early stages of embryo development have been identified. One such technique is *amniocentesis*, by which the genetic condition of the unborn child can be determined in some respects by examining the amniotic fluid in which the fetus floats in the womb. Another technique is *chorionic villi sampling*, in which a plastic catheter is inserted through the cervix to biopsy villi, the hairlike projections in the placenta. Because this is rapidly growing tissue, the results of chromosome tests are available in a few days (Kuliev et al. 1996). The chorionic villi test may be performed about eight weeks earlier than amniocentesis.

Why such advances are medically important is evident from the following statistics. There are approximately four thousand different diseases in the single-gene disorder group, all of which are caused by different abnormal genes (Trent 1993). Today, 33 percent of infant deaths are related to genetic causes. More than one hundred genetic conditions can be diagnosed before birth. Parent carriers of defective genes may have as much as a 50 percent risk of generating offspring with a genetic defect. The polygenic conditions, such as diabetes mellitus, gout, and some allergies, occur in 1.7 to 2.6 percent of all live births. There seems to be approximately a 3 to 4 percent incidence of genetic disease in all live births (Sharpe-Stimac et al. 2004).

In view of these facts, some scientists, in the name of preventive medicine, advocate prenatal or postnatal *genetic screening* of the whole population for four purposes: (1) to advance scientific research, because such research is necessary to achieve full understanding and control over human inheritance; (2) to assist responsible parenthood so that carriers of genetic defects may not pass them on; (3) to make possible early therapy before the malfunctioning of defective genes has caused extensive damage; and (4) to give the parents the option of aborting the child when the defect is serious and no therapy is yet known (Macklin 1985; Murray and Pagon 1984).

We have already given reasons why this last purpose is ethically unacceptable, but the first three are certainly legitimate. However, the tests involved are not problem free (Capron 1984). The research purposes of genetic screening must be regulated in the same way as any other type of research on human subjects (section 4.6). Thus, because amniocentesis involves risk of spontaneous abortion (although the risk has been reduced with the help of sonography to less than 1 percent), it cannot be used unless there are also proportionate benefits for the fetus. At present, therapeutic help for a genetically deficient fetus is limited, but more progress in this field is noted each year (Hendren and Lillehi 1988; NIH 1987). Some ethicists maintain that amniocentesis benefits the fetus because it helps the parents prepare more adequately for the birth (Duke 1983). In sum, amniocentesis is indicated only when a pregnancy is thought to be at increased risk for a particular disorder (Kahn 1987).

Genetic Screening

Most screening techniques done postnatally involve the withdrawal of an insignificant amount of body fluid or tissue and are harmless. Nevertheless, informed consent is required in all such cases, and it is highly questionable that it is legitimate to enact laws that require compulsory screening for research purposes alone. Even when consent is given, care must be taken about how the information is used (Brody 2002). If the results are made known to subjects, there is danger that they may misunderstand or exaggerate the seriousness and possible consequences of their condition or the condition of their children (Lehrman 1995). If others know the results, there is danger of stigmatization, that is, that victims will be regarded by others as humanly inferior or dangerous. For example, it is unfair to label those African Americans who are carriers of the sickle cell trait, or those of Jewish descent who are carriers of the Tay-Sachs disease, as inferior persons.

Caution is necessary, however, in the face of programs of *negative* eugenics advocated by certain enthusiasts who argue that modern medicine has upset the ecological balance by saving the lives of more and more defective persons who formerly would have died before they could reproduce (Pernick 1997). If only those persons who themselves suffer from a particular genetic disease are prevented from reproducing, this still does not eliminate heterozygous carriers who will continue to transmit defects dependent on recessive genes. At present, technology is far from being able to detect all these carriers. Even if science had this ability, such elimination would extend to many people. This would probably also mean the elimination from the gene pool of many desirable traits, because the same persons carry both good and bad traits, which sometimes are genetically linked in ways still very obscure. Thus programs of negative eugenics based on present knowledge would achieve their goals only very slowly, over many generations, and might have side effects worse than the evils they remedy. Moreover, as defective genes are eliminated from the gene pool, they are constantly being replaced by mutations caused by environmental factors (Gratzer 2000). It seems, therefore, that such information cannot be used to compel persons to refrain from reproduction, but it may be supplied to them to enable them to make responsible personal decisions. Even here, however, some public caution is needed.

Some states have adopted compulsory screening of newborn infants to detect those afflicted with phenylketonuria (PKU; Koch 1997) or other genetic anomalies. It is claimed that these compulsory genetic testing programs are justified by reason of the common good, but this is true only if this does not encourage abortion and provision is made for the treatment of children who may be affected by this condition. Caring for genetically afflicted infants is a heavy financial burden for the community and may often be avoided through care that will obviate development of future disabilities. The effects of mental retardation that often result from PKU may be prevented by diet. Therefore, such genetic testing programs have to be carefully designed. Public policy in regard to genetic testing or screening should be concerned with the following (Parker and Lucassen 2002):

1. The general principles in regard to research on human subjects must be observed, including informed consent and protection of privacy (section 4.6).
2. Information concerning genetic disabilities should be made available to those not involved in the study who might be affected by the findings, that is, relatives of the participants, if they so desire.
3. Counseling should be available for those who are revealed to have genetic disabilities or disease and provision made to ensure treatment.
4. Ethics committees of the institutions where testing takes place should monitor genetic testing programs.

Genetic Counseling

If such screening and testing programs are to be well constructed, the main concern is to counsel those who participate in the program, whether as parents of infants who have been found to have genetic anomalies, or as adults who attempt to decide how to use the information resulting from the tests. Genetic counseling may be characterized as a process of communication that attempts to deal with the human problems associated with the occurrence, or the risk of occurrence, of a genetic disorder in an individual or family (Atkinson and Moraczewski 1980). This process involves an attempt by one or more appropriately trained persons to help an individual, couple, or family do the following:

1. Comprehend the medical facts, such as the risk of occurrence or recurrence of a disorder, the probable course of the disorder, and the available therapies.
2. Appreciate the ways in which hereditary and environmental factors contribute to the disorder and the extent to which specified relatives are at risk for being affected.
3. Understand the options for dealing with a positive diagnosis.
4. Choose the course of action that seems appropriate, in view of the client's own values and goals, other than abortion, which may never ethically be advised or condoned as abortion is always a violation of human rights.
5. Make the best possible adjustment to the disorder in an affected member of the family.

Parents come to a genetic counselor because of fears about possible defects in children already in existence or about their responsibilities for future pregnancies. These fears may have arisen because of positive test results in mass screening, or because of a record of genetic disease in parents, previous children, or close relatives. Prenatal genetic testing is not usually useful, because there is still a slight risk to the infant in utero when amniocentesis is performed (Bennett 2001). However, the possibility of being better prepared to care for a genetically affected infant might justify the risk. Recent developments resulting from genome studies seem to indicate that analysis of fetal plasma may be possible from maternal plasma (Harper et al. 2004), thus obviating invasive procedures upon the fetus.

If the parents declare a firm intention to abort, the counselor should not cooperate in any way with them. The reason is that counselors should protect the right of the fetus to life—exactly as they would protect the rights of a child already born—against the infringement of these rights by the parents, no matter how well intentioned the parents may be. A counselor, however, in doing whatever is possible to avoid abortion, should exercise great prudence, avoiding threats, pressures, and recriminations, as these will only aggravate the situation. Indeed, undue persuasion may lead to a malpractice claim (Howlett, Avard, and Knoppers 2002). In sum, if abortion is in question, the counselor should respect the conscience of the parents while doing everything possible to protect the child.

Is it permissible for a counselor to give information to parents when the counselor suspects they may resort to abortion? In the present ethical climate this suspicion always exists, and it has deterred Catholic health care facilities from instituting genetic counseling centers. Parents, however, have a right to such information, which has good as well as bad uses, and the counselor who supplies it cooperates only materially and remotely if the parents use it for a purpose the counselor considers unethical. Moreover, counselors may be legally liable if they do not inform parents that an unborn child may be suffering from a genetic defect and that it is possible in some cases to make sure of this by amniocentesis or other prenatal tests. In our opinion, Catholic health care facilities have a duty to provide such counseling in accordance with Christian moral standards, because otherwise parents will be forced to obtain information from centers where abortion will be an accepted and even encouraged solution (Cole-Turner 2000).

A child certainly has a right to be free of every defect that medicine has the power to prevent or correct. It is paradoxical, however, to believe that destroying the child who has not been saved from defect protects this right. If parents knew that they would generate genetically impaired children, they may decide not to generate children, but having generated them, they have the duty to care for them. They cannot lighten their burden by destroying an unborn child any more than they could by destroying an infant or adolescent. Some secular humanists approve such destruction, but it is not consistent with a Christian view of the value of a person or the true meaning of human life (DeMarco 1999, 2000). However, couples do have the duty of responsible parenthood, and society has a legitimate concern to support and encourage this responsibility. The genetic counselor, therefore, has the function of helping prospective parents prepare themselves for the possibility that a fetus will be defective and to plan ways to provide for this eventuality. The counselor also has the task of helping them decide whether they will or will not generate children. For counselors or society at large to encourage in parents the attitude that they should not have children unless the children are perfect and require the least care possible is as reprehensible as it is to encourage parents to reproduce fatalistically.

Parental Responsibility

In the past, some would have argued that a person or a couple at risk of begetting a defective child or children, or of transmitting defective genes to future generations, should fatalistically marry and beget children and "leave it to God." This fatalism has not been damaging to society because it did not upset the ecological balance established by evolutionary selection. Nevertheless, Christian teaching does not favor fatalistic attitudes, but rather advocates parental responsibility. Prospective parents, therefore, have to consider these factors: (1) their own need to have children as the completion of their mutual love, (2) their own capacity to care for these children, and (3) the risk that each particular child may suffer from grave handicaps requiring special care, including the possibility that this child will be faced in turn with the question as to whether he or she should pass on defective genes to the next generation. Some significant risks of defect exist for *every* child and could not be eliminated even by the most radical use of abortion. Thus in all cases parents must decide whether they have the capacity to care for a potentially defective child. Furthermore, the counselor and society have the duty to assist the parents in accepting and meeting reasonable risks. Certainly, the correct professional attitude for genetic counselors is to give the parents reliable, objective information as to the probabilities of defect and its consequences and the type of therapy and care that will be required. Counselors should also help them (directly or by referral to other competent professionals) to deal with personal, economic, and social factors that determine the parents' capacity to meet the demands of care if a child has a particular defect. They should also inform the parents about the social resources that may be available to help. On the basis of this objective information and counseling support, the individual or couple must make their own decision about whether their need for children justifies taking the risks involved. Such decisions must be made not merely by some persons but by all prospective parents, because begetting new life is essentially a risky business. The reason that genetic counselors are needed today is that now more information is available about the risks involved in reproduction and more help is needed in dealing with the complexities this information discloses.

4.4 ORGAN TRANSPLANTATION

Two types of organ transplants are possible, one involving an organ or tissue taken from a dead person and given to a living person, and the other involving an organ taken from one living person and given to another living person. Transplanting an organ or tissue from a dead person to a living person in itself presents no ethical problem. With few exceptions, religious groups as well as humanistic ethicists have recognized the worth and ethical validity of such transplants (John Paul II 1995, 2000; Veatch 2000). Pope Pius XII (1956) summed up Catholic teaching on transplants involving an organ from a dead person: "A person may will to dispose of his body and to destine it to ends that are useful, morally irreproachable and even noble, among them the desire to aid the sick and suffering. One may make a decision of this nature with respect to his own body with full realization of the reverence which is due it. . . . ['I']his decision should not be condemned but positively justified" (646). If some serious question arises concerning transplant from a dead person to a living person, it stems from factors other than the transplant itself. For example, concern was expressed at first about the worth of heart transplants, most of it arising from the great expense of money and personnel involved in the procedure and from the fact that it brings little substantive value to human society in general (Ramsey 1970; Thorup et al. 1985). These concerns have been obviated, however, due mainly to a better survival rate from heart transplants. There also has been an ongoing related concern on the part of some that patients who are declared brain-dead have not truly died (Byrne 2005). One group even maintained that organ transplants are contrary to Catholic teaching because brain death criteria were not valid and thus transplants often cause death to sustain life (Bruskewitz et al. 2001), in spite of a papal statement to the contrary (John Paul II 2000); this group's opinion was rejected explicitly by a Vatican official (Steinman 2002). Recently, a method of excising organs from donors whose heart has stopped beating, but upon whom no efforts at resuscitation have been made, has also caused some concern (Rigali 2003). This method of obtaining organs, called non-heart-beating organ donation (NHBD), however, is compatible with the Uniform Declaration of Death Act and the ethical norms that correspond to Catholic teaching (DuBois 1999a, 1999b, 2001, 2002; Panicola 2003; Institute of Medicine 2000). John Paul II summed up Catholic teaching in regard to the signs of death when he stated (2000, 12), "It can be said that the criterion adopted in more recent times for ascertaining the fact of death, namely the *complete and irreversible* cessation of all brain activity, if rigorously applied, does not seem to conflict with the essential elements of a sound anthropology. Therefore health care workers professionally responsible for ascertaining death can use these criteria in each individual case as the basis for arriving at that degree of assurance in ethical judgment which moral teaching describes as 'moral certainty.'"

Transplants from Living Donors

Far more difficulties arise, however, with organ transplants between living persons. Prior to 1950 the morality of transplanting an organ from one living person to another living person was discussed by Catholic theologians from a theoretical point of view (Cunningham 1944). Although an interesting question, it was somewhat impractical because transplants between living persons were generally not yet technically feasible. Many theologians who considered the subject did not approve of it. These theologians argued that the principle of totality and integrity would justify mutilation or injury to one part of the body only if it was done to preserve the person's own health or human life. The principle would not justify a transplant to another person, however, because one person is not related to another person as means to end or as part to whole. Thus one person's bodily integrity could not be sacrificed for another.

Whatever the theoretical discussions, organ transplants from living donors began to be performed in the early 1950s. Because of genetic similarity, identical twins were the first subjects of kidney transplants. Many early transplants were not successful because the transplanted organ often was rejected by the reaction of the recipient's immune system (Murray 1986). Yet as some succeeded, scientists began to argue that unless there was freedom to undertake such experiments, medical progress would be hampered (Fox and Swazy 1978). Thus ethicists and moralists gave the problem closer scrutiny. Gerald Kelly, a leader in this development wrote, "It may come as a surprise to physicians that theologians should have any difficulty about mutilations and other procedures which are performed with the consent of the subject but which have as their purpose the helping of others. By a sort of instinctive judgment we consider that the giving of a part of one's body to help a sick man is not only morally justifiable, but, in some instances, actually heroic" (1956, 246). In developing the rationale for a more liberal opinion, Kelly maintained, "It is clear from reason and papal teaching that the Principle of Totality cannot be used to justify the donating of a part of one's body to another person. Moreover, since man is only the administrator of his life and bodily members and functions, his power to dispose of these things is limited."

Kelly, however, sought to delineate as clearly as possible the limits of this dominion, especially concerning organ transplants. Further, he asked, is there any other way in which this seemingly worthwhile and Christian action can be justified? He suggested that the principle of fraternal love or charity would justify the transplant provided that there is only limited harm to the donor. Although Kelly's opinion was not unanimously accepted, some theologians agreed with it and developed it more clearly. Distinguishing between anatomical integrity and functional integrity, they stated that the latter, not the former, was necessary to ensure human or bodily integrity (McFadden 1976).

Anatomical integrity refers to the material or physical integrity of the human body. *Functional integrity* refers to the systematic efficiency of the human body. For example, if one kidney were missing from a person's body, there would be a lack of anatomical integrity, but if one healthy kidney were present and working, there would be functional integrity because one healthy kidney is more than able to provide systemic efficiency. If a cornea were to be taken from the eye of one living person and given to another, however, the case would be different. Not only would anatomical integrity be destroyed, but functional integrity would be destroyed as well. The loss of sight in one eye severely damages vision, especially depth perception. Thus in this case, more than anatomical integrity is involved. For the most part, the transplant of a cornea from living persons is no longer a problem because transplanting a cornea from a dead person has been perfected.

This distinction between anatomical and functional integrity explains why blood transfusions and skin grafts are acceptable and why theologians approve elective appendectomy if the abdominal cavity is open for another legitimate reason. In these situations loss of anatomical integrity may occur through loss of blood, skin tissue, or an internal organ, but no loss of functional integrity occurs.

Thus the concept of functional integrity is the key factor in addressing the morality of transplants between living persons. Certainly a risk is involved if a donor surrenders an organ to another person, even if the donor has two of them. Aside from the risk involved in the surgical procedure, such donors take the risk of serious illness themselves if the one remaining organ becomes damaged or diseased. The risk, however, although serious, is deemed to be justified by the fact that donors share in the common good of the community to which they contribute by helping another, that is, by love.

Clearly, organ donation is not an obligation; rather, it is something chosen in the freedom of charity. Motivated by the same charity, one could decide not to offer an organ. Such a decision would not be unethical. For this reason, it is imperative that informed consent of both the donor and the recipient, or their proxies, be obtained (John Paul II 2000, 3). Given the fact that the more successful transplants are between members of the same family, familial or social pressure to offer oneself as a donor may at times be severe (Siminoff and Leonard 1999), but the courts (rightly, we believe) refuse to compel such donations. Because of the charitable motivation that justifies transplantation of an organ by a living person, it follows that selling organs is unethical. The federal government has prohibited the sale of all organs in the United States, but sale of organs by living donors in some countries is a common practice (Rothman 1998). As a result, efforts are being made to justify compensation for organ donation in the United States (Taylor 2002; Brock 2001). Kelly was certainly right in holding that organ transplants between two living persons are licit if the donor's functional integrity is maintained. Yet organ donation is not a problem-free procedure, especially on the part of the recipient for whom physiological and psychological problems might develop (Sharp 1995). The federal advisory committee on organ transplantation estimates complication rates between 15 and 30 percent, and the death rate at two in one thousand donors. Yet a review in the *American Journal of Transplantation* reports complications as high as 67 percent, and an article in a clinical journal by a surgeon at the University of Minnesota estimated the death rate as high as one in one hundred (Shelton 2005). Hence consent should not be given unless the prognosis for both the donor and the recipient is good. In some cases it is necessary to weigh the value of a brief prolongation of life for the recipient against the lifelong risk to the donor.

The development in the last forty years of the moral teaching of theologians concerning organ transplants between living donors and recipients is of more than antiquarian interest. First, it shows clearly that the opinion of theologians can evolve. Second, it shows that by refining accepted principles, and not denying them, new conclusions can be drawn from long-established principles. Third, it demonstrates that starting with intuitive judgments helps solve many ethical problems, but then an examination of whether this intuitive judgment is consistent with sound moral principles is still necessary. In summary, the transplanting of organs or tissues from a dead person to a living person does not offer any intrinsic ethical problem. Transplanting organs from one living person to another is also ethically acceptable provided that the following criteria are met:

1. There is a serious need on the part of the recipient that cannot be fulfilled in any other way.
2. The functional integrity of the donor as a human person will not be impaired, even though anatomical integrity may suffer.
3. The risk taken by the donor as an act of charity is proportionate to the good resulting for the recipient.
4. The donor's and the recipient's consents are free and informed.

Problems Due to Success

The success of organ transplantation, largely due to the use of cyclosporin and other drugs that suppress the activity of the recipient's immune system, has produced the following new problems (Bicknell et al. 2000): First, how can organs be fairly allotted? Because so many different organs and tissues are now subject to transplantation—not only heart and kidneys, but lungs, liver, pancreas, spleen, skin, and bone marrow as well—there is a continual shortage of suitable organs and tissue for transplant. In 2005 the number of people awaiting donation of suitable organs was more than eighty thousand (OPTN 2005).

At present, the system of obtaining organs and allotting them is not well defined (Gubermatis and Kliemet 2000). Regional transplant centers, funded in part by the federal government, publicize the need for organ donations, maintain waiting lists of those who need transplants and of possible donors, and assist physicians in allotting the available organs. Recent legislation has set guidelines for national sharing of available organs based on genetic matching between donor and recipients. In general, the organs are allotted to those in most grave need who at the same time have some chance of survival if the transplant is successful. Thus medical criteria are the main basis for allotment, but there is room for subjective judgment. Because all potential recipients are registered, a "first come, first served" allotment is followed in theory.

Should available organs in the United States be allotted only to U.S. citizens, or should aliens be allowed to benefit from the transplantation program? In 1986, the Department of Health and Human Services recommended that a quota system be established that would put foreign nationals on a quota list, but to date, this has not been done. Thus foreign nationals who can pay for the surgical procedure are often a source of profit for transplant centers (Cherry 2000).

A second ethical question emerging from the success of the organ transplant program concerns the financing of organ transplants. At present, either Medicare or Medicaid finances most kidney transplants. But in most cases, the medical and postoperative costs are well above the means of the average family. Some private health insurance plans fund heart transplants, but the tendency is to limit this type of benefit. Often families seek to raise funds for the required surgery and recovery costs through public appeals. Moreover, many states limit Medicaid expenditures to "basic" health care benefits and will not fund such procedures as liver or bone marrow transplants. In response to the growing desire for organ transplants and the need for donations to increase, there seems to be a need for a comprehensive policy in regard to the funding of organ transplants (Davis 1999). Of course, such a policy should be part of a renewed health policy for all aspects of health care in the United States. As we will see in chapter 7, the method of providing health care in the United States is highly discriminatory and needs a thorough revision and renewal. Clearly, although the percentage of the gross domestic product (GDP) in the United States devoted to health care in the last thirty years has increased dramatically, so has the complexity and sophistication of medicine and health care.

Increasing the Supply of Organs for Transplantation

A third question arising from the success of transplant surgery concerns increasing the supply of organs suitable for transplant. As organ transplantation has become more successful, the issue of organ supply has become more of a national priority. How can organs be procured without violating the rights of families and dying patients (Kaserman and Barnett 2002)? In addition to increased public appeals made by voluntary groups, the Joint Commission for the Accreditation of Health Care Organizations has requested each hospital to frame a policy that stipulates the procedure for requesting organ donations from the family of a dying or deceased person. At present, the Anatomical Gift Act has been approved in each state (Sadler, Sadler, and Stason 1968). This allows persons to sign their driver's licenses and indicate their desire to donate organs after death. However, the custom in most states requires the family of the deceased person to confirm such a donation. If the family were to disagree with the statement the patient made before death, it is unlikely that physicians or hospital administrators would approve surgery to remove organs for fear of ensuing malpractice litigation.

Basing argumentation on the common good and the fact that transplantation after death would not harm a patient in any way, a proposal to presume permission to transplant an organ should be agreed upon (Boyle and O'Rourke 1986). Those who have religious or other motivation for refusing donations of organs could express their refusal before death, in the same way that people are requested to express permission for retrieval of their organs after death. If no objections are verified, the organs could be removed for transplant, even if no positive statement granting this permission was made beforehand by the deceased person. Although changing the presumption in regard to organ donation by the deceased may seem rather radical, it corresponds to the practice in some countries. Some, however, question whether this method of procurement allows for informed consent.

Using organs from animals (xenotransplantation) has been attempted, but to date not with much success (Cooper and Lanza 2000), and overall it seems to be in accord with ethical norms as long as the animals from which the organs are removed are treated ethically (Pontifical Academy of Life 2001; Sgreccia, Calipari, and Lavitrano 2001).

Another effort to increase the supply of organs has been made by some who challenge the present criteria for brain death. Must the person's total brain be dead before organs are removed (Veatch 2003)? In the case of anencephalic infants, for example, the higher brain (cortex) will never develop, yet their brainstem is still functioning, although they will soon die. Nevertheless, determining that a person is incapable of higher cortical functions is quite different from certifying that a person is dead. The physical evidence clearly shows that the development of the cerebral cortex does not constitute a "marker event" between prehuman and human development; thus because brain death is the standard criterion of death, absence of the higher brainstem does not constitute death (Furton 2002).

The President's Commission for the Study of Ethical Problems in Medicine and Biomedical and Behavioral Research (PCEMR) stated this as one of the principles of organ retrieval in the first stages of bioethical investigation for the study of ethical problems in medicine and biomedical and behavioral research (1981): "First . . . it is not known which portions of the brain are responsible for cognition and consciousness; what little is known points to substantial interconnections among brainstem, subcortical structures, and the neocortex. Thus, the 'higher brain' may well exist only as a metaphorical concept, not in reality. Second, even when the sites or certain aspects of consciousness can be found, their cessation often cannot be assessed with the certainty that would be required in applying a statutory definition" (40).

Therefore, although the anencephalic infant may not develop in a manner that fulfills the full potential usually associated with "person," there is no scientific justification to consider anencephalic infants as dead (Sytsma 1996). Rather, they should be considered living human beings until total brain death occurs. True, an anencephalic infant is a severely debilitated human being and a human being who will not live for long. But it is not dead and may not be used as a transplant donor nor may any other person, however debilitated, before death of the total brain has been proven.

4.5 RECONSTRUCTIVE AND COSMETIC SURGERY

Without resorting to transplants, modern surgery is capable of remarkable feats of repairing bodily defects and injuries (Mathis 1997). Sometimes accidentally severed fingers or hands have been successfully reconnected to the body and restored at least to partial function. Self-transplants such as skin-plants and the transfer of blood vessels from the limbs to be used in a bypass in heart surgery have become common. Recently there have been advances in restoring severed nerves. Such reconstructive surgery raises no special ethical questions, other than general ones such as free and informed consent and cost/benefit issues, as long as the purpose is clearly one of restoring or improving normal function. Questions may be raised, however, in at least two types of cases.

What if the purpose of the surgery is not normal function but the destruction or inhibition of certain normal functions (Hardin 1997)? We have already discussed contraceptive sterilization whose purpose is the destruction of normal human fertility. Other types of deterrent mutilation of criminals, such as blinding criminals, cutting off their hands, or excising their tongues, have been used and even now are used in some countries. Such procedures violate human dignity and are therefore unethical. What, however, about such procedures as bariatric surgery that control obesity by surgically constricting the size of the stomach? In such procedures, as in contraception, the purpose is to solve a behavioral problem by a mechanical mutilation. If the cause of obesity were a malfunction of the digestive system that could be remedied by surgery, then such an operation could be ethically justified. If, however, obesity is due to a deliberate failure to control diet, resort should be had to addiction counseling before surgery is justified, as this type of surgery is not free of problems (Grezon and de Jong 2000).

Alternatively, cosmetic surgery is not directed at restoring normal function, but at improving *appearance* (Parens 1998). While human appearance can hardly be called a "function" of the body, it is certainly very important in human life, both with regard to sexual attraction and with regard to all our social relationships and sense of personal worth. We can therefore grant that it is ethically justified if the purpose is to acquire, when lacking, what is generally regarded as a normal, attractive appearance for one's gender or even to enhance it. Certainly when the defect in question is real and serious, and especially when it is associated with some functional defect, such as cleft palate, deformation of facial features, unattractive birthmarks, and so forth, such surgery is wholly reasonable.

When, however, the purpose is simply the enhancement of sexual attractiveness or the concealment of normal aging, such as face-lifts, breast enhancement, liposuction, and so on, it is pertinent to ask whether the expense, risks, and rationale of such procedures can really be justified (Ringel 1998). Society and style often promote stereotypes of youth and beauty that are illusory and harmful. It is to be feared also that some physicians promote such expensive procedures simply for their own profit and not the real welfare of the patient. The fact that people request such procedures and are willing to pay for them is not a sufficient ethical justification for physicians to cooperate. While this is not one of the major problems of bioethics, it is symptomatic of mistaken priorities in the promotion of human health. The Christian attitude, from New Testament times, has always been that it is wrong to promote the idea that human worth is to be measured by appearances rather than by character. Certainly it is unjust for a society to devote so much of its resources to vanity when the poor lack necessities.

Sexual Reassignment

As was shown in chapter 3 (section 3.1), *The Diagnostic and Statistical Manual of the American Psychiatric Association* in 1973 removed homosexuality from its list of disorders, but it retains gender identity disorders defined as "Disorders characterized by a strong, persistent cross-gender identification and by continuous discomfort about one's anatomic (assigned) sex or by a sense of inappropriateness in the gender role of that sex" (APA 1994, 24). It states that normally, even if the child is physically gender ambiguous, a child satisfactorily adopts the male or female identity supported by its parents, and if a disorder is to arise it usually appears by two years of age and manifests itself by its preference for cross-dressing, games usually played by the other sex, and negative feelings toward the actual genitalia.

Prominent among these gender disorders is transsexualism (gender dysphoria), described in *The Diagnostic and Statistical Manual of Mental Disorders* (*DSM-IV*) as involving the following five criteria (APA 1994):

1. Sense of discomfort and inappropriateness about one's anatomical sex.
2. Wish to be rid of one's own genitals and to live as a member of the other sex.
3. The disturbance has been continuous (not limited to periods of stress) for at least two years.
4. Absence of physical intersex or genetic abnormality.
5. Not caused by another mental disorder, such as schizophrenia.

Thus transsexualism should not be confused with transvestism, a condition in which a person, usually heterosexual in orientation, is more comfortable sexually while wearing clothing symbolic of the opposite sex. This is probably a form of fetishism (Fehlow 2002).

The anxiety felt by the transsexual is so severe that some 50 percent of victims die before they reach the age of thirty, often by suicide. Its occurrence is about 1 in 30,000 male births and 1 in 100,000 female births. A diagnosis of this disorder, which usually begins in early childhood, should not be made unless the feelings are continuous for at least two years (Bockting and Coleman 1993; Hausman 1995; Ramsay 1996; Breedlove 2005; Gender Trust 2005).

Though the evidence for such neurological differences is still not conclusive, it has led some to argue that it is ethical for persons, regardless of their genetic sex, to decide on the basis of their own feelings of gender to decide to be male or female and to use hormones and surgery to achieve as much conformity to their choice as possible. Although some researchers claim a 60 to 98 percent rate of success, this depends a great deal on the criteria chosen. In a careful review, Leslie M. Lothstein (1982) argues that such figures should be taken with caution and leaves the question open to further study. From this debate we would conclude that genetic sex remains the best determinant of true gender. To hold that persons can choose their gender in order to overcome their preferences is to succumb to the current denial of human nature and its intrinsic teleology.

Because, as we have just argued, surgical and hormonal alteration of the human body to solve behavioral rather than functional problems is ethically very dubious, the issue of "sex change" as it is popularly called, or "sexual reassignment surgery" as it is technically termed, is even more questionable. Sexual reassignment is a type of reconstructive surgery by which the sexual phenotype of a male is altered to resemble that of a female, or vice versa (Cohen-Kettemis and Gooren 1999). Such surgery, along with hormonal treatments and psychotherapy, is often used to treat transsexualism when psychiatric treatment fails. Transsexual surgery involves radical mutilation: castration and construction of a pseudo-vagina for the male, mastectomy and hysterectomy (sometimes also the construction of a nonfunctional pseudo-penis and testes) for the female, along with hormonal treatments with possible serious side effects (Huang 1995). Transsexual surgery is very expensive, yet it produces only an imperfect physical gender, especially for females and furthermore renders the transsexual infertile.

Arguments in Favor

The argument of psychotherapists and surgeons who perform sexual reassignment as a remedy for this dysphoria is that the situation is very painful and victims often find no relief in psychotherapy and are often insistent on surgery even to the point of threatening suicide. Many of those who undertake sexual reassignment also seem to be satisfied with its results. At present we do not accept these arguments. First, it has not yet been established that the cause of gender dysphoria syndrome is biological, although some have suggested this theory (Monteleone 1981; Van Spengen 1995). No such cause is evident at the genotypic or phenotypic level, and as yet the evidence is tenuous that the reason transsexuals believe from early in their lives that they have "a soul different from their bodies" is caused by some developmental accident in the central nervous or hormonal systems. At present, it remains more probable that the determining causes are at the psychological level of development, although there may be some biological predisposition (Sugar 1995; Oldham 1999). Consequently, the gender ambiguity in question is primarily psychological and should be treated psychotherapeutically.

One study of the problem (Lothstein 1982) shows that the condition is much more common in males than females and that, of those males applying for sexual reassignment surgery, only about 10 to 25 percent can be diagnosed as having *primary* gender dysphoria, that is, of the type that "has an obvious, lifelong, profound disturbance of core gender identity." A pioneer in the field, J. K. Meyer, went so far as to state, "I have seen any number of men who would like to live as females and vice versa; I have not seen one with a reversal of core gender identity" (1974, 280). Other candidates for surgery can only be diagnosed as suffering from *secondary* gender dysphoria, which is stress related and results from "failures of other gender identity adaptations, such as transvestism, effeminate homosexuality, and gender ambiguity." Thus the arguments for biological rather than a psychological etiology of this syndrome will hold (if at all) only for a very restricted group of patients.

Second, contrary to what is often stated, when candidates for surgery are required to undergo psychotherapy in preparation for surgery, many are found to be ambiguous about really wanting it and in the end decide against it. Moreover, most transsexuals who have been carefully diagnosed appear to be suffering from serious psychological problems, sometimes subtle and not immediately recognized, other than their gender dysphoria (Bodlung et al. 1993). Even after surgery they continue to need at least some psychotherapeutic support, although their frequent difficulty in forming stable personal relationships makes this follow-up difficult.

Third, although when this type of surgery was first introduced there were enthusiastic reports of its success, as experience accumulates there is less agreement that it does much good. The latest survey of studies evaluating the outcome of transsexual surgery concludes that previous studies have indicated more people being satisfied with the overall results of the surgery than dissatisfied (Lawrence 2003). The success rate for sexual transformation claimed by its most optimistic proponents is high, but the success they claim is an amelioration of the victims' dysphoria rather than a return to normalcy. Moreover, the paucity of control groups for this type of survey makes attribution of either improvement or deterioration to the surgical intervention scientifically questionable. Johns Hopkins University, noted for its leadership in early research in this field, announced the suspension of its program for further reassessment as a result of a report by J. K. Meyer (1974) that concluded this type of surgery offers no advantage over psychotherapy (McHugh 1992). Another study in regard to Medicaid funding of sex-reassignment surgery affirms this conclusion (Jacobs 1980).

Fourth, from a theological point of view, it is clear that surgery does not really solve these persons' life problems because it does not enable them to achieve sexual normality or to enter into a valid Christian marriage and have children. Because many of these individuals are somewhat asexual (Snaith 1994) their problem is not primarily sexual satisfaction but the relief of the burden of anxiety, which can usually be at least considerably lightened by psychotherapy. We would invoke the consideration that the good of the person cannot be achieved at the expense of the destruction of a basic human function, in this case the sterilization of the person, except to save the person's life. Furthermore, the studies reported by no means give assurance that sexual reassignment solves the more general problems of personality from which most of these victims suffer.

We conclude that, based on the present state of knowledge, Catholic hospitals or health care professionals are not justified in recommending or engaging in this type of surgery (Guevin 2005). Certainly compassion should be extended to this small but greatly suffering group of human beings, but it should take the practical form of psychotherapy and pastoral guidance. It is unfortunate that the widespread publicity given to sex-change surgery and the exaggerated reports of its success have created an increasing demand among troubled people, most of whom would not be accepted for such surgery by any reputable clinic.

Pastoral Considerations

How should such cases be dealt with pastorally? The fundamental aim of the therapist, as well as of the pastoral counselor, in these cases should be to restore the patient's sense of personal self-worth. He or she must be helped to see, as should homosexuals and those having other sexual problems, that today's culture is grievously mistaken in its exaggerated stress on sexual identity and activity as a primary determinant of human worth. They must be assisted to find interests—spiritual, intellectual, and social—that will enable them to escape their preoccupation with their sexual identity and discover their more fundamental value as human persons. As for persons who have already undergone surgery, we believe they should be counseled not to attempt marriage and should be supported in their efforts to live chastely with the assistance of the sacraments and the respect and fellowship of the Christian community.

A very different problem is that of the child born with ambiguous genitalia, a condition once called hermaphroditism (from the Greek god Hermes and the goddess Aphrodite), but now termed *intersexuality*. According to one estimate, one in every one hundred children has a body whose gender is somewhat defective, and one or two in one thousand have surgery to normalize their appearance (Blackless et al. 2000). Up to six weeks of gestation human embryos have the primordial elements of both sexes and on the whole appear feminine, but from the seventh week embryos that are genetically male develop testes and begin to produce testosterone, and the mullerian ducts, which in genetic females develop into the fallopian tubes and uterus, are suppressed by another testicular hormone.

When a newborn appears sexually ambiguous, its parents have the problem of choosing in what gender to raise it and have generally been advised by physicians in the past to raise the child in the gender in which it is most likely to be able to function best (Sultan et al. 2002a). Very often this resulted in the child being raised as a girl. Catholic moralists have agreed with this solution in general. Although in the previous discussion we have opposed "sexual transformation" of adults, there seems to be no objection to the use of surgery or hormones to improve the normal appearance or function of sexually ambiguous children before puberty in accordance with the sex in which they are to be or have been raised. The reasoning behind this traditional position is that a person must "live according to nature" insofar as this is humanly knowable.

Recently, however, this practice is meeting serious opposition because evidence is accumulating that when such persons attain puberty they often bitterly resent that the decision to raise them in the sex other than their genetic sex has been made without their free and informed consent (Reiner 1996; Reiner and Geaarhart 2004). Thus parents faced with this situation should not give proxy consent until they have given the risk thorough and informed consideration. The victims themselves need counseling that will enable them to accept their actual condition or, if they prudently decide that their parents made a mistake, assume the gender that is most appropriate and practical. If surgical or medical treatment, cosmetics, or clothing that enables them to assume the chosen gender role is feasible, it is ethically justified, but they must remain celibate if their condition makes valid and successful heterosexual marriage impractical.

4.6 EXPERIMENTATION AND RESEARCH ON HUMAN SUBJECTS

When science takes man as its subject, tensions arise between two values basic to Western Society: freedom of scientific inquiry and protection of individual inviolability.

These words introduce a major study by Katz, Capron, and Swift-Glass (1972, 1) on the legal and ethical issues involved in research on human subjects, which may be defined as seeking generalizable knowledge concerning human function or behavior through empirical studies (Belmont Report 1978). Katz's report states: "Human experimentation in the practice of medicine is as old as the practice of medicine itself, but only during the last hundred years, since the age of Pasteur, has medicine become aware of the need for deliberate and well-planned experimentation" (1).

Human experimentation not only affects the rights of human persons now and in the future, but may also condition and change the very core of human nature itself (Shapiro et al. 1986). As the realization of this problem has grown, the U.S. federal government has established the National Institutes of Health (http://ohsr.od.nih.gov/), which has a special office that has developed an ethical code on the Protection of Human Subjects (OHSR 2002).

That this growing research on human beings is often useful and often necessary for the common good is undeniable. Many beneficial vaccines and other therapies, such as smallpox and poliomyelitis vaccines, open-heart surgery, and successful treatment of certain birth defects, could not have been developed without research with human subjects, and the whole world attests to their value. At the same time, research on humans undoubtedly has also been abused (Weyers 2003). The world should never forget the horrors of the human research experimentation carried out on innocent human beings in the name of scientific progress in Nazi concentration camps (Lifton 1986). Aside from such atrocities, other egregious violations of human rights have occurred in the United States, such as the withholding of newly discovered penicillin from patients in the Tuskegee syphilis study (Jones 1982; Gamble 1997); the Willowbrook experiments, in which retarded children were used as experimental subjects; and the injection of live cancer cells in unknowing subjects in the Jewish Chronic Disease Hospital case (McCuen 1998). Psychological experimentation has also given rise to serious debate about behavior control (Eaton 2002).

Such abuses are not the product of demented or perverted minds; rather, they result from lack of care and ethical sensitivity on the part of well-motivated researchers who overlook the rights of human beings in an effort to ensure scientific progress or academic advancement. The public media today often contradicts itself by waxing indignant over unethical use of human subjects, while at the same time promoting research that kills human embryos to obtain their stem cells. For many years, in an effort to obviate excesses and facilitate progress in research, the federal government required that every institution that carries on research projects with public funds establish an institutional review board (IRB). The federal government will not fund research projects unless they have been first approved by an IRB (Institute of Medicine 2003).

Research and Therapy

Several categories of human subjects may be involved in research programs: (1) normal healthy adults, including the investigator, and elderly persons; (2) adults suffering from some malady, including the acutely and terminally ill; (3) prisoners, soldiers, members of religious communities, and any group living in a highly controlled community; (4) children, both healthy and ill; (5) mentally incompetent adults and children; (6) unborn children or still-living aborted fetuses; and (7) the aging. Each of these categories presents special problems. Efforts are made by the federal government to limit the risk to these various populations involved in research protocols (NBAC 2001).

Research on human subjects should be sharply distinguished from therapy, because the primary purpose of research is not to heal but to learn. Hence it has become customary to classify research as either therapeutic or nontherapeutic. *Therapeutic research* studies the effects of using diagnostic, prophylactic, or therapeutic methods that depart from standard medical practice but hold out a reasonable expectation of success. Such research may actually give greater benefit to the human subject than standard treatment. Thus what begins as human research may later become standard medical practice or therapy. *Nontherapeutic research*, conversely, is not designed to improve the health of the research subject; rather, it seeks to gain knowledge or develop techniques that in the future may benefit people other than the subject. This type of research is often called experimentation, but there is no hard and fast separation of the terms.

The proper manner of conducting these types of research on the various categories of human subjects has become one of the most discussed bioethical questions of recent years (Emanuel et al. 2003). Through seminars, studies, and the work of the various federal commissions, some ethical principles have been developed to serve as a guide for researchers and for those who support research. As a result of such studies by legal, medical, and ethical groups throughout the world, especially in the generation after World War II, these principles have become widely accepted. Interestingly, the norms produced by medical and legal experts of the World Health Organization (WHO), such as the Nuremberg Code (1946) and Helsinki statements (1964), are largely in harmony with the teaching of the Catholic Church on human dignity. More recent statements of research groups, such as the Warnock Committee in Great Britain and various statements of study groups in the United States, however, are not in accord with Church teaching because they follow a proportionalist method of reasoning, that is, while they may state general statements that predicate respect for human subjects, they also will often allow exceptions to these norms in order to gain knowledge that is otherwise difficult to obtain.

Principles of Research on Human Subjects

The basic norms for research on human subjects that are formulated and discussed here derive chiefly from three ethical principles: the principle of totality and integrity, which is especially relevant to therapeutic experimentation; the principle of human dignity, which relates to the limits of nontherapeutic experimentation; and the principle of free and informed consent, which relates to the capacity of the various categories of human subjects to participate freely in research programs.

1. The knowledge sought through research must be important and obtainable by no other means, and qualified people must carry out the research.

2. If possible, appropriate experimentation on animals and cadavers must precede human experimentation.

3. The risk of suffering or injury must be proportionate to the good to be gained.

4. Subjects should be selected so that risks and benefits will not fall unequally on one group in society.

5. To protect the integrity of the human person, free and informed (voluntary) consent must be obtained.

6. At any time during the course of research, the subject (or the guardian who has given proxy consent) must be free to terminate the subject's participation in the experiment.

In the following pages we investigate briefly the meaning of these norms. The first three of these norms are necessary if human subjects are to be used at all. Because the principle of double effect is used to justify the possible ill effects of human experimentation, the relation between risk and potential benefit is most important. Of course, predicting the degree of risk with certitude is seldom possible. Moreover, sometimes, as in the case of poliomyelitis inoculation in 1954, when the use of some poorly prepared live vaccine resulted in the death of children, some risks are far greater than predicted. Thus absolute certainty in regard to the nature and degree of the risk cannot be required. To demand such certitude would paralyze all scientific research and would very often be detrimental to the patient. Care must be taken, however, to predict as accurately as possible the nature and magnitude of risk from any particular human experiment, and the bias of enthusiastic researchers in favor of the promise of some new procedure must be subject to review by an institutional review board (Prentice and Gordon 2001).

When determining the degree of risk that a person might undergo, one must also keep in mind the difference between therapeutic and nontherapeutic research. If research is therapeutic, persons may ethically choose to undergo greater risk, and possibly even death, from the illness or malady that the researcher is aimed to cure. In nontherapeutic research, because one person is not related to another person or to society simply as part of the whole, the same degree of risk is not justified. Each individual person is an end to herself or himself and cannot be sacrificed for another. This is the basic reason why the public authority has no right to sacrifice individuals for "the interest of the state or for scientific progress" (John Paul II 1986). Although it is sometimes fitting that researchers themselves participate in experiments, they are bound by the same restrictions as other subjects. Pope Pius XII (1952) expressed this view accurately: "He [the doctor or researcher] is subject to the same broad moral and juridical principles as govern other men. He has no right, consequently, to permit scientific or practical experiments which entail serious injury or which threaten to impair his health to be performed on his person, and even to a lesser extent is he authorized to attempt an operation of experimental nature which, according to authoritative opinion, could conceivably result in mutilation or even suicide."

Experimental Controls

Special ethical issues arise in double-blind or randomized research or when placebos are used in clinical studies (DeMets 1999). The objectivity of scientific research depends largely on the use of controlled experimentation in which a group of subjects is divided into two subgroups, one of which receives the experimental therapy while the other, the control group, receives the standard therapy or a placebo. Sometimes three groups are used, one group receiving the experimental therapy, one receiving a placebo, and one receiving standard therapy or no treatment at all. To ensure even greater objectivity, *double-blind control* may be used: not only are subjects not informed as to which form of treatment they are receiving, but even those researchers who evaluate the effects of the treatments do not know which subjects have received which therapy. Only the double-blind technique can eliminate the *placebo effect*, that is, the improvement frequently experienced by patients who expect it and the effect of bias on the part of scientists.

Double-blind studies raise questions of justice, however, because it may be that those subjects who do not receive the new therapy are at a therapeutic disadvantage and that they may not have given free and informed consent to receive only placebo treatment. Thus in double-blind experiments the subjects should be informed that, if they consent to the experiment, some will receive the new treatment and others will not, but that none of the subjects will know (Moreno 1999). The potential subjects will then be free to consent to these experimental conditions or to refuse to participate.

If the clinical trial involves a placebo for the control group and the project aims at finding an agent that will mitigate or cure a lethal or disabling disease, a special ethical issue arises, because the control group may not be receiving adequate therapy for their illness or disease. This is especially true if there is some justification for thinking that the new therapy might be much more effective than previous ones. Thus the same protocol may be therapeutic for some and nontherapeutic for others. Researchers and review boards therefore must be particularly cautious when a double-blind placebo protocol is being designed or reviewed. If the new therapy proves to be effective, the protocol must be modified and the new therapy made available to all (Quitkin 1999). Of course, a rush to judgment concerning the efficacy of a new therapy must be avoided.

Impartiality and Consent in Selecting Subjects.   The fourth and fifth of the previously listed norms require that experimental subjects not be selected if they are subject to social or other pressures that limit their freedom of consent, as justice demands that the burdens associated with human progress be shared equitably. In recent years, the poor of the world, especially in the United States, have borne an unequal burden in relation to medical research. The causes of this situation are psychological as well as economic (Macklin 2003). Research protocols must be designed to offset this imbalance and ensure that when the poor take part in an experiment, their human rights are respected, and they are given the freedom that their human dignity demands (Resnik 2003). While it may often be easier to obtain subjects from the poor than from other groups, for this very reason special care must be taken to protect their rights. The same consideration holds for those categories of subjects who are chosen because they live in restricted and controlled circumstances where the researcher has easy access to them, such as prisoners, soldiers, or those confined to rest homes or mental institutions.

The fifth norm requiring truly free and informed consent by the experimental human subject is perhaps the most important and the most debated of all the principles involved in human research. More bioethics articles seem to be devoted to this topic than to any other. One of the first pivotal statements on informed consent, the Belmont Report (1978), declared that the essential elements of informed consent on the part of the patient are knowledge, understanding, and freedom. Despite extensive descriptions of informed consent published in ethical literature, serious discussions and disputes still arise concerning the concept and its application. Many question, for example, whether prisoners can ever give *free* consent because of their confinement. Others question whether double-blind procedures, an integral part of some experiments, can ever be employed. We believe, however, that both experimentation on prisoners and double-blind procedures can be performed if sufficient care is taken in obtaining their free and informed consent.

Proxy or Vicarious Consent.   A most difficult problem occurs in situations in which one person gives consent for another for whom the first is morally responsible. The need for such consent occurs when unconscious people are dying, as well as in research involving infants, children, or mentally impaired persons. Such substitute consent is usually called *proxy consent*, perhaps an unfortunate term, because in legal terminology a proxy is an agent acting on behalf of another with the consent of the other person. Perhaps a better term for those occasions when one must speak for another without being explicitly designated by the second person would be *vicarious consent*.

Vicarious consent should be distinguished also from *implicit* consent and *presumed* consent. Persons consent implicitly when they explicitly consent to some general line of action, which implies more detailed permissions, as when a patient consents to surgery without specifying what anesthetic is to be used. Consent is presumed when it is highly probable that someone who is not able to give consent because he or she is unconscious would have given it if present or conscious. Thus in emergency situations consent of injured patients to undergo surgery is often presumed.

Decisions of vicarious or proxy consent must be made in view of the good of the individual person, not for a higher good, for a class good, or for the good of another person, which would amount to manipulation of the person as a mere means. Thus, if the experiment were therapeutic, there would be reason for the proxy to allow risk in proportion to the person's best interest.

If nontherapeutic experimentation is involved, however, the decision is more difficult. Must the one giving vicarious consent avoid all risk to the subject of research? Would it be reasonable to suppose that children would want to contribute to the common good by exposing themselves to risk (Harris and Holm 2003)? We follow a protective opinion in regard to vicarious consent, maintaining that it is not licit to expose a ward to other than minimal risk in nontherapeutic research. Guardians have responsibility for wards that cannot care for themselves. The theories of presumed consent based on what the ward *ought* to do if the ward *could* consent are weak. If the risk is minimal, it may be allowed, because in moral theology there is a time-tested principle, "little counts for nothing" (*de minimis non est disputandum*).

Termination of Experimentation.   The reason for this sixth norm, which requires that human subjects be permitted to withdraw from the experiment at any time, in spite of their initial consent, is that the consenting subject or proxy may not have been able to anticipate correctly the subjective factors, amount of suffering, or the anxiety or depression involved until these begin to be actually experienced. Also, the subject or proxy may even discover the information given was inadequate or deceptive or imperfectly communicated, or the subject or proxy may have second thoughts about his or her own understanding or freedom when the consent was given. The subject or guardian cannot consent to give away the primary responsibility for defending the subject's own health and integrity, because this is an inherent right and obligation. Consequently, if during the course of the experimentation the subject or proxy begins to see that serious risks to the subject's well-being may be involved, the subject or proxy is ethically obliged to stop participation.

Psychological Experimentation

Special problems are involved in psychological research (Macklin 1983; Szasz 1982). To discuss these problems more fully, we defer the topic until chapter 5, where the nature of psychotherapy and its distinctions from medical therapy are more thoroughly explained. At this point, however, we can state that in such research all the precautions necessary in medical experiments must be preserved, especially informed consent, careful calculation of risks and benefits, and precautions against the bias of researchers in favor of their own freedom. We must also add the following three special rules in addition to the six rules already given:

7. In psychological research, which shades imperceptibly into social research, the researcher should work *with* rather than *on* the human subject (Morrison, Layton, and Newman 1982; Sider 1983).

That is, the researcher must gain the cooperation of the subject in the experiment so that subjects will participate with the purpose of gaining greater insight into themselves as persons in order to become freer and more realistic in coping with life's problems and also with the purpose of sharing this knowledge and freedom with others.

This principle is based on the fact that psychological experiments with a human subject are also psychological *experiences* for the subject that can be healthy and psychologically therapeutic or traumatizing reinforcement of bad behavior patterns. In very few cases can such experiences be merely neutral. Even the experience of filling out a questionnaire can be educational or terrifying. Any experience in which the patient is treated as a passive object rather than as a person cannot be a beneficial experience. It is questionable whether such treatment can even be experimentally useful, because in such a situation the human person is no longer acting humanly, but subhumanly. Thus persons should not permit themselves to be treated in this way because those who seek to reduce them to objects are violating their human rights. Psychological experimentation must involve the human, active cooperation of the subject and produce some learning and growth benefits.

8. The researcher must avoid breaking down human trust by lying or manipulation, although subjects can give free and informed consent to experiments in which they have to learn to interpret ambiguous communications or meet puzzling situations.

In many psychological experiments, the experimentalist does not seem to have any qualms about lying to subjects. Not only is lying (in our opinion) intrinsically wrong and contrary to professional ethics (see chapter 5, section 5.2), it is also psychologically harmful to the subject because it breaks down the social trust on which human relations are built. Commonsense proof of this is that those who have been subjected to such manipulation often react indignantly when they discover the deception and believe they have been treated unfairly (Sieber 2001). This is especially true when dealing with mentally disturbed patients, because elements of distrust, withdrawal, and paranoia present in most forms of emotional disturbance can only be reinforced by deception from professionals who claim to be especially trustworthy and authoritative (Thompson 2002).

This rule against lying, however, does not prohibit experiments in which previous warning is given that the experiment may involve games or tests with ambiguous clues and the subject's possible embarrassment and defeat. These are risks of the experiment to which the subject must have a chance to give free and informed consent or refusal. Deception in such a case is not what moral theologians define as a "lie," because traditional moral theology has always insisted that it is permissible to use ambiguous clues or language in situations where others are forewarned either explicitly or by the very nature of the situation.

Such games do not usually break down trust if the experimenter sticks to the rules. Moreover, they may be highly educational for the participant, because through them the subject gains insight as to how important it is to base one's interpretation of reality on solid evidence rather than on ambiguous evidence or subjective feelings.

9. Researchers must not take serious risks of reducing the subjects' ability to perceive reality as it is or to make free choices except as a temporary experience through which the subjects can learn to cope with distortions of truth and attacks on their freedom.

This rule states more exactly the special risks involved in psychological experimentation. It excludes permission for any more than temporary damage to patients' ability to remain or become free in managing their own lives. Thus an experiment would be forbidden if it might cause organic brain damage or induce drug addiction. This also applies to experiments that might make the subject unduly liable to hypnotic control or to compulsive patterns of behavior or that might create recurrent hallucinations. A special case of psychological research that may involve risks to freedom is research in dealing with human sexuality. This issue is discussed in chapter 5 in connection with therapy for inadequate or perverted sexual behavior.

These nine norms for ethical research are founded in the Christian concept of respect for persons and in the concept of responsibility that individuals have toward human community. On the part of researchers they require that the researchers' laudable desire to advance the cause of science and of the medical art should not tempt them to forget the interests here and now of the unique and irreplaceable human person they are studying.

Research upon Human Embryos

Before discussing this topic it is necessary to explain what is meant by a "stem cell." In the adult human body there are many types of cells, all of which have originated from the original one-celled human zygote by cell-division and differentiation as different portions of the genome are turned off. As was explained in chapter 3 (section 3.2), the cells of a human embryo in the first few divisions are *totipotential,* that is, they retain the genome in its full power, and this is why twinning can take place. As development continues, however, various powers of the genome are turned off, and the cells become different in each of the organs or fluids. When such embryonic stem cells are no longer totipotential, they at first remain *pluripotential,* as in the umbilical cord of newborns, and thus are still able to differentiate into many types of cells, but as this power to differentiate becomes limited, they are said to be only *multipotent* (NIH 2000). Even in the adult some few cells remain multipotent (or perhaps rarely even pluripotent), and these are what is meant by "adult stem cells" (PCB 2004a).

"Decades of research [on stem cells] have already yielded some 70 diverse therapies and clinical applications in treating diseases and disorders, including heart damage, spinal injury and several kinds of blood diseases" (Berg 2005; Korbling and Estrov 2003). Much of this work, however, has used cells that are only multipotent. Hence scientists are now eager to work more with pluripotent cells that supply more possibilities for therapeutic use and the testing of therapeutic drugs. Perhaps in this way many of the human ailments, such as Alzheimer's disease and multiple sclerosis, that to date have resisted successful treatment may be overcome.

The research use of umbilical cord cells, cells (called adult stem cells because they are not harvested from blastocysts) gathered from early miscarriages, or adult stem cells taken from organs in adults, is not controversial, but bitter dispute has arisen about whether researchers should be free to use "spare" embryos created through artificial in vitro reproduction and never implanted in utero, but preserved by freezing, or embryos, also artificially produced in vitro, but through the process called "cloning" (O'Rourke 2004).

Whether cloning and related processes are ethical will be discussed in the next section. As for all research that produces human embryos artificially in vitro, it has been already argued in chapter 3 that every human person has the moral right to be conceived through committed marital intercourse. Hence artificial reproduction in vitro, and all research that involves it, is seriously immoral.

Cloning

Cloning, as a form of assisted reproduction that is asexual, involves transferring the DNA of one cell into an ovum from which the nucleus has been removed. In some way still not fully understood, factors in the cytoplasm of the ovum cause the resultant new cell to revert to totipotentiality (Singer and Kuhse 1988; Silver 1997; PCB 2002, 6–15; Berg 2005) so that it is capable of twinning. When this totipotent new cell is electrically stimulated, it becomes a biological duplicate of the adult who provided the original DNA genetic material, that is, the adult's identical twin. For a time, cloning of animals was thought to be impossible, but in 1997, Ian Wilmut and his team of research scientists in Scotland succeeded in cloning a sheep, Dolly (Wilmut 1997; Kolata 1998). Speculation then, of course, arose concerning the cloning of human beings. The reaction to such a project was negative throughout the world, as this seemed an obvious threat by "mad scientists" against the value of personal individuality (Connor 2002). The notion of a *doppleganger*, or double, and of zombies has often been the subject of horror stories. Recently (2004) some South Korean researchers have claimed to achieve human cloning (Berg 2005), but only with the intention of using the produced embryos to obtain stem cells and then destroying these embryos at a very early stage of development.

Consequently some scientists, ethicists, and politicians are now arguing that cloning is ethically acceptable if it is not for reproduction but for strictly "therapeutic purposes," that is, if the cloned individuals are destined only for biomedical research in order to produce totipotent or at least pluripotent stem cells (Burley 1999; NIH 1994). These extracted stem cells would provide replacement cells or be developed into organs for sick people that their bodies would not reject because they would be genetically identical with their own. In order to avoid the opprobrium connected with human cloning, proponents of therapeutic cloning prefer to call it "somatic cell nuclear transfer" (SCNT). Such a change in nomenclature is problematic, "Although . . . somatic cell nuclear transfer may accurately describe the technique that is used to produce the embryonic clone, these terms fail to convey the nature of the deed itself, and they hide its human significance" (PCB 2002, 46).

Therapeutic cloning amounts to creating life in order to destroy it, and many leading ethicists strongly oppose it (Kass and Wilson 1998; Ahmann 2001; Kass 2003), and some oppose reproductive cloning (EGE 1998; Jaenisch and Wilmut 2001). Yet in most countries there have been few limitations placed upon retrieval and research upon embryonic stem cells, save the prohibition of cloning embryos for reproductive purposes (Royal Society 2000, 2002). In the United States, however, at present the federal government will not fund the retrieval of stem cells that involves the destruction of human embryos, but it does fund research on adult stem cells and research upon a limited number of cell lines developed from embryo stem cells (PCB 2002).

Ethical Issues

Moreover, recently several prominent scientists, politicians, and public figures have been lobbying to change the federal laws in order to eliminate the limits on embryo stem cell retrieval and research. Yet the extravagant claims made for stem cell research are similar to the claims made in the early 1990s for fetal cell research and transplantation. The promised results of this effort never materialized (Doerflinger 2001), although significant progress has been made in the therapeutic use of adult stem cells (Korbling and Estrov 2003). Much of the exaggerated publicity given to legalizing embryonic research is, sad to say, generated by groups interested in receiving government funding for their research projects (Taylor-Corbett 2001).

While the Catholic Church has affirmed the effort to improve therapeutic options by the use of adult stem cells, even to the extent of generating organ replacements, it opposes the use of embryo stem cells for either reproductive or therapeutic purposes. The Church opposes reproductive cloning because it devalues the person who is cloned, and as we argued in chapter 3 (section 3.1) because this mode of reproduction is asexual and therefore unnatural and contrary to human dignity and the rights of the child (CDF 1987). Cloning for research (XCNT) has also been decried because it creates life in order to destroy it. Therapeutic cloning of embryonic cells is also rejected as even far more unethical than reproductive cloning because it involves the killing of human embryos who are human persons. The position of the Catholic Church in regard to cloning was stated in a position paper presented to the United Nations in August 2003 (Migliore 2003): "The Holy See strongly supports the advancement of human biological sciences and agrees with the procurement of human stem cells as long as they are harvested from adult stem cells and not from live embryos. . . . The difference between 'reproductive' cloning and 'research' cloning consists only in the objective of the procedure . . . to ban reproductive cloning only, without prohibiting research cloning, would be to allow the production of individual human lives with the intention of destroying these lives as part of the process of using them for scientific research." John Paul II also stated in his encyclical *Gospel of Life*: "This evaluation of the morality of abortion is to be applied to the recent forms of intervention on human embryos which although carried out for purposes legitimate in themselves, inevitably involve the killing of those embryos. This is the case with experimentation on embryos that is becoming increasingly widespread in the field of biomedical research and is legally permitted in some countries" (1995, no. 63).

The Bush administration as a compromise permitted the funding of research using stem cells derived from already destroyed "spare" embryos resulting from artificial reproduction. The Pontifical Academy of Life also has asked (2001), "Is it morally licit to use embryo cells, and the differentiated cells obtained from them, which are supplied by other researchers or are commercially available?" but responded, "No, since prescinding from the morally illicit intention of the principal agent, the case in question entails a proximate material cooperation in the production and manipulation of human embryos on the part of those producing or supplying them." While we agree in general with this opinion, we could envision some researchers being so far removed from the "production and manipulation" of this process that their material cooperation would be mediate and remote. Thus some Catholic bioethicists have approved the use of vaccines produced from such cell lines when vaccines from better sources were unavailable. For Catholic health care facilities, however, Directive 66 of the *Ethical and Religious Directives for Catholic Health Care Services* (ERD) must be observed: "Catholic health institutions should not make use of human tissue obtained by direct abortions for research or therapeutic purposes" (ERD 2001).

New methods have recently been proposed to obtain pluripotent stem cells similar to those in human embryos, while avoiding creating and destroying human embryos. Dr. William Hurlbut has recently proposed obtaining stem cells from teratomas (Hurlbut 2005). These sometimes occur naturally as germ cell tumors and may contain several types of tissue, such as hair, muscle, and bone. Some such tumors, but not all, are malignant. Because it is doubtful whether some of these tumors might have originally been embryos, their origin is still so obscure that in our opinion Hurlbut's proposal cannot be accepted, because where there is doubt the benefit must be given to human life (Ponnuru 2005).

More promising is a method known as oocyte assisted reprogramming (OAR), in which the nucleus that is inserted in the ovum is first genetically altered so that it allegedly cannot produce an embryo (Walker 2005). A group of reputable and renowned scientists, theologians, and philosophers recently affirmed their conviction that this is an ethically accepted manner of producing human stem cells (Furton 2005). However, this method has been attacked on the grounds that the result may still be an embryo (Walker 2005).

Our conclusion at this time, therefore, can only be that until this process is better understood through animal experiments, it may not be used in experiments with human eggs (oocytes) until this difficult debate is resolved (Ponnuru 2005).

4.7 CONCLUSION

The ethical use of technology must always be within the limits of human nature and its innate needs. Hence the advance of genetics and surgery must be used for genuine human betterment. The use of genetics for therapeutic purposes is ethical, but the proposals to use it to enhance human nature threaten the survival of the human species. Genetics cannot ethically be used unless their effects are well understood and their intent is to perfect not change human nature. Also the testing and counseling of persons concerning their genetic health and defects must have genuinely therapeutic aims. Surgical organ transplantation from the dead and even from living donors is ethical provided that the donation is made with free and informed consent and does not seriously threaten the functional health of the donor. Cosmetic surgery can also be ethical but is too often unethically promoted and performed for insufficient reasons. The use of human subjects for experimentation demands their genuinely free and informed consent, which they should refuse unless there is reasonable hope of proportional benefit. Finally, research, including stem cell research that entails artificial reproduction and/or the destruction of human embryos, is seriously immoral.

Chapter Five

MENTAL HEALTH: ETHICAL PERSPECTIVES

OVERVIEW

A NERVOUS OR HORMONAL DYSFUNCTION, sometimes with genetic roots, is often the cause of mental dysfunction because human intelligence and freedom cannot operate normally without their bodily instruments. A factor in such mental illness, or even its principal cause, can also be the limitations set on the exercise of realistic human thought and freedom by cognitive habits or emotional disorders acquired during the course of early life, adolescence, or maturity, of which addictions are typical cases. The medical aspects of mental illness are today more and more effectively dealt with by pharmacotherapy and less often by psychosurgery and electroconvulsive therapy. Such medicotherapy usually needs psychotherapeutic support, and when there is no physical factor in mental illness, psychotherapy is paramount. The different current modes of psychotherapy are based on three main theories of human personality: psychoanalytic, humanistic, and behaviorist. That form of behaviorism called "cognitive therapy" is the one that today has the best empirical confirmation, but most therapists are in practice eclectic. The Christian view of the human person can assimilate these modern therapeutic methods, but it adds to them the spiritual dimension without which human freedom based on a true and essential understanding of reality is neglected. Thus the goal of psychotherapy is not merely adaptation to the prevailing culture, but a true understanding of human nature, its intrinsic needs, and the happiness—temporal and eternal—that is our real goal. The pursuit of this goal is facilitated by physical and emotional health. The ethical problems that occur in this field are often due to an inadequate view of human freedom, such as excessive behavior control, undue confinement of patients, the development of codependency with patients, and even their sexual abuse. A delicate problem is drawing the line between psychotherapy, which aims at freeing the patient to make ethical decisions, and the task of the ethical counselor or spiritual director. Problems in this field dealing with free and informed consent are discussed in chapter 2 (section 2.5).

5.1 WHAT IS MENTAL HEALTH?

The dualistic conception of the human person as a "mind" fallen into a "body" goes back to Plato and has influenced modern thought since Descartes revived it. Such dualism has raised the question whether the "mind" as a spiritual entity can become ill, as the body obviously can. At the end of the last century a group of "antipsychiatry psychiatrists" made a strong, if exaggerated, case against the whole concept of mental disease and the medical model of psychiatry (Laing 1976; Torrey 1972; Brody and Engelhardt 1980; Glymour and Stalker 1983; Perl and Shelp 1982). Richard M. Restak in *Pre-Meditated Man* (1975) claimed that most of the problems of psychiatry are not really ethical in the ordinary sense, but political, that is, questions of power as to whose will concerning human behavior is to prevail. The line between normal behavior and abnormal behavior thus would be only a question of who is deciding what they want us to do.

Similarly, in *The Myth of Mental Illness* (1974), Thomas Szasz argued that the concept of mental illness is completely invalid and that the greater numbers of psychiatric illnesses are really social maladjustments between the behavior of a nonconformist individual and the demands of a social system (Szasz 1998). The cause of these maladjustments is found in the modern social system, which is unable to deal with individual differences. Szasz even compared modern psychiatry and mental hospitals to the medieval religious Inquisition, that is, to an institution whose purpose supposedly was to enforce conformity of more highly individualized personalities to a rigid and oppressive social system through a cruel process of interrogation and torture. One group of psychiatrists call themselves "radicals," and they see the whole mental health establishment as an instrument of oppression (Erwin 1978; Haafhems, Nijhof, and Vander Pool 1986). This group has also been attacked as fundamentally antireligious (Bowman 2000; Webster 1995). The Antipsychiatry Coalition denies the reality of mental illness on its website (www.antipsychiatry.org).

Evidence that these accusations are not without serious foundation is shown in the actions of some governments such as the former Communist regimes (Medvedev and Medvedev 1971; Stover and Nightengale 1985) that have confined dissidents to mental institutions under the pretext that anyone who criticized the regime must be insane. Even the American Psychiatric Association (APA), by appointing a task force to study the use of seclusion and restraint in psychiatric therapy (APA 1985), has admitted that such ethical problems can arise. The novel of Ken Kesey (and even more the classic movie based on it) *One Flew Over the Cuckoo's Nest* (1962) dramatized the way in which patients, even those self-committed to a mental institution, can be reduced to robotlike conformity by the "system." The tragedy of this story was that the "monster" Nurse Ratched was in fact a dedicated, well-meaning, and highly professional person who quite unconsciously had become a manipulator of people. Clearly in such cases it is not the individuals who are sick, but a system that fits both patients and health care professionals into a mutually destructive gestalt.

This accusation is further strengthened by realization of the effect of the "total institution" on human beings (Goffman 1962; Rothman 1980), which shows the dangers of a closed social system where people live so far within a rigid set of man-made ideas and behaviors that they are cut off from contact with a reality beyond and different from their limited perception. This often leads to a distorted, paranoid way of perceiving and interpreting the world. But not only can an asylum, a prison, a monastery, or a hospital become a "total institution." Modern society itself, with its technological organization, its mass media of brainwashing, and its all-seeing surveillance, can act as a total institution, so that there is no escape except (as in Kesey's novel) to sail out to sea in a boat.

Prevalence and Variety of Mental Disorders

In spite of these criticisms of the very notion of "mental illness," every counselor knows that people suffer from many conditions of emotion and thought that are far more intense than average and are contrary to objective reality. In the United States in any year, an estimated 22 percent of persons eighteen or older in age, that is, about one in five adults, have a diagnosable mental disorder. Of the ten leading causes of disability in our country four are mental disorders. According to the APA (1994) *Diagnostic and Statistical Manual of Mental Disorders*, fourth edition (*DSM-IV*), the "bible" of clinicians, there are more than two hundred kinds of mental disorders, and more are constantly being recognized. Of these four are the leading causes of disability: *major depression, bipolar disorder, schizophrenia,* and *obsessive-compulsive disorder.* The fact, cited by some critics (www.antipsychiatry.org), that it is difficult to define these illnesses exactly or to assign their precise causes is no more convincing than it would be to claim on the same grounds that cancers do not exist.

Axis I of the *DSM-IV* lists the principal illnesses of which the major ones can be grouped as follows:

1. *Adjustive disorders* first evident in infancy, childhood, or adolescence: attention-deficit hyperactivity disorder (about 4 percent of children and adolescents, two to three times as many boys as girls); autism and its milder form, Asperger's disorder (one in five hundred children but increasing and in about four times as many boys as girls, but more severe in girls), oppositional defiant or conduct disorder, separation anxiety disorder, Tourette's syndrome (tics), and elimination disorder.

2. *Anxiety disorders* that include panic disorder, obsessive-compulsive disorder, post-traumatic stress disorder, generalized anxiety disorder, and phobias. Panic disorder affects 2.5 million, post-traumatic stress disorder affects 5 million (almost one-third of the veterans of the Vietnam War), generalized anxiety disorder affects 4 million, agoraphobia and other phobias affect 3 million. The two sexes are equally affected by obsessive-compulsive disorder (3.5 million) and social phobia (5 million), but in general anxiety disorders affect almost twice the number of women as men.

3. *Eating disorders*: pica (a tendency to eat unusual things), anorexia nervosa, and bulimia and binge-eating affect as high as 3 percent of women and some men. Sleep disorders, sleeplessness, disturbed sleep patterns, and parasomnia (sleep walking, nightmares).

4. *Depressive disorders*: major depressive disorder, bipolar disorder, and the milder cyclothymic and dysthymic disorders affect some 19 million U.S. adults of which

two-thirds are women and which can be connected with anxiety disorders and substance abuse and result in some thirty thousand suicides a year (men kill themselves
four times as often as women).

5. *Sexual disorders*: the paraphilias such as exhibitionism, fetishism, sexual masochism
   and sadism, voyeurism, pedophilia, transsexualism, and sexual dysfunction. Homosexuality was formerly included here but has been removed for reasons to be discussed
   later.
6. *Organic-based disorders*: delirium, vascular dementia, alcoholism-related dementia,
   Alzheimer's dementia, which affects about 4 million Americans, most commonly after
   age seventy-five and endures for eight to ten years before death.
7. *Schizophrenia delusional disorder*: brief psychotic disorder, schizophreniform disorder,
   schizoeffective disorder, and psychotic disorder shared by two or several persons,
   malingering, and hypochondria. These are conditions of mental confusion, halluci-
   nation, and lack of normal affectivity suffered by 2.2 million Americans. Affecting
   about 20 million, schizophrenia occurs equally as often in the two sexes but often
   affects men in their teens and women in young adulthood.

Axis II describes personality disorders more difficult to treat than Axis I problems and these
include:

1. Mental retardation and also the paranoid, schizoid and schizotypal, antisocial
   borderline, histrionic, narcissistic, avoidant personality, dependent, and obsessive-
   compulsive personality disorders.
2. Finally, there are problems of substance-related disorders of various types, including
   alcoholism and other addictions.

Axis III of the *DSM-IV* deals with current medical conditions that may affect the client,
Axis IV deals with psychosocial and environmental factors affecting the client, and Axis V
deals with the estimation of the client's overall level of functioning. Thus the range and
complexity of problems of mental health is staggering yet understandable in view of the
complexity of the human person with its biological, psychological, ethical, and spiritual
dimensions, as shown in chapter 2.

The Reality of Mental Illness

From this discussion of the nature of mental illness, the following four conclusions can
be drawn:

First, mental illness, in the strict and proper sense, results from faulty development and
use of human sensitive and affective capacities (Gert, Culver, and Clauser 1997). Physical
and physiological impairments may contribute to this faulty development and function
because they inhibit the adaptive capacity of the person.

Second, it is necessary to hold firmly to the fact that dysfunctional forms of human behavior caused by organic and physiological defects do exist (Boyle 2002). Lesions of the
central nervous system, as well as a wide variety of physiological disorders, can make it
difficult or impossible for human beings to sense and perceive the world correctly, to live
in a state of emotional balance and sensitivity, to think clearly, and to make decisions free

from uncontrollable impulses. The evidence for a genetic basis for some mental illnesses (U.S. Surgeon General 1999) is undeniable. Yet the tendency to consider genetics as the cause or the source of all mental illness must also be resisted (Udry 1995).

Third, it is essential to keep in mind that these physical disabilities (except in the most severe cases) do not automatically lead to highly abnormal behavior. Rather, it is a matter of tension between the innate capacities of the individual and the demands of the environment. For example, a patient with a respiratory disorder may be relatively comfortable under some atmospheric conditions and intensely uncomfortable under others that would not greatly distress a normal person. This disparity may also prevail among people with an inadequate or impaired capacity to adjust to certain environmental and social stresses. Clearly this suggests that the mental health of a society is to be achieved not only by treatment of the individual but also by political and social readjustment of the environment to more adaptive lifestyles. It would seem that modern society should have enough social control to be able to tolerate varied human capacities.

Fourth, prolonged hospitalization of the mentally ill is not only costly but often bad therapy. Nevertheless, it is a serious injustice to dismiss them to wander, distressed and distressing, perhaps suicidal or dangerous, homeless in the streets (Lezak and Edgar 1998). While those with mental illness need an environment that is as normal and open as possible, they also desperately need care, support, and guidance to cope with reality. A large number of people in society require psychiatric care that is impossible without hospitalization. Extreme caution must also be taken within practical limits to protect the human rights of mental patients, especially as to both voluntary and involuntary commitments and retention, the right of treatment during the patient's stay, and even the right to refuse some forms of treatment. They are so common that, in 1992, the United Nations passed a resolution to defend the rights of mental patients.

It is also essential that psychiatric care include an effort to help patients develop skills to cope with the social situation in which they must live after leaving the hospital, a situation they ordinarily cannot much alter. The patient's family must share in this process to assist in the patient's reentry into normal living, or a halfway house should be available to facilitate this difficult transition. It is essential, moreover, that Christians recognize and respond to the need for a profound social transformation of culture so that it will be able to meet the needs of so-called deviants who are among the "little ones" for whom Jesus taught us to be advocates.

Fifth, a special question is raised by the Bible accounts of demonic possession and exorcism. It is evident that in Jesus's time conditions that would today be judged to be mental illnesses were interpreted as possessions by evil spirits that Jesus "cast out," and also empowered his apostles to do so (Mk 17:17). Consequently, the Catholic Church continues to practice the exorcism of evil spirits. If God has created pure spirits with free will, as Jews, Christians, and Muslims all believe, it is reasonable to think that some have misused their freedom to gain power in rivalry to God, as we humans have done throughout our violent history.

For such reasons, the modern Catholic Church is very cautious to distinguish extraordinary events from mental illnesses that have probable natural explanations (CCC 2000, no. 1773). The Catholic Church only permits exorcisms in the name of the Church in rare circumstances, although Christians can pray for deliverance from demonic powers.

5.2 MEDICAL/SURGICAL THERAPIES

Because organic defects and physiological malfunctions underlie some forms of mental illnesses, their healing requires correction of these defects. Over the years, three medical/surgical methods of treating mental illnesses—psychosurgery, electroconvulsive therapy, and pharmacotherapy—have been developed.

Psychosurgery

Arguments on the ethics and merits of psychosurgery vary from severe condemnation to considerable enthusiasm (Black and Szasz 1977; Kleinig 1985; Valenstein 1987). The psychosurgical procedure that attracted the most attention was the prefrontal (or transorbital) lobotomy performed on people with severe psychotic disorders (Sabbatini 2004). The Portuguese surgeon Ega Moniz was awarded a Nobel Prize for the invention of psychosurgery in 1937, and it was introduced into the United States by doctors William Freeman and James Watts Freeman, who performed more than three thousand lobotomies in twenty-eight years. Freeman became notorious as the "ice pick surgeon" because of the instruments he used (El-Hai 2001; Jansson 2004).

The use of lobotomy increased in the United States from 1947 to 1949 from five hundred to five thousand annual procedures (McManamy 2005). It was a procedure that in some cases was done under local anesthesia and consisted essentially in severing the white nerve fibers that connect the frontal lobes of the brain with the thalamus in order to blunt abnormal human emotional responses and thus calm patients' antisocial behavior. Many hoped it would solve the severe overcrowding and understaffing in state-run mental hospitals and asylums. During a period in which about fifty thousand Americans were treated by this technique, studies showed that 41 percent of patients so treated had recovered or were greatly improved, 28 percent were somewhat improved, 25 percent showed no improvement, 2 percent were worse and 4 percent had died. But by 1950 there was a strong reaction against its use.

Psychosurgical techniques today are chiefly aimed at the connections between the limbic system located on the inner side of the cerebral cortex, which is believed to regulate human emotions, and the frontal cortex that is believed to serve higher thought processes. Bilateral cingulotomy has replaced lobotomy and is used mainly for major depression, bipolar disorder, or obsessive-compulsive disorder and sometimes also to relieve chronic, intransigent pain in cancer patients. Because, however, the long-term effects of such surgery are still not clear, cingulotomy should be used only after careful screening of patients to determine if these conditions have not responded to less drastic forms of treatment and if the patients have given free and informed consent to the risks of the technique.

In cingulotomy there is not, as in lobotomy, any destruction of large sections of the frontal lobe of the brain. A computer-based process called stereotactic magnetic resonance imaging is used to guide a small electrode to the limbic system, and an electrical current burns a small lesion only about a half-inch in diameter. In a bilateral cingulotomy the excision is in the cingulate gyrus that connects the limbic system to the frontal lobes. Sometimes an instrument known as a "gamma knife" is used to focus beams of radiation that without surgical invasion converge within the brain and destroy the small area. A 1997 report from Massachusetts General Hospital reported significant improvement in somewhat more than one-third of its cases treated with this procedure. After lobotomies, some patients exhibited bizarre behaviors and profound changes in personality, but the newer techniques do not seem to result in loss of higher level thought or memory.

Electroconvulsive Therapy

Even in Hippocrates' time and again in the Middle Ages, physicians noticed cases in which high fevers, especially those produced by malaria, might result in improvement of mental health in the insane. In the period 1917–35 this type of therapy was rediscovered in Europe in four forms (Abrams 1988; Sabbatini 2004).

1. Dr. Julius Wagner-Jauregg in Vienna in 1917 used malarial fever to treat syphilitic patients.
2. Dr. Manfred J. Sakel in Berlin in 1927 used insulin coma and convulsions to treat schizophrenia.
3. Dr. Ladislaus von Meduna in Budapest in 1934 used the chemical Metrazol to treat schizophrenia and affective psychoses.
4. Drs. Ugo Cerletti and Lucio Bini in Rome in 1937 began to use electroconvulsive shock therapy.

The popularity for a time of these "shock treatments" and the controversies it generated resulted in the split between the "psychological school" and the "biological school" of mental therapy that still persists.

The theory on which such shock treatments were based was that this violent stimulation of the brain would cause the readjustment of disordered neural patterns. While it was sometimes effective, it could be dangerous, causing broken bones or heart attacks, and when used repeatedly was said to leave the patient in much the same condition as lobotomy. It was also greatly dreaded by some patients who were frightened by its violence, risks, and aftereffects. The sometimes dramatic efficacy of his procedure led to further research, and when Jose Delgado (1969) and the Schwitzgebels (1973) devised the much milder electrical stimulation of the brain (ESB) as a neurological research tool, the way was opened for electroconvulsive therapy (ECT).

After ECT began to be widely used, it came to be regarded as more destructive than therapeutic by some scientists and physicians (Carroll and O'Callaghan 1984). Chief among these critics was Peter Breggin (1972, 1979), a practicing psychiatrist whose scathing denunciation, based mainly on ethical considerations, reprinted in the *Congressional Register* (March 30, 1972), gave rise to national debates. Legislators became so involved in this medical-moral issue that two bills to prohibit psychosurgery, or to limit it severely, were introduced in Congress. Today, ECT is generally accepted as the preferred treatment for severe depressions that have not yielded to drugs or in cases when the patient cannot tolerate drugs, or the patient's condition is very difficult to manage without a quick improvement (NIH 1999), yet this report was not accepted by all (Goode 1997). The reasons for its efficacy are still problematic. What is most certain is that these procedures produce a temporary but often severe loss of memory and general state of psychic disorganization. Apparently this makes it possible for some patients to break out of fixed patterns of fantasy and feeling and to begin to respond in a more normal way.

Significant improvements in the technique of ECT have been made since then, including the use of synthetic muscle relaxants, such as succinylcholine, the anesthesia of patients with short-acting agents, pre-oxygenation of the brain, the use of electroencephalogram (EEG) seizure monitoring, and better devices and shock wave forms. Despite these advances, the popularity of ECT greatly decreased in the 1970s and 1980s, due to the use of more effective psychoactive drugs and as a result of a strong anti-ECT movement. The famous novelist Ernest Hemingway and the noted poet Sylvia Plath received this treatment, yet both ended by committing suicide.

More recently, however, ECT has regained some of its favor due to its efficacy especially in treating major depression in older people. It is the only somatic therapy from the 1930s that remains in widespread use today. Between 100,000 and 150,000 patients are subjected to ECT every year in the United States, but under strictly defined medical conditions.

The obvious lesson that needs to be drawn from this period in the history of medicine is that it is unethical to popularize healing techniques until their effects can be carefully studied with small experimental and controlled groups and for a considerable period of time (Jansson 2004).

Pharmacotherapy

The "biological school" has in the main turned from the hopes of psychosurgery and shock treatment to the use of psychoactive drugs. A drug is *psychoactive* when it has some psychological effect such as altering thoughts, imagination, perception, or emotions; causes alertness, drowsiness, or feelings of anger; and so forth. Such drugs are also called *psychotropic*, and the study of these drugs is called *psychopharmacology*. Some forms of psychoactive agents, such as alcoholic beverages, have been used since the beginning of civilization, although the distilled liquors were medieval inventions. Opium in one form or another has been used as a pain reliever for centuries. Aspirin, the first of the "wonder drugs," has been used for more than one hundred years to treat pain and anxiety. Of course a distinction must be made between the use of psychotropic drugs for therapy for mental illness and for behavior modification in children or adults.

Early in the history of medicine it was believed that an imbalance of "humors" was at the root of all illnesses physical and mental. Researchers in the last half of the twentieth century showed that many emotional problems either are biochemically caused or at least are intensified by accompanying biochemical effects. Today the range of psychotherapeutic drugs is vast and constantly increasing, partly because of their profitability for the booming pharmaceutical industry. They are also advertised under a confusing number of trade names. Leaving these trade names aside, except for a few examples (Quitkin 1998; Bezchlibnyk-Butler and Jeffries 2003), the principal types are as follows:

1. Antidepressants: (a) tricyclics and tetracyclics, (b) monoamine oxidase inhibitors, and (c) serotonin-specific reuptake inhibitors, which include the well-known Prozac and Zoloft and miscellaneous other brand names.
2. Antianxiety medications (anxiolytics, minor tranquillizers) that often have the side effect of drowsiness, but patients can adapt to this. Xanax and Valium are examples.

3. Antipsychotic medications (major tranquillizers or neuroleptics) used for schizophrenics, major depression with psychotic features, and patients who become violent or extremely agitated. These are very powerful drugs and have many serious side effects; a well-known example is chlorpromazine (Thorazine).
4. Antimanic medications such as Lithium.
5. Sedatives and hypnotic medications that include barbiturates, such as Nembutal, Luminal, and Seconal.
6. Medications that offset side effects of the previous medications that include beta-blockers and antihistamines.
7. Medications used for attention deficit disorder (hyperactivity), notably Ritalin.

Although today there is such an impressive range of psychotropic drugs available for therapy, the potential for the future is both frightening and promising (Ray and Ksir 2003). As Klerman said, "As knowledge of the relationship between brain and behavior increases, it is likely we will develop knowledge of the neurochemical and neuropharmacological bases of memory, learning, mood, aggression, appetite, and sexual lust" (1991, 4). Thus not only must psychoactive drugs be evaluated as therapeutic agents, but also future ethical evaluation must consider their potential to improve capabilities and enhance personal pleasure and enjoyment of life.

Therefore the increasing extent to which psychoactive drugs are used in our society must raise serious ethical concerns (Beitman and Klerman 1991; M. Smith 1991). Antipsychotic, antidepressant, and antianxiety drugs are used not only by people who are severely ill and unable to manage their emotions without medication but also by relatively normal people attempting to control anxiety, tension, depression, insomnia, and other states arising from the stress of life in modern society (PCB 2003). Since 1988 there has been a 20 percent increase in the number of visits to a doctor that have resulted in the prescription of a psychotropic drug (Pincus et al. 1998). Moreover, for 2002 in the United States 8.3 percent of the population used some illicit form of psychotherapeutic drugs, 6.2 percent used marijuana, and 2.6 percent used some nonmedical psychotherapeutic drug other than those sold without prescriptions (Faststats 2004). In addition, many use nonprescription or over-the-counter drugs for relief from headache, tension, insomnia, anxiety, and other "lesser" maladies of life. Much anxiety among parents has been caused by the controversy over the use of drugs in public schools to control hyperactive children.

Psychotropic drugs have proved highly effective in psychotherapy in (1) tranquilizing patients in manic states or in uncontrollable anxiety; (2) reducing the condition of mental confusion and dissociation, especially in schizophrenia; and (3) lifting certain types of depression (Beitmann and Klerman 1991). These effects may be symptomatic rather than truly curative, yet they raise the hope that as the underlying organic causes are understood, more successful therapies and preventatives for mental illness can be developed. It is also clear, however, that drugs can never be the total answer to the problem of mental health, which also involves factors of social, environmental, and psychological development.

There has been a major shift from psychotherapy to pharmacology in treating most illnesses since the 1970s and 1980s. Scientific judgment increasingly questions the evidence supporting psychotherapy. Double-blind studies seem to demonstrate the greater efficacy of pharmacotherapy. Beitman and Klerman (1991) discuss the possible clinical effects of this shift. To summarize their studies, the introduction of drugs into psychotherapy may do the following:

1. Convince the therapist and patient to become dependent on faith in the "magic" of drugs rather than to seek genuine insight into psychological processes.
2. Reduce the patient's anxiety and therefore the motivation to seek help and change.
3. Reduce the patient's symptoms only to generate new symptoms in their place.
4. Make patients feel that they are being given drugs because they do not have the capacity to attain self-understanding through psychotherapy.

Positively, the use of drugs may effect the following:

1. Make patients more accessible to psychotherapy.
2. Improve "ego function," that is, "influence verbal skill, improve cognitive functioning, improve memory, reduce distraction, and promote concentration," so that the client is better able to cooperate in psychotherapy.
3. Promote "abreaction," a basic element in psychotherapy, the ability to relive and confront past traumas and fixations.
4. Replace the feelings of despair and stigmatization associated with mental illness with the optimism and normality of getting medical help.

Alternatively, psychotherapy can have both negative and positive effects on drug therapy. Negative effects may consist of the following:

1. If the illness is the result of a single physiological factor correctable by drugs, psychotherapy is irrelevant.
2. Psychotherapy may disturb the patient and aggravate symptoms.

Positive effects may consist of the following:

1. Rehabilitation of the patient after drugs have done their work.
2. Psychotherapy helps patients accept and be consistent in use of the drugs.

Thus pharmacotherapy is based on the hypothesis that the mental disorder is the result of a neurophysiological malfunction that may or may not have a genetic basis and that the administration of drugs will correct this imbalance or at least mitigate its symptoms. Psychotherapy cannot correct this underlying problem, although it may assist in enabling the patient to cope with its disturbing effects in daily life. If this is the case, then to subject the patient to extensive psychotherapy is not only a waste of time and money but unethical, because it must be motivated by either prejudices against the use of drugs, ideological attachment to unproven psychological theories, or simply an exploitative desire on the part of the psychotherapist to keep control of patients and the fees they pay.

Thus, on the one hand, it is ethically wrong for therapists not to explore the genetic, physiological, and hygienic condition of their patients in an effort to determine whether there is in fact a neurophysiological basis to their symptoms before they engage in what may be a prolonged, expensive, and useless course of psychotherapy. On the other hand, it is also unethical for a therapist to be content to prescribe medication without attempting to determine whether there are other purely psychic factors that require psychotherapy. For example, it would be poor medicine but also unethical neglect to continue to dismiss a patient with manic-depressive symptoms with prescriptions for Lithium when this proves only partially effective, and there is evidence that the patient's lifestyle is a source of severe pressure.

In summary, from an ethical point of view, the increasing reliance on pharmacotherapy seems justified by its results, but requires on the part of therapists the following:

1. Not to succumb to the temptation to give pills, rather than to carefully diagnose and monitor the patient.
2. Not to let prejudices in favor of the "medical model" of therapy lead them to neglect psychotherapy as indicated.
3. Not to neglect assessing and monitoring possible side effects of the drugs to be used and observing the principle of free and informed consent before prescribing them.
4. Promote and keep informed of continuing research to determine scientifically the value of the drugs in question and to continue to improve them and increase their safety.

Psychotropic Drugs for Behavior Modification.   In addition to therapy for mental illness, psychotropic drugs are also used widely to modify the behavior of children who are restless, inattentive, or hyperactive and for adults who suffer from anxiety. When children are impulsive or have difficulty concentrating or learning, and if the difficulty is chronic, they are often diagnosed as suffering attention deficit/hyperactivity disorder (ADHD). There is no definitive biological marker for this diagnosis. Family and teachers usually make the conclusion that a child suffers from this condition as a result of observation. Thus there is a strong subjective element involved in the diagnosis. In order to be diagnosed with ADHD, the patient must exhibit inattention, hyperactivity, and impulsivity for six months or more to a degree that is inconsistent with his or developmental level (APA 2000). The frequency of this diagnosis is rising rapidly in all sections of the United States (Zito 2003). Several critics attribute the behavior to normal difficulties involved in growing up in our modern stress-filled society. However, it does seem that attentiveness and overall conduct do improve if psychotropic drugs are prescribed, especially those with the brand names Ritalin and Adderall. These drugs, closely related to amphetamines, from which these commercial products are derived, were originally used to support blood pressure and have a definite effect upon the central nervous system. In addition to aiding the focus and attention of the person who uses them, they also diminish fatigue and enhance concentration. Because amphetamines often have addictive effects when used promiscuously by adults, they are classified as controlled substances; hence the Federal Drug Enforcement Administration (DEA) monitors their production and sale.

The use of psychotropic drugs by adults who would not be described as being afflicted with mental illness is also on the increase. Antidepressants such as Prozac and Zoloft have become a commonplace prescription in modern America. The ethical concern raised by increased use of drugs among children and adults is twofold: Do they cause addiction or other psychophysiological harm, and do they dispose the users to avoid confronting the normal difficulties of daily life?

To date, there is no evidence that the use of Ritalin or Adderall for children has caused physical maladies or addictive behavior. However, there are several reports that children do not welcome being assigned to the ADHD category and seem to look forward to vacation periods when they are free from taking their medicine. Moreover, the tendency to make children meet the expectations of their parents, whether academic or athletic, by means of psychoactive compounds had been decried consistently in recent times.

Insofar as the use of pharmaceuticals to control the emotional state of adults is concerned, there is need for caution and prudence. To some extent, using psychoactive drugs to control unwelcome reactions to stress and strain is similar to taking aspirin for a headache. But conversely, psychotropic drugs have more impact than aspirin, and their use seems to be more habit forming than aspirin. In sum, the use of these pharmaceuticals whether by children or adults is not a problem-free practice, even though their use cannot be declared unethical in itself.

5.3 PSYCHOTHERAPIES

Psychosurgery, shock treatments, and pharmacotherapy fit easily into the "medical model" by which physical diseases are usually treated, but psychotherapy as such is a strikingly different mode of treatment (Sider 1983). To treat patients by talking with them or guiding them in recalling and reenacting past experiences or changing unreal ways of solving life's problems is very different from giving them a pill, cutting out a tumor, regulating their diet, or even directing their physical exercise. It is more similar to education or reeducation (Ursano and Silberman 1988), if "education" means not the mere acquisition of information but rather the learner's own growth toward self-understanding and control, which the therapist facilitates but cannot originate.

Psychotherapy is based on the assumption that the mentally disturbed person has at least some capacities for normal mental life, but that these capacities have not been properly developed, are malfunctioning, or are being poorly used. In other words, the mentally sick person has to a degree the capacity to cope with situations satisfactorily, but he or she has not learned how to use this capacity effectively or is inhibited from such use by abnormal fears and faulty perceptions of reality.

There is, however, an important difference between psychotherapeutic or mental health education and other types of education. Education, in the usual sense as a function of an academic institution, is the development of human capacities at the rational or conscious level. Psychotherapy deals with psychic processes less conscious and less free than rational thought, just as education at the spiritual level deals with psychic processes that transcend the level of discursive rational thought.

At present, there is a plethora of psychotherapeutic methods, and we must first sort these out according to the different theories of human personality on which they are based. We then compare these to the classical theory of St. Thomas Aquinas (1225–74) on which the Catholic view of ethics described in chapter 2 is based. Authors Maddi (1996) and Monte (1999) give complicated divisions, but for our purposes the three given by George Boeree (2004) will suffice:

1. *Psychoanalytic* theories that explain human behavior through experiences suppressed into the unconscious. Sigmund Freud pioneered this approach.

2. *Humanistic* theories that explain human behavior in terms of conscious experience and the natural orientation of the human person to integral self-fulfillment. Abraham Maslow and Carl Rogers typify this approach.

3. *Behavioristic* theories that explain human behavior in relation to its external environment. A radical form that ignored introspection originated with J. B. Watson and B. F. Skinner, but now in a more moderate form it has become *cognitive therapy*, which, while attentive to introspective processes, emphasizes that behavior is influenced by learned thought patterns through interaction with the external environment. Neal Miller, John Dollard, Albert Bandura, and others promote this approach.

To understand why the differences between these theories arose and why they have not yet been fully resolved it is necessary to review briefly their historical origin. Wilhelm Wundt, generally considered the father of modern scientific psychology in his *Theory of Sense Perception* (1961) and *Principles of Physiological Psychology* (1904), began the use of scientific techniques in the study of psychological phenomena. He argued that psychology must be based directly on experience, but for him this meant controlled introspection. He founded the first psychological laboratory (1879) and the first journal of psychology (1881). The rooting of this approach in the dualistic Cartesian "turn to the subject" that initiated modern philosophy is obvious. Wundt's introspective method proved scientifically unreliable because even trained observers of their internal mental processes often disagree.

It was the Russian Ivan Pavlov (1849–1937) who in his study of the behavior of dogs experimentally established the laws of classical conditioning and the stimulus-response (S-R) model of explanation that became the basis of radical behaviorism as it was taken up by the American J. B. Watson in his 1913 lecture, "Psychology as the Behaviorist Views It" at Columbia University in New York in which he rejected all introspection as scientifically unverifiable. B. F. Skinner (1971, 1985) further radicalized behaviorism by ignoring explanations based on the internal state of the nervous system.

Meanwhile the Austrian Sigmund Freud (1857–1939), a secularized Jew as committed to scientific reductionism as Watson and Skinner, in 1900 had published his *The Interpretation of Dreams* and in 1901 his *The Psychopathology of Everyday Life* that, like Wundtian conscious introspection and in sharp contrast to behaviorism, sought to explain human behavior in terms of instinctive drives hidden in the id, or unconscious part of the human psyche, that manifest themselves only symptomatically and symbolically, though they can be partially explored through the technique of psychoanalysis.

Freud, a physician, had come to this view from his work with Joseph Breuer (1842–1925) on patients diagnosed as "hysterical." He himself says in the first of these books that in his dreams he identified himself with Hannibal. He interpreted this as meaning that Hannibal and Rome symbolize "the opposition between Jewish tenacity and the organizing spirit of the Catholic Church" with which he was fascinated but which stood for him as symbolic of his suppression of his hatred of his father and of his core human drives (Bakken 1975; Vitz 1994).

While for Freud the core of the human psyche is the unconscious id, he did not consider the ego to be identical with consciousness because much of the contents of the ego become hidden by defense, as we must conceal our antisocial instincts not only from others but also from ourselves. Thus defensiveness—the tendency to ignore, forget, and repress the fact of one's inherent selfishness so as to seem, even to oneself, to be a good citizen, "a decent person"—for Freud, marks all human behavior even at its best. It hides the excessive demands of our three core needs—"life, sexual pleasure, and death"—that society restricts. Yet in the process of psychoanalysis some contents of the id emerge and can be checked against reality and social demands, although it never becomes conscious in its totality (Webster 1995).

Thus threefold division of psychotherapies can even be reduced to two very different conceptions of human psychological development. Perry London, in *Behavior Control* (1979), named these "insight therapy" (psychoanalytic theories) and "action therapy" (behavioristic theories), while the third or humanistic school can be seen as an attempt to synthesize the insight and action approaches. Certainly in practice these therapies overlap, especially in the moderate behaviorism of cognitive therapy, but they have different theoretical and clinical sources.

The insight therapies derive largely from Freud and the psychoanalytical school, although they have now moved on to include a great variety of therapeutic methods other than psychoanalysis, especially to include the social-group aspect of behavioral disorders (Engel 1981). What characterizes these therapies is that they aim at helping individuals understand ("have insight into," "get in touch with") their own behavior and its affective sources and thus learn how to deal with life situations in an effective way (figure 5.1).

Insight therapies assume that mental disorder means simply that (1) patients lack this insight or the skill to deal with their emotions and interpersonal relations; or (2) as with the obsessive person, they have much insight and little skill; or (3) as with the psychopathic person, they have much skill and little insight because during the course of their psychosocial development they have been traumatized or wrongly guided. Thus psychotherapy of this type deals with the lack of coordination between the rational level, and in the case of the therapy of Jung (1984), perhaps also with the spiritual level (Arraj and Arraj 1984) and the psychological level of the personality. Normal persons coordinate their rational and subrational processes satisfactorily, whereas neurotic or psychotic persons do not.

Figure 5.1   Freud's Personality Concept

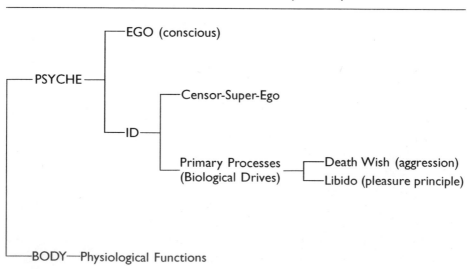

Alternatively, action therapy is the outcome of the behaviorist school of psychology, which rejects or bypasses the whole notion of the subconscious because it does not consider the notion of consciousness to be of any great help in psychological theory (Agras and Berkowitz 1988). While most action therapists do not go in theory to this behaviorist extreme, they do seek to understand human behavior primarily in terms of "operant conditioning." Human beings behave as they do because they live in a physical and social environment that has educated them to behave in a certain way. This education consists in an ordered series of rewards and punishments (positive and negative reinforcements) that favors some forms of behavior and eliminates others.

It should be noted, however, that action therapies not only include reeducation by means of external rewards and punishments (e.g., by administering painful electric shocks) but also extend to reeducation of the person's fantasy life by *desensitization*, as when a patient overcomes a phobia by imagining painful situations and gradually comes to feel less anxious about them. Thus methods that rely on suggestion are considered action therapy, although they may appear similar to methods in insight therapy.

More related to the insight therapies, yet sharing with action therapy a reluctance to explain behavior by unconscious processes, is *cognitive therapy,* which tries to reeducate the way clients reason about themselves and their problems. For example, depressed persons think about reality in a pessimistic, defeatist way that fails to give attention to the options open to them among which they can select more positive creative ways of acting. As long as they continue to live in a defeatist mental atmosphere, failure is inevitable. Cognitive therapy aims to enable such persons to recognize that this hopeless round of thought can be broken and new thought patterns learned. Other persons habitually live, like Dickens's Mr. Micawber, in a rosy but merely fanciful future, ignoring their real possibilities of decision and action. This daydreaming, too, is a sure recipe for failure, and cognitive therapy aims to bring the dreamer down to earth. Its technique is to help clients analyze the ways of thinking that have caused them to fail in living and to reeducate them to think logically and realistically.

Insight and Action Therapy Reconciled

The controversy between insight and action therapies still continues and is often obscured by bitter polemics, but it reflects two aspects of human psychology that are not necessarily contradictory. Action therapy reflects the fact that human behavior, which at first may be conscious and deliberate, quickly takes on a pattern and becomes automatic and subconscious. Thus when a person is learning to drive a car or play the piano, each motion is conscious and deliberate, but once the habit is acquired, these actions can be performed without conscious attention. This applies also to motivation, because in general it is easier and more pleasant to perform in a habitual manner and more difficult and even painful to go against a habit or routine response. The advantage of such automatization of behavior is obvious; it frees one's attention from the details of routine behavior and permits concentration on decisions about new or unusual situations, problems to be solved, and new skills to be acquired. Without this capacity to form habits, a person's energies would be wasted on the routine acts rather than concentrated on the adaptive and creative ones.

Furthermore, in psychosocial development, the formation of such habits in the child precedes the time when the human person is mature enough to have full self-consciousness and control. No wonder, then, that children who have been badly trained by their social environment arrive at the stage of self-control with many faulty and perhaps disastrously restricted or inconsistent and conflicting patterns of behavior, whose origin and even existence they do not understand. These may operate both in the conscious and at the unconscious levels of the psyche. Thus children may have developed irrational fears by associating fear reactions with harmless stimuli, but they no longer understand why they are afraid. Or the extreme pessimist or optimist may, at the conscious level, have developed patterns of noticing only the dark or the light side of situations.

The action therapies, based on a highly developed theory of learning through conditioning, seek to reeducate the patient by extinguishing undesirable patterns of behavior and establishing or strengthening desirable ones. Included are not only external behaviors but also undesirable emotional reactions, especially the hampering and disorganizing type of fear called neurotic anxiety.

The insight therapies agree that the human being has many automatisms and that aberrant adult behavior is often rooted in faulty conditioning in early childhood, when the organism is highly impressionable and the power of the ego to resist environmental influences is low. The emphasis of insight therapies, including cognitive therapy, is on the emergence of the ego or self as controlling behavior in an adaptive manner in the face of the natural and social environments. Consequently, if the therapist simply corrects faulty habits in the client, this only treats the symptoms. The real problem is to help patients develop a strong ego and to understand how they came to have faulty habits of thinking and acting so they will be able under their own choice to form better ones. Thus it requires at least some measure of exploration of the past and a growing insight into one's own personality structure (Kolb and Brodie 1982).

Apparently, therefore, the two therapies can complement each other (Karasu 1982). In fact, the latest behavioral theories go beyond Skinner and postulate an interaction between environment, behavior, and cognition processes to explain human behavior (Bandura 1986). Moreover, clients who have acquired insight into their own behavior and unconscious motivation may still need to be taught how to recondition themselves and to be aided by others in so doing. Freud and the psychoanalytical school too quickly assumed that a person who understands why he or she acts irrationally will then spontaneously be free to act rationally. This failed to take into account that psychological restructuring in the form of breaking old habits and forming new ones is a complex task. In this case, cognitive and learning theory is extremely important.

In contrast, the goals of action therapy seem too limited because they are based on a narrow and behaviorist conception of human life. Such learning theories have been developed from animal experimentation and have proved themselves most practical in dealing with subnormal intelligences, just as insight therapies are most successful with highly intelligent, verbal, and creative personalities. Learning good habits is not all there is to having an integrated personality. It is also necessary to develop an autonomous ego.

Thus, insofar as it is distinct from medical therapy, psychotherapy is not so much a process of healing a defective organic structure, as of reeducation, not at the level of fully rational behavior but at the level of automatic, conditioned, or subconscious behaviors. Its purpose is to free the individual from undesirable patterns of behavior, especially those that are inconsistent, so that rational free life becomes more possible. The criteria of successful psychotherapy of any type can be summarized as follows:

1. Relief of undesirable symptoms (e.g., excessive anxiety).
2. Increased productivity in the person's work.
3. Adjustment and satisfaction in sexual relations.
4. Better interpersonal relations.
5. Increased ability to endure the stresses of life.

The Empirical Validity of Current Models

Because all but the psychoanalytic school, and the ego psychology closely related to it, arose historically in opposition to Christian teachings, the first question that needs to be answered is whether psychoanalysis, today under severe criticism as scientifically unsound and therapeutically ineffective (Criticisms of Psychoanalysis: Bibliography 1999), has anything that needs to be retained in a Christian psychotherapy. The fundamental notion of psychoanalysis is that the ego is *defensive* against the id (Maddi 1996). The id is the basic, self-centered drive of the organism that "wants what it wants when it wants it, without regard for what other people may need, prefer or insist on." It is wholly "uncivilized," but is also wholly ineffectual in the external world and necessarily requires the ego to obtain its real satisfactions, which otherwise would have to be content with mere fantasies (primary processes).

Maddi (1996) shows that research has provided ample evidence that humans do in fact have defensive tendencies, but gives little support to Freud's view that all behavior is defensive. In fact, research shows that "some people do not appear to appreciably distort reality, even when pressured and threatened" (261). The later versions of the psychoanalytic model have attempted in various ways to mitigate the darkness of Freud's classical version of that model, but, as Maddi in criticizing them concludes, "Both versions of conflict theorizing [the psychosocial, classical model of Freud and the ego psychology model of Anna Freud, Erik Erikson, and the intrapsychic version of Rank and Jung and so on] adopt a tragic view of the human condition in which there is no singular, triumphant way to live" (264). Today, although there are still some twenty thousand psychoanalysts practicing in the United States, long-term psychoanalytic therapy has not demonstrated its effectiveness. Yet there are elements in it that are still viable and of practical value. Freud alerted modern thought to the complexity and obscurity of human thought and behavior, a truth, however, not unknown to past ages, as is evident from the words of the Hebrew prophet Jeremiah (17:9): "The heart is deceitful above all things, and desperately sick; who can understand it?" Cartesian rationalism, with its mathematizing notion of "clear and distinct ideas," had obscured this rather obvious truth that now in our postmodern age is being pushed to the other extreme.

The behaviorism model in its several versions stands in sharp contrast to that of Freud and his disciples, yet it too, at least in its radical version, is largely discredited. As our knowledge of what goes on in the brain and central nervous system and in the hormonal system is rapidly increasing, Skinner's refusal (1985) to include this biological and neurological data seems absurd. Consequently, Aaron Beck (2004) and others have turned to cognitive therapy (CT), which is based on a study of how the way people think influences their behavior and can be altered by learning experiences. This has also been integrated with behavioral conditioning techniques to form cognitive behavior (or behavioral) therapy (CBT). CT and CBT can be tested experientially not simply by the kind of pure introspection that Wundt unsuccessfully tried to employ but by observing verbal and nonverbal expression of thought in its relation to other kinds of also external behavior and stimulation. Thus these systems have been empirically validated in the treatment of a number of mental disorders. Most forms of psychotherapy have some degree of success, but a success more dependent on the skill of the therapists in relating to the client than in verifying the theoretical model of personality.

It should be noted, however, that as radical behavior therapy has given way to cognitive therapies, these therapies fit better into a humanistic model than into a behaviorist model of personality. If we grant that humans can learn to control their behavior by the way they think, it becomes evident that central to human personhood is the striving for the realization of its potentialities and even for creative transcendence of its present limitations. There has been a great effort in recent years to experimentally test all these different therapies.

Because the classical Catholic model of the human person considered both as to nature and to grace is obviously a fulfillment model, it would seem that at least it is not incompatible with present empirical data. What we must consider is both whether it adds anything to that model and whether it can also assimilate the verified features of the other models. The Christian model is sufficiently grounded in centuries of counseling experience and commonsense observation of human behavior as its consequences that such research will probably support that model and make it again generally available for therapists (McMinn 1991).

Monte (1999) sums up his own evaluation of current theories of personality thus: "No theory, in the present state of the art and certainly none of the so-called grand theories from psychology's history, can both comprehensively and irrefutably account for the wholeness, the uniqueness, for the universality of human propensities, foibles, drives, abilities and desires" (218).

Psychoanalytical methods are extremely time-consuming and expensive. Hence there is increasing reluctance on the parts of HMOs and government agencies to pay for such extended treatment whose outcome is difficult to evaluate. The action therapists have argued that the insight therapists have very little objective proof that their methods succeed better than natural processes; furthermore, the success they have seems largely independent of the mode of therapy and mainly dependent on the personal relation with a therapist who is a sensitive, realistic, and caring person.

The action therapists claim to have a better and more demonstrable record of success, but on examination, this success mainly appears in rather restricted areas of neuroses, and its permanence is often questioned. Furthermore, action therapy fails to achieve the ultimate aim of developing a strong autonomy in the patient. At present, it must be concluded that this type of problem is very complex, and knowledge about it and the ability to cure it still very limited. Nevertheless, therapy usually produces moderate improvement and sometimes is very successful. Perhaps this is not so different from any other area of medical care, or of ethical and spiritual guidance. It can never be stressed too much that all modes of therapy are only of service to facilitate the inherent power of human beings, as organisms and persons, to heal them.

Clearly, the goals listed by Wolpe (1966) and Harper (1959) are rather modest. Other therapists speak in terms of "the mature personality." These terms, however, as well as the popular "autonomous person," are ambiguous (Edwards 1981). If "mature personality" means that therapy extends to total development of the human person—that is, to the development of what once was called "the virtuous person," who is morally excellent and also spiritually profound and creative—this clearly goes beyond the psychological level and touches on the ethical and spiritual levels. It is true that some therapists, particularly those of the Jungian and existentialist schools (May 1983), have come to be not only therapists in the usual sense but also something similar to gurus or spiritual guides. Their work more closely resembles that of a philosopher, educator, or spiritual director than that of a health care professional. Although we do not deny the great value of the work of some of these persons, it seems that some limit must be put on the task of psychotherapy. Its work is complete when the person becomes psychologically normal (i.e., in a state of normal adult health). After this form of normality is attained, the individual should achieve even more growth in all the dimensions of human nature; however, guidance of this growth seems to exceed the work of psychotherapy and to demand ethical and spiritual counselors.

Drawing a Line

How, then, can this line be drawn? A look at the insight therapies provides the answer. Psychoanalysis, for example, is terminated when patients are sufficiently free to manage their own lives realistically, independent of the therapist, and are no longer hampered by unconscious motivations or self-deluding excuses that would prevent them from perceiving the world as it is; they can make free choices and carry them out effectively (Menninger 1958). In short, the patient now has a self-determining ego, which realistically recognizes its own emotional complexity, its innate needs, and its limitations. It also realistically recognizes the practical and human situations of life to which it must accommodate itself to satisfy its needs. This does not mean that all clients who terminate therapy will live their lives well in an ethical sense. A psychologically healthy person can, theoretically at least, also be an ethically bad person and a spiritually undeveloped person, but this is caused by his or her own free choices, not from compulsions imposed by personal background or social situation. At the point when the client can live by free choice, he or she no longer needs the therapist or therapy. Of course, a client may later regress under new stresses and have to return to treatment.

This notion of autonomy or freedom as defining the term *therapy* is not so acceptable to action therapists. Influenced by behaviorism, they often reject the notion of freedom altogether. Thus B. F. Skinner and his followers carry on a systematic war against the whole notion of human free will (Skinner 1971, 1976, 1985). As many critics (Gaylin 1973; Machan 1974) have pointed out, however, Skinner and other behaviorists unconsciously contradict themselves. They assert that the therapist can assist the client to behave more realistically, that is, as the therapist behaves. This makes sense if the therapist is free to choose between alternative modes of behavior for himself or herself and for the client, whereas the client, although still not yet free, wants to become free. This makes no sense, however, if both are equally not free and merely conditioned by their environment.

Therefore mental health is psychological freedom based on a realistic perception and understanding of the world. It involves self-understanding, self-consistency, and self-control. By self-control, however, we mean a realistic self-control, that is, one based on a realistic recognition and practical provision for one's intrinsic needs as a human being. Mental health must be considered before the ethical questions of moral right and wrong, because only when a person is free can there be a question of moral choice and moral responsibility.

Human Freedom

In view of the multidimensional and integral character of human personality, it is important to emphasize that no human being is totally free. Human freedom is limited (1) by innate biological structure, determined genetically, and by various accidents of development, with its innate needs or drives; (2) by unconscious conditioning of the sort already described and that therapy deals with; and (3) by one's knowledge of the world and self, set largely by the culture in which one lives, and the scope of one's experiences and education. Psychotherapy deals principally, but not exclusively, with limitations of human freedom that arise from the level of unconscious conditioning (Holt 1980).

At the psychological level, the area of freedom is very limited in the psychotic person who is out of touch with reality. Most psychotic persons, however, probably have some areas of freedom, at least sometimes; this is why they can be reached by psychotherapy or chemotherapy (as the case may be), which aim to gradually extend these free areas. Neurotic persons are decidedly more free but have some areas of nonfreedom that do not occur in normal persons. The normal person also has a limited area of freedom, but its limits lie near the level of the necessary determinisms of automatic and routine behavior that are compatible with normal freedom.

Also, the areas of freedom among normal individuals undoubtedly differ widely. Highly creative and adaptive persons have much greater freedom in their lifestyle than normal, but this freedom is limited in unimaginative, rigid people who operate best only in routine situations. Even here there is a question of whether therapy (e.g., of the Jungian type) may lead such people to greater freedom. Modern therapy has tended to move from the treatment of sexual neuroses, common as a result of the Victorian refusal to recognize basic biological needs, to the treatment of anxiety, as a result of excessive demands on a work-oriented society, which fails to recognize human needs for leisure and human intimacy (Masters and Johnson 1976; Masters, Johnson, and Kolodny 1986). Thus therapy deals more and more with neuroses of emptiness or lack of meaning as a result of society's failure to recognize the creative and spiritual sides of personhood. In all these cases, psychological therapy can only go so far to awaken the person's full capacity for freedom.

Freedom demands not only trust between persons but also within social groups. Recently, methods of group therapy are becoming common, not only because of the shortage of therapists but because mental illness is partly a disturbance of social relations and can be adequately treated only through learning social communication skills. In particular, family therapy, in which a family is treated as a dynamic system whose malfunction is reflected in the psychological problems of individual members, gives promise of a radically effective approach to many mental problems that originated in the family.

Such methods raise some special ethical issues, chiefly those of confidentiality and of adequate professional control. The frank communication required within the group can easily lead to an abuse of the privacy of individual members; if the therapist does not remain fully in charge and sufficiently sensitive to the needs of every member, some especially fragile participants may be more hurt than healed by the experience (Schmid et al. 1983). The therapist has the responsibility not to permit the psychological condition of any member of the group to be destabilized to a degree that the therapist is not willing or not able to see that it is resolved before the process is terminated, even if this means additional one-to-one sessions with the disturbed patient or at least proper referral for further therapy.

5.4 THE CHRISTIAN MODEL OF MENTAL HEALTH

How then do these current views of personality and its mental illnesses square with the classical Christian account of personality referred to in chapters 1 and 2 and that may be diagrammed as shown in figure 5.2?

First, we must insist that mental illness is not, as such, an impairment of the *spiritual* faculties of human intelligence and free will. The intellect is subject to error and the free will to sin, but because these faculties are spiritual and hence cannot be acted on directly by physical forces, they cannot be "diseased," except in a metaphorical sense. Yet because our human intelligence and will cannot operate without the instrument of the brain to supply the intelligence with the information we obtain through our bodily senses, these spiritual faculties can be inhibited and distorted in their action by illnesses, malfunction, or miseducation of the body, especially of the internal senses and the hormonal system. Mental sickness, therefore, has its source in the malfunction of the internal senses and human affectivity, as these prevent the intelligence from rightly perceiving reality and the human will from acting freely. Intelligence and free will can contribute by the refusal to face reality or to use one's power of rational control over bodily impulses.

Second, the classical Thomistic analysis of the human person resembles behaviorism in that it does not begin with introspection in the Platonic manner, but with the Aristotelian empirical approach in which one (a) proceeds from external *acts* (behavior), (b) to infer internal *powers* or "drives" by which these acts are performed, (c) to finally infer the structure of human *nature*. Introspection enters this analysis only insofar as this analysis takes into account that humans are self-conscious of their own acts, but this self-consciousness is manifest in behavior through communication with others by language and gesture. Our powers and nature, however, are not directly known, but only through the acts or behavior that manifest them.

Third, the classical analysis of the human powers based on such behavioral observation but without the techniques of modern controlled and statistical experimentation is surprisingly more revealing and exact than that of modern psychology, although it is supported by what modern psychology has established by such techniques. Note in figure 5.2 the clear distinction between the inanimate chemicals of the human body and the animate functions: (a) those we have in common with plants, namely, nutrition and growth; (b) those we have in common with animals, namely, conscious sensation and affective drives; and (c) those that are specifically human, namely, abstract intelligence and free will. Note also the distinction between cognitive powers and affective powers at both the animal and the strictly human levels. Furthermore, note the careful distinction of four types of internal sense cognition, often confused in modern terminology: (a) the sense *memory* that stores the images derived from the five external senses; (b) the *common sense* that combines the information from the five external senses into a complete image of some object; for example, our image of a dog is not only visual but includes

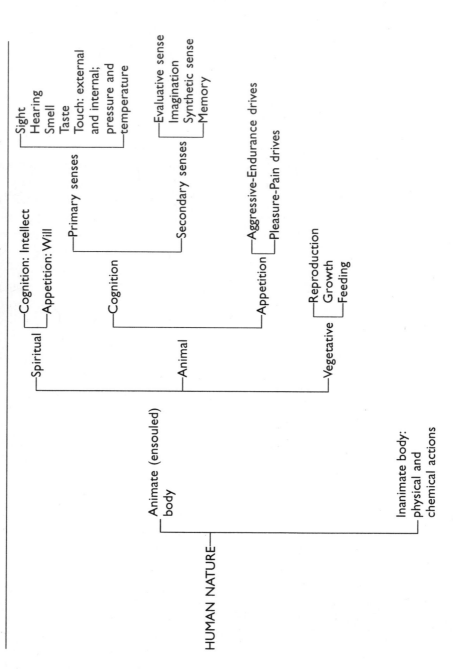

Figure 5.2   The Aristotelian and Thomistic Model of Human Personality

its bark, its smell, and the texture of its skin or fur; (c) the *imagination* that can recombine in a variety of ways the images provided by memory and the common sense; and (d) the *evaluative* sense (also called the *vis cogitativa*, instinct, animal intelligence, or discursive sense) that relates the images provided by the imagination to the affective powers so that they appear pleasant or painful.

This evaluative sense in animals is called "instinct" and is often, as for example, in the migratory instincts of birds, very remarkable. Animals have very specific instincts, although they can learn still more about pleasant or painful experiences; but in humans the instincts are very generalized in order to make possible greater flexibility in learning. Because this internal sense is directly related to the animal's affective drives by which it seeks pleasure and avoids pain or in spite of pain endures and fights against obstacles, it is very directly related to behavior. Current psychology, therefore, is largely a matter of dealing with the way our evaluation of experiences as painful or pleasurable, threatening or arousing to attack, has become distorted by trauma, whether from poor education, experiences of failure, or from the bad effects of drugs. Thus the Thomistic model fully agrees with modern psychology that healthy sense organs and especially a healthy nervous system and brain, which are the organs of the internal senses, are needed for mental health.

The Thomistic model, however, is much more explicit than modern psychology about human *freedom*. We discussed in chapter 2 that we are free because our intelligence can see the relation of alternative *means to a goal*. Animals act as a result of the evaluative sense (instinct, natural or trained), but by our intelligence we can transcend the judgment of the evaluative sense and attain an objective view of the relation of means to ends that is not limited to our instinctive drives or previous training. If this were not so, we could not create cultures, languages, science, art, and technological inventions, but like the lower animals would go on generation after generation within a very limited range of behaviors. Thus the damage of mental illness is above all that it restricts or even destroys our freedom, because we cannot be free unless our intelligence is served by a healthy evaluative sense that leaves the intelligence open to objective reality. At the same time, the restriction of freedom that results from mental illness lessens the responsibility of the sufferer, as we will see in section 5.5.

Fourth, Freud and not a few later psychotherapists have treated what is now called "spirituality" as a form of mental illness because it seems to be based on mere feelings or illusions. The term *religion* is often used to include both the ethical and the spiritual levels of human personality that figure 5.2 distinguishes. While the ethical is concerned with the choice of means appropriate to the goals of human existence, religion—although, of course, concerned with ethics—is primarily concerned with the nature of these ultimate goals. At this level, intellectual insight provides a vision of ultimate values, the realities that constitute the goals of authentic human living, while the will commits and moves the person to seek these goals.

Two mistakes are often made with regard to spirituality. Freud, who was a nineteenth-century materialist who, without being very scientific himself, put his ultimate faith in science, argued in *Totem and Taboo* (1913) and *Civilization and Its Discontents* (1930) that religion is a neurotic regression to the peace and security the child once experienced in its mother's womb. The mature, mentally healthy person, conversely, is ready to accept harsh reality in stoic resignation. While Freud's great disciple Carl Gustav Jung was able to give a more informed and positive psychoanalytical analysis of religion, he too confused intuitive knowledge with what he called the "collective unconscious." Many psychotherapists, both because of their narrowly scientific education and because they have often seen religion playing a sinister part in their patient's mental ailments, share with Freud this same prejudice against it.

Because spirituality relates to the ultimate goals that are central to human life, it is not at all surprising that mental illness often infects this life center with a neurotic, distorted religiosity. The schizophrenic, for example, who thinks he is God probably does not do so because he is deeply religious, but because he is deeply religious his schizophrenic illusions take a religious form, just as a schizophrenic soldier claims to be Napoleon. In particular, it is a mistake to think that the overwhelming guilt, scrupulosity, or anxiety that is frequently involved in neuroses is a genuine religious guilt. As Freud himself showed, neurotic guilt arises from the irrational superego, not from the mature, realistic ethics of a religious person who has achieved an objective self-understanding in terms of the ultimate goals of life. After all, who is more in touch with reality than maturely religious persons who live in the constant presence of ethical responsibility to their neighbors, of death, of judgment, and of the Creator?

Psychological studies of the Catholic saints often fall into either the error of reducing everything remarkable in their lives to mental illness or the other extreme of supposing everything in their lives was a sign of holiness. For example, we cannot be sure whether the inability to eat of the great St. Catherine of Siena was anorexia nervosa or a miracle of sustenance by the Eucharist alone (Walker 1987). Perhaps it was both. St. Therese of Lisieux seems to have suffered as a child from a hysteric illness, but as a young woman she faced death from very real tuberculosis with great courage and profound self-understanding (Görres 2003). The scrupulosity that St. Alphonsus Ligouri suffered to his dying day was perhaps due to an anxiety disorder, but he was a great church leader, scholar, and a very prudent counselor of others (Miller and Aubin 1940). Considering the complexity of human personality, mental disease is no less compatible with true human maturity than is physical disease. While mental disease is often a great obstacle to maturation, or to exercising one's maturity once attained, it can also become a source of maturation as a person struggles to overcome the limitations imposed by the illness. The biographies of great personalities often recount their struggles not only with physical disease but also with emotional problems that today we identify as mental illnesses.

Finally, the attitude of many modern psychotherapists toward ethics and religion fosters the tendency, exposed by Philip Rieff in his well-known book *The Triumph of the Therapeutic: Uses of Faith after Freud* (1968), to define the goal of psychotherapy not as true health but merely as "adjustment." Of course, it is often impossible for health care professionals to restore patients to true and perfect health, but they should never be satisfied merely with "adjusting" them to their life situation, which is in fact often itself sadly in need of healing. Even when a particular person suffering from illness or disability cannot be restored to normal life, the healing profession must work tirelessly to discover better remedies for future patients.

5.5 ETHICAL PROBLEMS IN MENTAL THERAPY

There are several problems that may arise in the process of mental therapy. In this section we treat two of the main ones: behavior control and codependency.

Behavior Control

Behavior control might be described as "getting people to do someone else's bidding." In this sense, behavior control has existed since the beginning of time. In the more restricted sense, however, and the sense in which we use the term in this section, behavior control is any medically indicated treatment, procedure, or process that is intended, with or without a person's consent, to cause a person to discontinue a personally or socially undesirable activity (Agras and Berkowitz 1988; Kerlanger 1986). As this description indicates, behavior control is not necessarily contrary to a person's intention or desires, but it signifies that some force over and above internal human motivation has been used in the interest of changing an activity pattern. The purpose of this control may be therapeutic (e.g., the use of drugs can sometimes actually correct a physiological malfunction producing abnormal behavior), or it may simply be aimed at controlling antisocial actions (Clark 1987).

For example, a person trying to overcome the habit of alcoholism may use Antabuse (disulfiram) to help conquer the habit. Although the use of this drug is in accord with this person's desire, it is still a form of behavior control. From an ethical point of view, behavior control has become a serious problem because of the increased efficacy of surgical procedures in controlling behavior, the vastly increased panoply of psychoactive drugs that modify emotional responses, and the increased tendency to impose conforming societal norms. Not only are these procedures comparatively new but also they are swift and efficient, and their effect on a human person can be deep and lasting. Thus they have greater potential for good or evil than many of the techniques of scientists and physicians in the past centuries. Also, a temptation exists to attempt the solution of problems by altering the person rather than attempting to transform the social environment.

Given these examples of behavior control and modification methods that are prevalent and becoming more common every day, we suggest several ethical principles that should govern their use and which require that social control enhance the dignity of the members of the community, not reduce them to mere means of political manipulation (Ingleby 1980).

1. No form of treatment may be used that will destroy human freedom. Pius XII (1952) stated this well when he wrote,

   In exercising his right to dispose of himself or his faculties and organs, the individual must observe the hierarchy of the scale of values and within an identical order of values the hierarchy of individual goods to the extent demanded by the laws of morality, so, for example, man cannot perform upon himself or allow medical operations, either physical or somatic, which beyond doubt do remove serious defects or physical or psychic weaknesses, but which entail at the same time permanent destruction of or a considerable lasting lessening of freedom, that is to say, of the human personality in its particular and characteristic functions. (no. 371)

   Thus any form of psychosurgery, personality manipulation, or use of psychoactive drugs that would remove or severely limit human freedom or destroy human personality could not be permitted and may need legal control (Guydish and Kramer 1982; NIH 1985).

2. If the purpose of the behavior control is therapeutic, the benefit to the patient must be the purpose of the action, and the damage or risk must be accidental to the therapeutic action. A frontal lobotomy, for example, should be performed only as a last

resort and with some indication that there will be an overall benefit for the patient. Above all, lobotomy and ECT should not be considered as ordinary treatments for prisoners and others who have displayed antisocial behavior. As a general rule, signs of organic brain pathology should be present before psychosurgery is approved.

3. If the purpose of the treatment is therapeutic, the long-term effect of the treatment must be considered as well as the short-term alleviation of some particular difficulty. Simply because a particular therapy alleviates or eliminates a symptom does not mean that it is ethically acceptable. Most of the drugs currently available for the relief of anxiety and tension carry some danger of dependency, habituation, and addiction (Freedman 1991; Lehmann 1979). Such dependency diminishes human freedom and dignity and thus is to be avoided. Therefore the very theory prevalent in the United States of using psychoactive drugs to treat psychological difficulties when the disorder lacks a physiological or organic basis must be questioned. Would it not be better to treat the causes of anxiety or depression through counseling or increased self-awareness rather than to depend on pills, which merely treat the symptoms? Questions such as this are fundamental in developing a philosophy of health care, and they are too often neglected in search of easier, but less beneficial, solutions.

4. If behavior controls are used, the rules of free and informed consent apply, including the right to refuse treatment (Gallant 1983; Gilbert 1981; Levine 1983). Thus operant conditioning, psychoactive drugs, and psychotherapy should not be inflicted on competent people or imposed on them (Annas 1989; Turnquist 1983). If they are incompetent, the norms for proxy consent for therapeutic treatment should be followed (Eth, Levine, and Lyon-Levine 1984). Moreover, children, prisoners, and people with a limited sense of awareness should not be subjected to experimental behavioral control, nor should proxy consent be given unless the treatment is truly therapeutic for them (Sprague 1978).

5. Professional confidentiality must be applied with special care in psychotherapy, because the trust of the patient in the therapist is of fundamental importance, even in group therapy or where peer review of the psychiatrist's performance is necessary (Arnstein 1986; DeKraai and Sales 1984; Schmid et al. 1983).

6. Experimental research on behavioral control should conform to the norms explained previously in the section on human experimentation (chapter 4, section 4.6).

7. Use of behavioral control procedures to improve human capabilities such as memory, intelligence, and sexual abilities would seem to be licit if free consent is given, if there is no other way to achieve the same goal, and if the action is in accord with the integrity of the human person. In itself, human betterment, or human improvement, is ethically acceptable and beneficial. Care must be exercised, however, to make sure that the basic integrity of the human person is not violated and that addiction does not result in the course of seeking self-improvement (PCB 2003).

8. Using alcoholic beverages or even psychoactive drugs for relaxation or pleasure is not in itself ethically wrong provided that freedom is not notably restricted. Such substances used moderately might provide needed and legitimate relief from the everyday strain and tension of life. Because there is a great tendency to abuse the use of drugs, however, even to become dependent on or addicted to them, and because of the potential bodily harm resulting from some drugs, great care is required in the use of any behavior-modifying substance for recreational purposes.

Given these general norms of respect for the human freedom of the mentally distressed, certain special ethical issues require attention.

Codependency

For patients whose psychosis is less "all embracing" and for neurotic patients, not only action therapies but also the insight therapies are feasible. The use of insight therapies, however, has raised a whole series of ethical problems (Moore 1978; APA 1981) that in the twenty-first century remain still largely unresolved. The first concerns the process of therapeutic transference (Marmer 1988; Menninger 1958). Psychoanalytic therapy depends in some measure on the dependence of the patient on the therapist for the duration of treatment. This dependency mirrors the child-parent relationship and involves not only trust but also, at least sometimes, an element of erotic love. Without this profound dependency, patients are not sufficiently freed from their anxieties and inhibitions to let themselves become conscious of their true motivations. The termination of therapy is indicated when the patient becomes sufficiently autonomous and under self-control that he or she no longer needs the therapist. He or she has become a healthy adult who still loves his or her parents (therapists) but no longer needs them.

This vulnerability of patients obviously invests therapists with special ethical responsibilities. The first of these is that therapists must not violate the trust placed in them (Schmid et al. 1983). This requires that a therapist carefully maintains professional secrecy, be truly concerned for the patient, be prompt in appointments, and be reasonably available for consultation. It means also that therapists are honest with patients and do not lie to them or break promises. Furthermore, the therapist must avoid all manipulation of the patient in the sense of seeking personal gratification from the treatment rather than seeking the patient's benefit. The therapeutic relation requires dependency of the patient but not codependency of therapist and patient. This does not demand that the therapist have a superhuman objectivity; rather, it simply means that the therapist must be worthy of trust.

Clearly, this excludes the therapist from having sexual relations with the client—although some have defended this as possibly therapeutic (Gartrell 1986). The idea that the therapist could engage in such relations merely for the patient's sake seems unrealistic, and the risk that the patient will then or later view it as exploitation is all too real. The principles of ethics adapted by the APA are clear in specifying that sexual relations between psychiatrists and their patients are unethical (APA 1981, 1986a, 1986b).

Some have raised the question as to whether it is permissible for patients to enter into therapy if they risk falling seriously in love with the therapist. It should be emphasized that the danger here seems no greater (and perhaps more consciously avoided) than the danger of a patient's falling in love with his or her medical doctor. The relation is rather that of parent to child than that of lover to lover, and its excessive erotic investment is the mark of the illness from which the patient is already suffering rather than its consequences. This risk seems no greater than the patient's coming to hate the therapist and seeking to harm him or her, as has sometimes happened.

A second issue sometimes raised by Catholics is whether the process of abreaction is not dangerous, because the patient in free fantasy revives the memory of former temptations or sins, of illicit sexual activity, or of hostility and destruction. Is it legitimate to again put oneself in the "occasion of sin" where sinful consent is possible? Similarly, some object to the process of abreaction, especially in the case of nondirective therapy, because the therapist may permit the patient to engage in objectively wrong actions. Such dangers may occur in therapy, but they are usually the result of poor therapy. The purpose of psycho-analytical abreaction is precisely to return to some sin or mistake of the past where the patient failed to resolve a problem correctly and to help the patient now face it in a clearer light. It is not likely that patients engaged in the therapeutic process will actually consent to what they consciously reject just because their rejection now becomes fully conscious. Also good therapists do not encourage their patients to act out their neuroses (Ornstein and Kay 1985). Even in psychodrama or venting of feelings, the reenactment is precisely a dramatic one, that is, a "make-believe" in which it is essential to the therapeutic process that it not be a real, freely willed activity. If the patient acts out a neurosis, it is generally recognized that this reinforces the neurosis rather than liberates the patient from it.

Changing the Patient's Value System

Perhaps the most controversial issue of all regarding psychotherapy is whether the thera-pist is permitted to change the patient's value system (Block, Chodoff, and Green 1999; Rokeach 1973). The common answer is that a therapist should not change this system but should try to adjust the patient to the present system. This answer, however, is somewhat disingenuous. As the existentialist psychoanalysts have pointed out, distortions in the patient's value system often underlie the disorder. Furthermore, the source of many prob-lems is what Freud called the patient's superego, that is, the value system of the parents or society that has been incorporated in the child's unconsciousness. Here lies the source of all the issues raised by the antipsychiatrists. Is therapy simply the adjustment of patients to the disordered value system of the society in which they live? Alternatively, if the psycho-logical and ethical dimensions of human personality are distinct, as we have argued, it clearly cannot be the role of the therapist to indoctrinate the patient in the therapist's value system.

In answer to this difficulty, we must say that there are certain values on which the very relation of client to therapist depends, and these must be reinforced by therapy (Clements 1983). Thus the therapist must help the client to become more trustful, more honest, more hopeful, more courageous, more patient, and more realistic. Such values are common to most recognized ethical systems, whether religious or philosophical. The therapist must adhere to these values and should not be reluctant to strengthen them in the client. If cli-ents submit voluntarily to therapy, they freely accept these values no matter how unfree they may be in other respects. This is the small area of mental health and moral virtue that must become the basis of recovery. Therapists teach these values primarily by their example in their relations to clients as they attempt to establish satisfactory therapeutic transferences. Consequently, the importance of a genuinely personalist education for psy-chiatrists is even more important than for other physicians (Light 1980).

The effort of the therapist is thus to extend the area of freedom for patients (Bartoli 2003). As patients become freer, they must make some unhampered ethical decisions and will do so according to their own conscious, rational system of values. At this point, the therapist is nondirective in the sense that it is not the therapist's task to give the patient ethical advice, but only to help the patient be free of illusion and neurosis in making de-cisions. This requires great delicacy and objectivity on the part of the therapist. Sometimes the therapist thinks that the client's decisions are not ethically good, objectively speaking. In such a case, the therapist may point out that the client's decisions are questionable or refer the client to an ethical counselor (clergyman, lawyer, friend), but the therapist should be careful not to take any responsibility for the client's decision. Thus the therapist ought to refer the client to ethical or spiritual advisers if it becomes apparent that the client's value system is inconsistent or inadequate.

Philip Rieff in his book of 1968, *The Triumph of the Therapeutic,* raises a deeper problem as mentioned earlier and by others. Is it possible that the whole system of insight therapy as it originated with Freud has a built-in system of values or ideology that it inculcates? Many have accused psychoanalysis of being essentially a product of the middle class in opulent capitalist countries. They argue that it has taken on the political function of adjusting this middle class to a social system riddled with inherent contradictions. Freud (1930) himself, as we have already noted, saw all of civilization as the imposition of social controls on human beings' infinite and even contradictory drives. Consequently, Freud held that every social system is a delicate balance between the repressive controls necessary for social life and work and the explosive drives of the id. In capitalist countries, as Rieff shows, the abundance of goods and the impersonal shape of social organization contribute to a much greater permissiveness, a society in which all types of behavior (between "consenting adults") is tolerable. Others, such as the proponents of radical sexual therapies, argue that as this permissiveness spreads, it will lead to social revolution.

Rieff predicts that we are embarking on a "therapeutic society" in which the "therapeutic man" will become typical. Such a person, whom Rieff pictures as the type successful psychoanalysis actually produces, is one who lives for a constant succession of intensely satisfying experiences, without any drive to realize some plan of life or some ultimate goal. Daniel Yankelovich (1998) calls this "expressive individualism," although he believes that it is beginning to yield to a great communitarian attitude. A person who is an expressive individualist is highly autonomous in the sense that he or she feels no guilt about seeking personal satisfaction in every situation, leaving the others involved to take care of themselves. Such an individualist is capable of satisfying intimate relationships but does not depend on any particular person for achieving these; thus he or she can move from one relationship to another without any sense of loss or feeling of guilt for infidelity.

If Rieff is correct, and certainly very different interpretations of the goals of psychoanalysis are given by Erik Erikson (1978), Erich Fromm (1975), Rollo May (1983), and others, the inherent ethic of psychoanalytical theory is to produce autonomous, hedonistic, goalless, conscienceless persons—the very sort ethicists have always condemned as selfish, loveless, and empty. Such persons are uncommitted to any social goals except the achievement of freedom to do what they please. Rieff's interpretation of psychoanalysis emphasizes Freud's belief that civilization, that is, social life, is always repression, not fulfillment, of fundamental human needs—a necessary evil. If this is the whole picture, it is difficult to see how a Freudian ethics could ever be compatible with a Christian value system. It is essentially an ideological defense of the style of life of those who profit from capitalism and who use their analysts to quiet their guilt.

Alan Bloom, in *The Closing of the American Mind* (1987), describes contemporary college students in terms similar to those employed by Rieff. Bloom finds his subjects, dominated by relativism, highly self-centered, and devoid of commitment to family, religion, or country. Although Bloom attributes the causes of this malaise to many different factors, he does maintain, "Once Americans had become convinced that there was a basement to which psychiatrists have the key, their orientation became that of the self, the mysterious, true, unlimited center of our being. All our beliefs issue from it and have no other validation" (160).

These accusations, offered by Rieff and Bloom, are very serious ones. They demand the following:

1. The community of therapists must make a serious examination of social conscience and a purification of the theory, training, and practice of therapists, who must become conscious that the goals of therapy must be related to higher social and spiritual goals.
2. Clients should trust their therapists not as omnipotent fathers, but only for their limited skills. Clients also should receive guidance at the ethical (political and social) and spiritual levels from others as soon as they become sufficiently free emotionally to do so (Van Kaam 1986).

Thus persons undergoing therapy should not change their system of values, divorce their partners, give up their religious vocation, or change their religion or their professional vocation merely under the influence of psychotherapy. The tendency to erect one of the many forms of therapy (including the various mystical cults now so popular) into a religion is a violation of the lines between the psychological level of personality and the ethical and spiritual levels doomed to end in disillusionment (Vitz 1994; Browning and Cooper 2004).

In recent years, some of the Protestant and Catholic clergy and members of religious orders have discovered the value of psychotherapy and have come to place an excessive faith in it to meet all the needs of people for counseling, to the detriment of their confidence in the value of their own special roles as ethical and spiritual guides (Murnion 1984). They have become preoccupied with getting in touch with their feelings, getting freed up, or developing a capacity for intimacy, and some have deserted the celibate life, the priesthood, or the ministry to become psychotherapists themselves so that they might "really" help people. The U.S. Jewish community has experienced a similar phenomenon, where psychotherapy has become a widespread substitute for the religious discipline of the Torah; the therapist has taken the place of the rabbi, and Freud the place of Moses.

Undoubtedly, religious people and the clergy in particular have sometimes been in real need of therapeutic experiences to correct an excessively repressive religiosity that disregarded their human emotional needs. Too often such persons have been discouraged from obtaining needed psychotherapy by the false notion that although morally good people may be physically ill, they cannot be mentally ill. Nevertheless, profound self-understanding and choice of one's life vocation require an exploration of the self that goes even deeper than psychology can penetrate and where ethical and spiritual guidance is of great value. Needed are ethical and spiritual guides who genuinely appreciate the contributions of psychotherapy to human wholeness but who pursue their own roles with a sense of their own mission. There is an important analogy between psychotherapy and spiritual purification, but it is an analogy, not an identity (Van Kaam 1986).

Addictions

Generally speaking, addiction or dependency is habituation to some practice harmful to the subject. Although the term *addiction* usually refers to habituation to drugs, one can also be addicted to other detrimental substances or activities, such as alcohol, tobacco, coffee, and excessive food, as well as too much sleep, too much work, and pursuit of sexual pleasure (Francis and Franklin 1988). Many people use all these things in ways that do not destroy human equilibrium, but some persons, for a variety of reasons not fully understood, become addicted to them. Their whole life is more and more absorbed by a single activity that distorts the personality, consumes physical and psychic energy, and often results in an intense self-centeredness, personality deterioration, and inability to communicate with others. Addiction or dependency on drugs and alcohol is more likely to result in such extreme symptoms. Thus this section addresses those addictions that are often referred to as "chemical dependency."

In 2001, 5.9 million Americans were using illicit drugs, about 7.3 percent of those were twelve or younger, and 5.4 percent were using marijuana, .07 percent cocaine, 1.5 percent pain relievers, and .07 percent tranquillizers. In 1999 deaths from such abuse reached 19,102 (legal and illegal drugs). Most were slow to seek treatment; abusers averaged fourteen years of use before entering treatment for the first time (SAMHSA 2002). Episodes requiring entrance into a hospital emergency department in which drug abuse was involved in 2002 were 1,100,539. This problem of addiction with its tragic personal and social effects is not confined to drug abuse but extends to all matters in which physical pleasure gets out of control, whether with regard to the ingestion of material into the body or the use of sex or the pleasures of acquisition and competition. In chapter 2 we showed that traditional ethics discussed this life problem under the heading of the cardinal virtue of Temperance or Moderation, which is fundamental to the whole life of virtue. Drug abuse, however, also causes physiological changes and can be so violent as to severely limit human freedom. The chemically dependent person soon comes to feel compelled to use a drug not simply for pleasure but for *relief* from a sense of painful deprivation. Moreover, the relief achieved becomes less as the addiction progresses so that larger doses become necessary to achieve the same result. Addiction thus involves a destructive *cycle* of behavior. The addict feels compelled to have a "fix," but the relief soon wears off and leaves an increasing profound sense of depression that is often worsened by feelings of guilt and shame as the person realizes their enslavement. Then, driven by this pain, the addict again resorts to the drug and the cycle continues and worsens. This cycle often ends in death, but in the meantime the addict's health and ability to live a normal life has decreased, he or she may have taken up crime to attain the enslaving substance, and human relationships to family, work, and society have been destroyed. This is, of course, the worse scenario, but even when addicts survive for years, their addiction really harms the quality of their life and prevents them from attaining their potential.

Addictions are often initiated by the bad example of associates who assure the beginner that a little experimentation is harmless. They can also arise from self-medication without the advice of a physician. The development of an addictive personality can be fostered by one kind of pleasure, which when recognized as dangerous, is then replaced by another equally or even more harmful. This is because the addict has become habituated to finding relief from sadness, "tension," or the stress involved in responsible and realistic decisions by seeking a pleasant oblivion from care. Thus the sexual indulgence of masturbation, which adolescents so easily experiment with, cannot only itself become an addiction but may set an addictive pattern of life that leads to other addictions later. Addictive patterns can also be found in uncontrolled aggression, as in gambling, competition in work, avarice, and a sadistic harming of animals and persons (Nakken 1997).

The ultimate and only fully satisfactory remedy for addiction is the acquisition of the virtue of Temperance, which places the pleasure drive under the control of the realism of a prudent, reasonable way of solving life's problems. As shown in chapter 2, natural temperance is acquired by practice and the use of an asceticism that resists indulgences, and this natural virtue is supported and elevated by the gift of a corresponding virtue in baptism and deepened by the other sacraments. The most effective treatment method for drug addiction is the famous Twelve Step Program (Humphreys 2000), practiced by support groups of 2 million Alcoholics Anonymous (AA) members in 150 countries, founded in 1935 by an addict, Bill Wilson, and Dr. Robert Smith. Wilson had attended meetings of the Oxford Group, which is now Moral Re-Armament, founded in England by a theologically liberal and social justice active minister Frank Buchman (1878–1971), but he was also influenced by writings of Carl Jung and William James's *Varieties of Religious Experience*, which he read while hospitalized for his addiction. In Akron, Ohio, on a business trip, he was about to enter a bar when he had a sudden inspiration that he might be cured by helping some other alcoholic. The twelve steps that he subsequently developed are the following:

1. We admitted we were powerless over alcohol—that our lives had become unmanageable.
2. Came to believe that a Power greater than ourselves could restore us to sanity.
3. Made a decision to turn our will and our lives over to the care of God, *as we understood Him.*
4. Made a searching and fearless moral inventory of ourselves.
5. Admitted to God, to ourselves, and to another human being the exact nature of our wrongs.
6. Were entirely ready to have God remove all these defects of character.
7. Humbly asked Him to remove our shortcomings.
8. Made a list of all persons we had harmed, and became willing to make amends to them all.
9. Made direct amends to such people wherever possible, except when to do so would injure them or others.
10. Continued to take personal inventory and when we were wrong promptly admitted it.
11. Sought through prayer and meditation to improve our conscious contact with God, *as we understood Him,* praying only for knowledge of His will for us and the power to carry that out.
12. Having had a spiritual awakening as the result of these Steps, we tried to carry this message to others, and to practice these principles in all our affairs.

AA has for sixty years proved its effectiveness, but its religious orientation, although theologically vague, has aroused opposition by secularists and presents some legal problems for government sponsorship. This has led to a countermovement called Rational Recovery (Trimpey 1997) that emphasizes self-help and independence from support groups and employs cognitive therapy, but whose effectiveness relative to AA remains to be established. One aspect of AA, however, requires special comment. It has made popular the view that alcoholism is a "disease" and that to emphasize this assists addicts by somewhat diminishing the social stigma of their addiction. Yet, although there is evidence that there may be genetic dispositions to this "disease," and it is certainly true that persons sometimes slide into addiction without full responsibility and that once addicted their culpability is greatly diminished, nevertheless, the moral aspect of addiction should not be ignored. In fact the Twelve Steps, at least, implicitly acknowledge this need for repentance. Every vice diminishes responsibility, but it is still a vice if it was incurred by deliberate actions against moderation. Thus alcoholism or any addiction is an illness only in relation to the physiological changes that, whether deliberate or not, result from the immoderate use of an addictive substance. Because such addiction originates in the human need for a moderate amount of recreative pleasure, a culture needs to promote healthful forms of recreation.

The use of drugs in the treatment of pain under professional supervision seldom leads to addiction. It is, however, also a responsibility of medical professionals to note signs of addiction in all patients and even to consult with their friends and relatives to get the addict to seek rehabilitation. This is not the place to discuss the question of public policy about governmental efforts to curb addiction and the drug trade. Prohibition did little for the elimination of alcoholism, and it is not clear that our antidrug laws work well either. The main effort therefore should be education of the public regarding the dangers of drug abuse and the provision of adequate treatment. It should be recognized, moreover, that drug abuse is promoted by poverty and homelessness and in turn augments these evils. Public policy, encouraged by the medical profession, must aim at breaking this vicious cycle.

One component of chemical dependency, and the most obvious, is its hedonistic character, although persons who are in other respects very ascetic may fall victim to it, precisely because they lack healthy pleasures in their lives. In the face of every difficulty of life, every tension or frustration, the chemically dependent person runs away from the loss of normal satisfaction and achievement by indulgence in the physical pleasure, relaxation, and euphoria of the addicting experience (Vaillant 1984). This search for pleasure, however, does not of itself constitute addiction; it also involves the increasing sense of guilt and helplessness that begin to accompany the addict's overindulgence. The result is that the incipient addict begins to indulge not for the sake of pleasure itself, but to blot out the guilt and remorse for the consequences of previous indulgences. Furthermore, this vicious circle is reinforced by the use of psychological coping mechanisms of rationalization and denial that victims need to suppress guilt and pain, so that they become increasingly unable to perceive the real consequences of their behavior. Alcoholic persons, for example, frequently suffer from blackouts, repression, and delusional euphoric recall that so distort their memory that they actually have a very incomplete picture of what is happening to them.

Addiction and Personality Types

Persons of very different personality types can become addicted, but a common feature is excessive dependency needs, sometimes masked by outward aggressiveness and competitiveness. Moreover, as addiction progresses, it tends to produce a pattern of behavior that overrides all temperamental differences. At one time addicts were thought to come mainly from the poorer classes (Barber et al. 1973), and undoubtedly addiction is common among some socially depressed groups. Recent research demonstrates, however, that chemical dependency can affect people of all backgrounds. Often gifted, talented, wealthy, and successful persons succumb to this severe personality problem (Smart and Murray 1985).

Chemical dependency or addiction may be broadly classified as physiological or psychological. Physiological addiction, which causes a modification or need in the addict's physiological system, usually requires increasing doses of the addicting substance to obtain the same physiological effect. Moreover, in physiological dependence, withdrawal from the object of dependency, for example, heroin, results in severe physiological disturbance, even death, because the body has become so adapted to the presence of the substance in the system that it cannot function without it (Kosten, Rounsaville, and Kleber 1985). In physiological addiction, however, the psychological component predominates; thus persons who lack this component can sometimes use even so highly addictive a drug as heroin without exhibiting the typical features of addiction. Psychological dependency itself results from a learned conditioned behavior pattern that leads the victim to anticipate the pleasure and release of tension, even when the substance does not notably modify the physiological system (Khantzian 1985).

Is this to say that the sense of moral guilt felt by the addict is merely neurotic? On the one hand, therapists speak of addiction as a "disease" in order to reduce its moral opprobrium and to achieve a more sympathetic attitude on the part of nonaddicts. On the other hand, an important part of therapy is to get addicts to accept moral responsibility for the harm they have done themselves and others through addiction. This ambiguity can be cleared up if two points are kept in mind. First, chemical dependency is always a psychological disease because it involves an abnormal behavior pattern accompanied by the neurotic coping mechanisms already described. It can also be a physiological disease because it sometimes produces physiological dependency and usually produces widespread organic changes that greatly aggravate the condition. Second, voluntary acts must be distinguished from free acts. Addictive behavior is voluntary in the sense that it proceeds from an inner compulsion, but it always involves a restriction of freedom, because the addict becomes less and less able to perceive alternatives of action or to choose among them. In times of addictive need, the practical conscience of the addict is concerned totally with the need for a drink or a fix. He or she acts voluntarily, compulsively, but without free choice.

Thus actual consumption of addictive substances by addicts is seldom in itself a morally culpable act, and the guilt felt afterward is unrealistic and neurotic. Even the acquisition of the addiction often proceeds so gradually and subtly that it is difficult to judge that the addict knowingly and deliberately chose addiction. Nevertheless, it would be a mistake to think that the whole guilt felt by addicts is illusory. If it were, it would be difficult to explain why admission of responsibility has proved so important a part of therapy. The truth seems to be that the real moral responsibility of the addicted person lies in the obligation to ask and receive help from others when this is offered, as therapy cannot be effective until the addict accepts help. Acceptance does not take place all at once but passes through stages: (1) admission into treatment, (2) compliance with treatment (with hidden defiance and resistance), (3) acceptance or recognition of real need for health (with unrealistic anticipations of cure), and (4) surrender, that is, realistic acknowledgment and acceptance of the responsibility for lifelong change. Thus it is a mistake to reduce this complex situation either to a purely moral question or to a purely sociological or medical one. To deny all moral responsibility or capacity to change is to degrade addicts as persons, yet to pass judgment on their degree of responsibility is to misjudge the many ways in which they are victims of forces beyond individual control.

Treatment outcome studies in alcoholism indicate that a variety of treatment programs yield benefit and may be cost-effective; however, few studies exist that differentiate which programs are best for which types of patients. "So far the outcome literature reflects that patient factors such as having a stable family, stable job, less sociopathy, less psychopathology, and a negative family history for alcoholism are more powerful predictors of positive prognosis than is type of treatment" (Francis and Franklin 1988, 320).

Family Intervention

Students of addiction emphasize that the earlier in the addiction therapy begins the better, but they also point out that family and employers often contribute to the problem by covering up, excusing, or attempting to endure addictive behavior, hoping that the addict will finally come to his or her senses. This spontaneous self-insight by addicts is very rare, and family, friends, and employers have a serious ethical responsibility to face the facts realistically and intervene decisively and persistently until the addict accepts treatment. Intervention is best done by those who can be supportive rather than judgmental, but who can also face the addict with detailed evidence of the seriousness of his or her condition.

Health care professionals sometimes are impatient with and contemptuous of alcoholics and other addicts, whom they regard as delinquents rather than as victims of illness. Such attitudes are intensified by unwarranted pessimism about the effectiveness of therapy. This is especially unfortunate because health care professionals themselves have an especially high rate of chemical dependency, caused not only by their relatively easy access to drugs but perhaps also by the ethos of the profession. This maximizes guilt feelings over breaches of professional standards, while doing little to support persons who may have high dependency needs, which they mask under professional self-assurance and pride. Therefore, it is important for professionals to acquaint themselves thoroughly with the nature and therapy of addiction, the ways of intervening to get addicts to accept treatment, treatment centers to which they can be referred, and ways to support them in their new life (Bissell and Royce 1987).

Perhaps an even more effective way for health care professionals to combat chemical addiction is through preventive measures. They can play an important role in combating the mentality in the United States that seems to predispose people for substance abuse and addiction (Miller 1983; National Institute of Drug Abuse 1986). Americans seem to think that every pain, every sorrow, or every frustration can be overcome with a pill, potion, or injection of some type. Pharmaceutical firms constantly push drugs through advertising, and health care professionals often are used by such agencies to promote unnecessary drug use. Christian professionals will not share in this promotion because they realize that human pain, frustration, and sorrow simply cannot be suppressed. Human beings grow as persons by facing the difficulties and struggles of life realistically, "bearing one another's burdens" (Gal 7:2) as free people, not as slaves to a pleasure ethic. In saying this, we are not proposing an exaggerated stoicism as the Christian ideal, but a realistic effort to overcome the real causes of suffering rather than an escape into unconsciousness. AA, which has led the way to the most successful methods of therapy for chemical dependency, has always emphasized that the addict cannot recover without a reaching out to a higher power and a willingness to repair damage done to the neighbor and to be of service to the neighbor.

We can sum up this section by repeating that mental illnesses often have a biochemical basis and that with the use of proper medications many of these conditions can be controlled. This has produced a revolution in the treatment and understanding of large groups of mental illnesses. Psychotherapeutic medications require that patients take them at adequate doses for a sufficient period of time; otherwise their effectiveness may never be realized. Also, some of these medications may have an addictive potential. However, the incidence of any addictive problems is quite rare when the medications are being properly used.

All medications have side effects, but these should not dissuade someone from using these medicines in their proper doses. The potential benefits of these medications far outweigh the possible side effects. Doctors usually proceed with an adequate trial of a particular medication in each patient to determine if it in fact produces relief from the undesired symptoms. Remember that side effects are not seen in most people who take these medications, and many of the side effects that occur early in the treatment often lessen or disappear as time passes. Also, when the medications work, people report that they gladly put up with minor side effects as the price they must pay for other therapeutic effects. The lists of side effects does not mention the percentage of people getting every side effect, and many times the incidence of a side effect can be the report of just a very few people. Also, some of the side effects are dose related or the result of a mixture of drugs, and sometimes the appearance of some side effects indicates that an adequate amount of the medication is being used. Some side effects require that the drug be stopped. Other side effects do not. Great care and clinical experience are needed in order to determine exactly what is causing a side effect. Any questions about side effects must be discussed with the prescribing physician.

5.6 CONCLUSION

For many years, psychiatry and religion were at odds with one another. Leaders in both fields criticized and cast doubt upon one another and the disciplines they represented. Although a few pioneers of psychology such as William James treated religion sympathetically, others such as Sigmund Freud treated religion at best as an illusion that society would some day outgrow. Similarly, theologians and philosophers often expressed a distrust of psychology and psychiatry that bordered on outright hostility. More recently, however, these opposing disciplines work hand in hand. For example, in an effort to encourage mental health professionals to view the religious experience of patients more seriously, the *DSM-IV* (APA 1994) includes a new entry titled "Religious or Spiritual Problems." By recognizing religious problems as a category of concern distinct from any mental disorder, the revision reflects a move away from earlier tendencies among psychiatrists to treat religion as a delusion or a neurosis.

On the side of religion, movements toward reconciliation have also been realized. In 1994, Joseph English, M.D., then president of the APA, led a delegation to meet with Pope

John Paul II. Dr. English asked the Pope to help overcome the myth that the mentally ill, even the homeless, suffer because of moral failure (Steinfels 1994). In fact historians have shown that, even in the Middle Ages, the distinction between mental disease and sin was recognized (Kroll and Bachrach 1984). On the part of the Catholic Church, Pope John Paul II took full account of psychology and psychiatry when writing encyclicals and moral exhortations. Thus in the encyclical *Veritatis splendor* (1993, 33) he said, "A number of disciplines, grouped under the name of the 'behavioral sciences,' have rightly drawn attention to the many kinds of psychological and social conditioning which influence the exercise of human freedom. Knowledge of these conditionings and the study they have received represent important achievements which have found application in various areas, for example in pedagogy or the administration of justice." Yet the Pope insists that the psychological and cultural limitations on human freedom do not remove the responsibility that all but the seriously psychotic have to seek greater freedom and to use it ethically. When mental therapies of any type are employed, their aim should be the enhancement of human freedom to make realistically informed and conscientious decisions.

Chapter Six

SUFFERING AND DEATH: A THEOLOGICAL PERSPECTIVE

OVERVIEW

THIS CHAPTER CONSIDERS SUFFERING AND DEATH, two concomitant realities of health care and medicine, from a theological perspective. We begin by considering the response of health care professionals to suffering and death, analyzing the phenomenon of fear of death from the viewpoint of Christian spirituality. In the present era we use two different sets of clinical signs to determine that human death has occurred: irreversible cessation of cardiopulmonary function and the criteria for brain death. Hence the ethical evaluation of brain death is considered. Next we discuss the responsibility in Christian care for the dying and dead person of truth telling and respecting the remains of the person after death has taken place, then we consider the ethical distinctions between suicide, euthanasia, and allowing to die and study various aspects of this last-mentioned reality. Finally, we consider patients who are in a permanently vegetative state (PVS), as well as the problem of pain.

6.1 MYSTERY OF DEATH

From time immemorial, human beings have viewed suffering and death and asked, Why? Why would a loving God allow people to suffer? Why would God allow a child to be born with Down's syndrome, or allow the father of a large family to undergo a mental breakdown, or allow a mother to be taken from her growing family when others, aging or without children, are left untouched? People both wise and callow have questioned the meaning of suffering and death since the beginning of time. In the Jewish and Christian traditions, some insight has been gained over the centuries concerning these concomitants of human existence (Lewis 1943; Kraemer 2000). Some of the knowledge and understanding is found in the scriptures; much of it is in the oral tradition of churches and families. However, suffering and death remain mysteries—mysteries that will never be unraveled clearly and completely in this life—because they are bound up in the intimate life and love of God. Admitting that suffering and death are mysteries that cannot be solved fully in this life may seem to be a denial or delimitation of the human desire and power to know the truth. Actually, it is not a denial of human potential and aspiration; rather, it is an admission that human beings are incapable of knowing everything and that God plays a very important part in the life of any individual person or any group of persons.

To say that suffering and death are mysteries does not take them out of the realm of human investigation, nor does it mean that we should stand in helpless awe of them. After all, some of the great moments in human history are the results of efforts and success in conquering illness and disease. There is, however, a point beyond which human beings cannot go. Suffering will never be eliminated as long as humanity continues, and each person must die. These ultimate truths are testimony to the power of the Creator, with whom humankind cooperates in the genesis and continuation of the human race, but who in the final analysis is the only ruler of the world, the Lord of the universe (John Paul II, 1979).

"Death was not God's doing; he takes no pleasure in the extinction of the living. To be—for this he created all" (Ws 1:6–14). "God had not wished to include suffering and death in man's destiny" (Pius XII 1944). What our Creator willed was that we should exist in his image and thus enjoy the gift of knowing the truth and having the free will to choose to live by it. From where, then, came suffering and death? St. Paul says, "Through one man sin entered the world, and with sin death, death thus coming to all men inasmuch as all sinned" (Rom 5:12; cf. also Aquinas 1920, I–II, 164, 1). Sin is the free choice of what we know is really contrary to our true nature and happiness but through which we prefer to achieve some apparent but ultimately false satisfaction.

Original sin was essentially a sin of pride, the will to be like God, not by using God's gifts to come closer to God in community, but to use these gifts to set up the human individual in self-centered domination of the world apart from God (*Summa Theologiae* I–II, 83, 3). It is this misuse of God's gifts from the beginning of the human race to this day that has prevented humankind from overcoming the natural causes of suffering and death. It is "original" not only in that it began with the first humans but also in that now every child comes into the world influenced from its conception by the physical and moral effects of all the sins of human history. This misuse of human freedom also introduced into the world countless social evils and transformed natural death, which might have been a joyful completion of this life and a serene passage into a greater life, into a blind, terrifying mystery.

Human injustice has produced a world where the environment is polluted and where poverty and war spread disease and death. Thus it is plain that in large measure human suffering is the result of human folly. God has not punished the human race by blasting the Earth with suffering like a thunderbolt from heaven, he has simply left us as a community to suffer the consequences of our own folly in hopes that it will finally awaken us to accept our responsibility to restore and preserve the good world God created for us and which we have made a world of suffering.

Suffering as Punishment?

"But does that mean that if I am sick, I must have sinned?" That is a question that many sick people ask in moments of depression, and their distress is increased by their fear of guilt. Of course, in some cases in fact our sickness is the consequence of our own misbehavior, and God permits us to suffer the consequences of our own misuse of his gifts. If we are sick because of drug abuse, gluttony or laziness, sexual promiscuity, or recklessness, then in all honesty we must admit we brought this on ourselves. If we are personally responsible for our suffering, we must then admit our responsibility and turn to a merciful God to help us repair our lives. But, as the Bible dramatically pictures in the Book of Job, innocent people also suffer and die. The birth-injured or genetically defective child, the hemophiliac infected by HIV blood, hard-working men and women exhausted by caring for their families—certainly such suffering is not a punishment from God. Yet it is ultimately a consequence of human sin, not of any sin of the victim, but of our human community past and present that could have prevented these tragedies or remedied them.

Human intelligence if properly used can ensure that the innocent cease to suffer from the sins of others. The innocent child is not responsible for being abused, but society is responsible for not rescuing the child. It is this responsibility that inspires all our efforts at medical research. We have already found remedies for many of these evils and can make progress in overcoming more. As we have misused God's gifts and brought suffering to the innocent, so we can also use these gifts of intelligence to repair the harm we have done. To have the patience and wisdom to repair the consequences of sin, however, we need the grace of God. Thus health care professionals play an important role in God's redeeming work, together with Jesus Christ, the Healer, the conqueror of sin and death.

Even when people have turned their backs on God, he has not turned from them but has offered them forgiveness and restoration. In his mercy, however, God cannot deny their human freedom but has called them to return to him, not simply by restoring them to their innocent beginnings, but by a long history of struggle and learning from experience, an experience in which suffering is inevitable. For the Christian and for all who travel by less clearly marked paths, God has revealed in Christ the direction of their journey and the power of grace by which it can be traveled (Melina 2002). In baptism, according to St. Paul (Rom 6:1–11), through the cross of Christ humanity has died and been reborn in a new creation that will be completed in the resurrection of the body in eternal life. Human beings live now in such unity with Christ that all the events of their lives take on meaning from his life and death. Consequently, both the joy and the suffering of this life have a Christian meaning: its joys are signs of the hope for everlasting life in his kingdom, which is already present here on Earth in promise, and its sorrows are a sharing in his cross through which a victorious resurrection is to be achieved.

Jesus came to Earth to conquer suffering and death. In what sense has he succeeded? People still get sick and continue to suffer, and death is inevitable. He conquered sickness, suffering, and death in the sense that he inspired us to overcome the evils that spread suffering and death. Even when we cannot escape suffering Jesus gave it a new meaning, a new power. By believing in Jesus as Savior, by joining our suffering and death to his, humankind overcomes their evil (Sheehan 2000). Although the results of original and actual sin are still present in life, they no longer dominate it. Rather, suffering and death are transformed into the very actions that help humankind fulfill its destiny.

Death is defined as the separation of body and soul, but it can be more than that. In their attempts to specify more clearly what it means to die, modern theologians have concentrated on death as a personal act of a human being, an act that terminates earthly existence but also fulfills it (CDF 1979). Thus the person is not merely passive in the face of death, and death is different for the just than for the sinner. In the view of Karl Rahner (1965), a view accepted and developed by many theologians, death is an active consummation, a maturing self-realization that embodies what each person has made of himself or herself during life. Death becomes a ratification of life, not merely an inevitable process (Boros 1965). It is an event beyond our control, yet also a personal act in which the freedom of the person is intimately involved. Dying with Christ is an adventure; it is a consequence of, but it need not be a condemnation for, sin. This is a new approach to death, yet it is thoroughly in keeping with the Christian tradition. Indeed, this view of death seems to describe more clearly the experience of Christ, who offered his life rather than have it taken from him, who completed his love and generosity in the final act of obedience to the Father: "It is consummated" (Jn 19:30). Not only pastoral care personnel but also those in other fields of the healing profession will enrich their own lives and the lives of their patients if they are able to communicate this notion of death.

This mystery of death has recently been exemplified for us in the suffering and dying of Pope John Paul II. As his successor Benedict XVI said of him in his funeral homily (2005):

> He interpreted for us the paschal mystery as a mystery of divine mercy. In his last book, he wrote, "The limit imposed upon evil 'is ultimately Divine Mercy.' And reflecting on the assassination attempt, he said: In sacrificing himself for us all, Christ gave a new meaning to suffering, opening up a new dimension, a new order: the order of love. . . . It is this suffering which burns and consumes evil with the flame of love and draws forth even from sin a great flowering of good. Impelled by this vision, the Pope suffered and loved in communion with Christ, and that is why the message of his suffering and his silence proved so eloquent and so fruitful." (706)

6.2 FEAR OF DEATH

Because health care professionals are human, they tend to retreat from any phenomenon that causes fear or wonder (Perez-Carceles et al. 1999). Death is such a phenomenon; it involves awe, fear, and mystery. For this reason, health care professionals, just as other people, are tempted to avoid facing the evil of death. The result of this fear has been studied by perceptive observers E. Becker (1973), Dekkers (2001), and Jansen (2003). When health care professionals are controlled by fear, they often deceive patients as to their true condition and neglect their need for understanding or comfort. Moreover, the occasion for personal spiritual growth is lost for both the patient and the health care professional, and the opportunity to help another human being prepare for death and eternal life is lost as well. Studies show that too many health care professionals retreat and cut themselves off from the dying patient completely (Doka, Rushton, and Thorstenson 1994). To put it another way, dying is not only a biological process but also a psychological process that involves the health care professional as well as the patient.

To overcome fear and to help people die well, the health care professional must learn to handle the emotional strain that accompanies suffering and death and to deal with the ethical dilemmas sometimes encountered (O'Brien 2001). Although many helpful books on these topics are available, some clinical training in this area is also necessary. Every hospital staff should include people who specialize in the care of the dying. Their purpose is not only to help the dying patient work through fear, anger, and depression but also to help the members of the healing team participate in the event of death in a way that is helpful for themselves (Burge et al. 2000; Lynn 2001). Otherwise health care professionals, no matter how well educated or technically expert, will suffer psychological harm from their constant involvement in death. Is the high rate of alcoholism, suicide, and divorce among health care professionals in some way connected with stress over their inability to express their grief and sadness at the constant sight of death (O'Connor and Spickard 1997)?

Given the power and prestige of the health care profession, acknowledging the importance of God in human life, the mystery of his presence as evidenced through suffering and death, is an important step in humanizing that profession. To accept limitation is to accept one's humanity. Health care professionals who assume a position of unlimited power in the process of healing have an outlook that is unrealistic. They think of themselves as the persons who cure, rather than realizing that it is God who cures and health care professionals who cooperate in this work by using the forces of nature.

Those who must deal with the dying have three options: (1) They can ignore the dying patient and thus become hardened and jaded, (2) they can relate to the dying patient in a sincerely personal manner without knowing how to deal with their own feelings, or (3) they may relate to the dying patient in a healthy way, recognizing the psychological strain that patient and professional undergo together. Taking this last option can teach a professional to value the experience of helping another fellow human being suffer and die in Christ, either with explicit Christian faith or perhaps simply with an openness to the mysterious future, which is the effect of Christ's grace in those who do not know him except under some other name or symbol. Few health care professionals, however, will be able to achieve this healthy, healing attitude without special training in the art of working with the dying (Bennet 2001).

The Art of Compassion

In learning this art of the care for the dying, three points should be kept in mind. First, because suffering and death are obstacles to the fullness of life that Christians affirm, we have not only the right but also the duty to try to overcome or mitigate them. Thus Christians should strongly favor medical research to conquer disease and to preserve and prolong life, for example, the crusade to eliminate heart disease and cancer or to make the environment more healthful. Medicine as a profession, as a science, and as an art has a Christian birthright of service. St. Paul, himself a miraculous healer, could say paradoxically (Phil 1:22–25),

> For to me life is Christ, and death is gain. If I go on living in the flesh, that means fruitful labor for me. And I do not know which I shall choose. I am caught between the two. I long to depart this life and be with Christ, [for] that is far better. Yet that I remain [in] the flesh is more necessary for your benefit. And this I know with confidence, that I shall remain and continue in the service of all of you for your progress and joy in the faith.

Second, efforts to overcome the evils of sickness and suffering by medical science have not eliminated the healing role of prayer, which is also a part of the Christian heritage. Jesus healed physical as well as spiritual ills and commanded his followers not only to preach but also to heal and drive out demons (Mk 3:14–15). The reference to demons indicates the forces of evil that must be overcome for complete human healing in all the dimensions of the human person, spiritual and ethical, as well as psychological and physical; these forces are greater than merely human intelligence, even with the aid of science, can ever hope to achieve. Thus to complete human healing necessitates turning to Jesus Christ, who, having died himself and risen, has conquered sin and death and who is the source of all healing powers, even those provided by modern medicine. Therefore health care professionals striving to help the suffering and the dying need to pray for and with them.

Third, although sickness and suffering have entered the world through sin, they are not themselves sinful, nor is the one who is suffering always the same one who has sinned. Jesus suffered because of the sins of others, and this is also true of innocent persons today. Again St. Paul says, "Now I rejoice in my sufferings for your sake, and in my flesh I am filling up what is lacking in the afflictions of Christ on behalf of his body, which is the church" (Col 1:24). Thus health care professionals should see the sick as victims rather than as responsible for their own condition, unless in fact this responsibility is obvious. Even if they are in fact responsible, sick persons must then be helped to understand the forgiving mercy of God by which the road of hope is always open. The real problem of caring for the suffering and dying, therefore, is to help them realize that they can bring good out of evil by making their painful and frightening experiences a means of personal growth and a witness of courage to others who someday will have to meet the same test. The current situation of patients with acquired immunodeficiency syndrome (AIDS) emphasizes the importance of helping patients to approach death with a sound theological outlook. Although the situation of AIDS patients may be hopeless in regard to their physiological condition, the mercy of God is always open for them. Caregivers should help AIDS patients realize that they have not lost their human dignity (Duggan 2002).

Christian health care professionals will best succeed in this difficult task if they themselves understand suffering and death in terms of the suffering, death, and resurrection of Jesus Christ, which provides the only help in living hopefully with this mystery. Many health care professionals feel utterly defeated by the death of patients whom they have cared for and by the helplessness of even their best efforts in many cases to restore normal health. Only Christian hope has an answer for that despair. The sign of the cross in Catholic hospitals stands for this profound attitude of hope (Bernadine 1995).

Clearly, it takes more than words to accomplish this transformation of suffering and death. One must be willing to surrender to God through the person of Jesus Christ every day if one wishes to give new meaning and power to suffering and death. The small deaths one dies every day prepare a person for the larger and more important deaths and finally for the ultimate moment of meaning and power. Nor can we forget the wise warning of St. Paul that although we ought not judge each other, "We shall all stand before the judgment seat of God" (Rom 14:10), because he who gave us the precious gift of freedom has in justice a right to require us to use it well. To refuse to face this fact is the final foolishness.

The perfection of Christian suffering and death is to ask God's mercy and accept it with hope and joy. This is not possible unless one works at it faithfully, relying on the unfailing grace of God. To communicate to patients effectively the meaning and power of death, health care professionals must have some experience of its reality themselves. Thus health care is more than a job, more than knowledge and technique. Basically, in its fullness it is a way of life that sees beyond the hurt, the sickness, the anguish; a way of life that enables one to look beyond the drudgery of daily reality, beyond the suffering in the hospital ward and the emergency room; a way of life that centers in God's love for his children, his ability to bring good out of evil, the suffering of Christ for all human beings, and his victorious resurrection.

6.3 DEFINING DEATH

When biologists speak of the death of any living organism, they refer to that inevitable and critical moment when an organism ceases to function as a specific, unified, homeo-static system and becomes disorganized into a mere collection of heterogeneous chemical substances (John Paul II 2000; DeGrazia 2005). Sometimes, however, even after this moment, some tissues or cells or even organs of the former organism may continue temporarily to carry on some independent minimal life functions. Thus recently a pregnant woman diagnosed as brain-dead was kept artificially in a condition in which the child in her womb was able to develop to a healthy, although premature, delivery by a Caesarian operation. If she was in fact brain-dead, this is possible because in complex organisms the various organ systems have a relative autonomy, which continues to function only briefly without unification by the brain, unless artificially supported. Thus from a biological point of view, the death of a human organism is similar to any death and is determined in much the same way, by various signs that the unifying life functions have ceased.

Yet the death of a human person is not just a biological event. Human death has a mystery about it because at death we lose touch irrevocably with a person who previously was able to communicate and to share our human community of thought, of love, of freedom, and of creativity (Kung 1984). Human death is not merely a decay of an organism; it is the departure of a member of the human community. People all over the world have interpreted this departure of someone known and loved as the separation of a spiritual principle of life from its body. Science cannot close the door on such an explanation. Christians believe that the departed will return in their bodily personhood in a transformed existence, as Jesus did (Lk 24:36–43).

In any case, people often have the painful responsibility of determining when the death of another has occurred, because the time of death influences many other human decisions, such as inheritance, legal and moral rights possessed by the dying person, spiritual care for the dying person, and possibility of organ transplantation.

Dying is a process, but death is an event (Corr, Nabe, and Corr 2000). We can be certain this event has not yet occurred as long as a person can communicate through speech or gesture. When such communication ceases, we can only judge by signs that are no longer distinctly and specifically human. We do not dare conclude, however, that death has occurred merely because such specifically human signs are no longer evident, as becomes very clear when we observe someone wake from sleep or coma.

Consequently, we are morally obliged to treat anybody who is apparently human (even in the fetal state) as a human person with human rights until we are sure that this body has become so disorganized that it no longer retains its human unity. To know this, we must be reasonably sure of three facts:

1. that the body does not now exhibit specific human behavior,
2. that it will not be able to function humanly in the future, and
3. that it no longer has even a minimal capacity for human functions because it has lost the basic structures required for integration of human functions, bodily and spiritual.

The third condition is required because medical experience has shown that persons who have been in apparent coma nevertheless have sometimes recovered human consciousness (CHA 2005; Carey 2005). Such resuscitation is possible as long as the essential structures of the human organism remain and the causes that inhibit their normal function can be removed.

At the same time, there is no reason to deny that after true human death some cells or even organs of the human body may for a time (perhaps indefinitely if artificially supported) continue to exhibit some life functions. These functions are not those of the human organism as a unified entity, but merely a residual life at a level of organization comparable to that of plants and lower animals. Thus the essential point about determining human death is not to decide whether *any* kind of life is present, but whether human life in the sense of a unified human person is still present.

Some signs of human death were always easy to identify in the past. If rigor mortis or putrification occurred, even nonprofessionals were able to recognize that the human organism was irreversibly destroyed. Other less conclusive signs of human death were the absence of breathing and heartbeat, although it was known that these might sometimes be revived by such methods of resuscitation as were then available. When such efforts failed, death was judged certain. Physicians were required to pronounce the patient dead on the basis of such evidence and certify the time of death for legal purposes such as inheritance. Thus irreversible cessation of spontaneous heart and lung function became known as the *clinical* signs of death.

New Clinical Signs of Death

In recent years, two developments have led to the proposal of a new set of clinical signs for determining human death (Furton 2002): First, machines have been perfected that artificially aid the function of the heart and lungs or that enable a person to be resuscitated after the heart and lungs have ceased to function for a short time. Often people recover full and spontaneous heart and lung function as a result of being temporarily assisted by such machines, proving that the essential structures of the unified human organism had not been destroyed. Alternatively, such machines may be able to maintain heart and lung function for a considerable time, even after this unity of the organism has ceased to exist, as the heart completely separated from the body can continue to beat, just as tissues in a test tube can continue to exhibit some residual life if nourished by an appropriate solution.

Thus such artificially sustained heart and lung action is not proof that human life still remains, yet as long as they are sustained, it is difficult to verify the traditional signs of human death. Therefore the following question has been posed: Are there other clinical signs that can be used, not to constitute a new definition of death, but rather as alternative criteria to establish the same essential fact, namely, that human life is no longer present because unified human function is not present and cannot be restored (Bernat 2001; Gallagher and Wijdicks 2001)?

The second, and perhaps more important, reason for seeking new clinical signs of death has been the recent advancement of techniques of organ transplantation (Dubois 1999a). Such transplants are more likely to be successful if the organs are retrieved from a body through which blood continues to circulate. Thus transplant surgeons prefer to keep the cadaver of a dead donor on a respirator and thus maintain cardiac function.

How, then, is it possible to be sure that the donor is in fact dead? First, the traditional cardiovascular clinical signs are basic and sufficient and should be utilized if possible when determining death. The new brain-death criteria, assessing function of the whole brain, should be employed only when traditional signs cannot be used because the dying person is dependent on a respirator or other form of artificial maintenance. In our opinion, patients in many cases are left on a respirator too long and thus must be declared brain-dead when a simpler determination would be possible. If brain death were permitted to become the exclusive criterion for human death, no one would be judged dead without elaborate tests in a hospital. Present moral dilemmas about how to determine death are caused largely by excessive reliance on technology, and that excess should be moderated rather than encouraged (Karakatsanis and Tsanakas 2002).

Second, well-trained professionals must ascertain the brain-death criteria. Human error and even carelessness must be anticipated and avoided. How can such errors be prevented when human life is at stake? Most criteria for brain death require more than one clinical observation of the patient. In the first set of criteria used to certify brain death, the "Harvard criteria," the observations were separated by twenty-four hours. At present, six to twelve hours between observations is considered sufficient (Wijdicks 2001). Moreover, persons applying the clinical criteria for brain death must be trained to recognize such conditions as hypothermia and drug-induced coma, which may produce a condition from which the patient can recover (Canada Law Reform Commission 1981). Other safeguards require that the physician who certifies death should not be a member of a transplantation team that might be overanxious to pronounce the donor dead. In some cases, the opinion of more than one physician is required before brain death is determined. One way or another, fail-safe procedures must be built into the process of using brain functions as the clinical signs to ascertain human death.

Third, and most serious, is the question about the nature of brain death itself (John Paul II 2000, 2004a; Pontifical Academy of Sciences 1985). It is critical that the criteria used to certify brain death establish that the person is dead, not merely dying or in a deep coma. Although the medical profession has accepted the general idea of using the activity of the brain as the main criterion in some cases to establish human death, exactly which specific signs should be used to determine that the total brain no longer functions have not been agreed upon by all (Halvey and Brody 1993). For the most part, the criteria center on clinical observation, such as response to pain, cerebral function, brainstem reflexes, and testing for apnea. These clinical observations are often confirmed by electroencephalogram (EEG) or blood-flow studies.

Controversy about Defining Death

The variance in opinion as to the validity of brain-death criteria primarily results from theoretical issues. Thus one group of physicians maintains that cessation of neuronal activity in the brain is not sufficient to signify human death unless the cessation is proved to be irreversible and indicates destruction of all cerebral function (Shewmon 2001; Byrne et al. 2000; Byrne 2005). We have considered these arguments in the section on transplantation (chapter 4, section 4.4). This argument seemingly has been obviated by studying the circulation of blood in the brain by means of an angiogram or isotopes rather than by using an EEG to study neuronal activity. If the angiogram establishes that blood no longer circulates into the brain, the brain is dead because there remains no way to restore activity to the brain when circulation ceases. The lack of blood circulation in the brain may also be proven through newer methods of imaging. Hence, when the whole brain is dead, the person is dead, because the organ that is the source of unified activity no longer functions, even though there may still be signs of residual cellular activity in the brain and other parts of the body.

Although it is not our purpose to settle any differences of opinion in regard to medical matters, we conclude that when total and irreversible function of brain activity is clinically proved, the person in question is dead because the form (soul) is no longer able to inform the matter of the body (Furton 2002). To date, many states have approved this method of discerning human death in so-called definition of death legislation, and the need for national legislation in this regard has been recommended. The legislation of the various states requires that the signs indicate that total, not merely partial, death of the brain has occurred (UDDA 2005).

Would it be possible to declare a person dead if only some part of the brain, that is, the higher or neocortical centers on which specifically human thought processes apparently depend, did not develop fully or ceased to function? This view was defended by some in the past who desired to use anencephalic infants as organ donors before total brain death occurs or who maintain that such infants may be aborted in the third trimester (Holzgreve 1987). While this opinion received support from the American Medical Association (AMA) Council on Ethical and Judicial Affairs (1994) for a time, eventually a substantial number of physicians objected to this opinion and it was later withdrawn.

While the tendency to declare that a person is dead if only the brain stem is functioning is not prominent in contemporary society, there is a tendency to declare that persons with impaired brain function have no rights or moral standing (Persson 2002). To refute this attitude, Pope John Paul II (2004a) declared:

> I feel the duty to affirm strongly that the intrinsic value and personal dignity of every human being do not change, no matter what the concrete circumstances of his or her life. A man, even if seriously ill or disabled in the exercise of his highest function is and always will be a man. . . . Even our brothers and sisters who find themselves in the clinical condition of a vegetative state retain their human dignity in all its fullness. The loving gaze of God the Father continues to fall upon them, acknowledging them as his sons and daughters, especially in need of help. (no. 3)

Therefore, although we accept total brain death as a sufficient criterion for human death, we do not believe that partial brain death is sufficient to declare that a person is dead or without moral standing. We do not believe that death should be certified as long as patients are able to maintain *spontaneous* breathing and heartbeat, because this constitutes strong evidence that the brain, as the seat of the essential unity of the human body, is still living, even if it is not evidencing its higher functions.

6.4 TRUTH TELLING TO THE DYING

"What to tell the patient" has been considered one of the more difficult and delicate ethical questions for health care professionals. Modern communication theory has shown that successful transmission of information from one person to another depends on good emotional relations between the communicators. Hence the importance of trust between patients, their families, and health care professionals. In past generations, some health care professionals thought that the less patients knew about their condition, the better would be the chances of recovery. In some cultures, this attitude still persists (Fainsinger, Nunez-Olarte, and Demoissac 2003). Moreover, some health care professionals would even withhold information of impending death, fearing that such knowledge might lead a person to despair. Because of an awakened moral sense by health care professionals and a sharper realization that patients have legal and moral rights that must be respected, today there is a much greater tendency to be open and honest with patients concerning their condition (Giesen 1993).

In general, patients have the right to the truth concerning their condition, the purpose of the treatment to be given, and the prognosis of the treatment (Annas 1998). This honest communication of diagnosis and prognosis is especially significant in the face of death. Clearly, information concerning serious sickness or impending death is to be furnished even if the individual does not ask for it. Legal precedent as well as moral concern prompts this honesty and frankness with persons who must prepare themselves for death. Thus physicians and other health care professionals may not defend their lack of communication on the grounds that the patient did not wish to know and did not ask questions. In some hospitals, a patients' representative helps patients understand their situation, especially when surgery is anticipated. Whenever possible, the leader of the health care team, not excepting the physician, should be involved in explaining the situation to the patient. *The Ethical and Religious Directives for Catholic Health Care Services* (ERD) declare: "Persons in danger of death should be provided with whatever information is necessary to help them understand their condition and have the opportunity to discuss their condition with their family members and care providers. They should also be offered the appropriate medical information that would make it possible to address the morally legitimate choices available to them. They should be provided the spiritual support as well as the opportunity to receive the sacraments in order to prepare well for death" (2001, D. 55).

Difficult Situations

Although health care professionals usually respect the rights of patients insofar as providing the proper information is concerned (Gordon and Daugherty 2003), difficult situations often arise, and health care professionals hesitate to tell patients their true condition (Elger and Harding 2002). In these cases the words of Dr. Eric Cassell (1976) are still relevant:

"The depression in patients that commonly occurs after the diagnosis of a fatal disease seems to stem in part from the conspiracy of silence. The physician can be a great help by simply making it clear to the patient that he is available for open and direct communication" (19). Interviews with seriously ill patients indicate that they do not want to be kept unaware of their condition. However, it is never helpful to inform patients in a brusque manner; they do not want painful information revealed to them in an abrupt or brutal manner. According to Dr. Elisabeth Kubler-Ross, who was the first person to expound the importance and technique of helping patients with terminal illness understand their situation (1969), "When we asked our patients how they had been told, we learned that all the patients knew about their terminal illness anyway, whether they were explicitly told or not, but depended greatly on the physician to present the news in an acceptable manner" (183). Howard Brody (1981), reflecting on this difficult situation, aptly assessed the practical solution when he stated,

> [T]elling a patient something takes place over a span of time and is not a one-shot affair. Thus, the shading of phrases used, whether the truth is delivered all at once or in small doses, and the kind of follow-up are all important parts of the ethical decision, as well as "tell" or "don't tell."
>
> A decision to reveal a grave prognosis, which may be "ethical" in itself, may become "unethical" if the physician tells the patient bluntly and then withdraws, without offering any emotional support to help the patient resolve his feelings. In fact, the assurance that the physician plans to see it through along with the patient, and that he will always make himself available to offer any comfort possible, may be more important than the bad news itself. In many of the "sour cases" that are offered as justification for withholding the truth, it may well be the absence of this transmission of compassion, rather than the telling of the truth, that produced the unfortunate results. (40)

Because physicians are not always able to convey information concerning serious illness or impending death in a fitting manner, every health care facility should have a trained pastoral care person trained in the dynamics of helping patients accept sickness, suffering, and death, and when they are open to the Gospel, in a Christian manner. The value of these pastoral care persons working closely with health care professionals is evident. On the one hand, crisis counseling is not an arcane art, but on the other hand, one must be adequately prepared to perform it well. Well-meaning but untrained people can do more harm than good when trying to help in crisis situations. Kubler-Ross maintained that to help others face death one must be at peace with death oneself. The normal training for health care professionals, and often for religious ministers, does not prepare persons well for this type of care. Several hospitals in the United States, however, have training programs to meet this need. The need for this service in hospitals is clear and has been recognized, but help in facing sickness and death is also necessary for people in noninstitutional settings, such as for the poor and elderly. In summary, increased knowledge of psychology and greater regard for the subjective process that accompanies sickness and dying has changed the ethical question in regard to truth telling. As Kubler-Ross declared: "The question should not be 'Should we tell?' but rather, 'How do we share this with the patient?'" (1969, 183).

6.5 CARE FOR THE CORPSE OR CADAVER

When a human being dies, the body is no longer vivified by the life-giving principle, form, or soul by which it was constituted a substantial element of the human person. The cadaver of a person, then, is no longer a *human* body in the proper sense of the word. As St. Thomas Aquinas explains (*Summa Theologiae* I, q. 89), the person is a living union of soul and body, and the spiritual soul, although it is naturally immortal and hence survives the body, cannot be called in the strict sense a "person" until at the Resurrection its own body is restored to it. Thus a dualistic conception of the human soul as simply "clothed" with a body that at death it dispenses with is very mistaken. While existing in this life, the human person is a substantial unity of spirit (form) and body (matter), not an accidental juxtaposition of two distinct entities. The remains of a human body may resemble the body of a living person, and this resemblance may be prolonged through embalming; however, the remains are not a *human* body, but a mass of organic matter, decomposing into constitutive, organic elements.

If the corpse of a human person is not a human body, why are people so concerned about proper care for the remains of the deceased person? Why treat the remains of a human body with the respect and reverence that it usually receives? Respect and reverence are due the remains of a human being because of the sacredness of the person who once was associated with the now inert mass, which are the remains of the person. For the Christian, the Orthodox Jew, and the Muslim this body will also be reunited with the human soul in the Resurrection and thus become eternal. As St. Paul says, "For just as in Adam all die, so too in Christ all shall be brought to life" (1 Cor 14:21). Jewish piety is expressed in the Old Testament book of Tobit, in which Tobit relates how one evening he was eating supper when news came of a man murdered in the street: "I sprang to my feet, leaving dinner untouched, and I carried the dead man from the street and put him in one of the rooms, so that I might bury him after sunset. Returning to my own quarters, I washed myself, and ate my food in sorrow. . . . And I wept. Then at sunset I went out, dug a grave, and buried him" (Tobit 3:4–7). And this concern is expressed in the New Testament by the account of the care of the holy women and Joseph of Arimathea for the body of the crucified Jesus (Lk 23:50–56).

But even for those who do not share this faith in bodily resurrection, to mourn the person who will no longer be present in the same human manner as before, certain reverential actions are performed, which express the love of the people who remain. Respect for the dead body, then, signifies respect for human life, respect for the Author of life, respect for the person who once existed in human form and who will exist again in the transformed body. Thus the actions and ritual that people follow when caring for the body of a deceased person have a meaning beyond their mere utility.

Although the commercialization of wake, funeral, and burial has been criticized for its excesses (Mitford 2000), the ritual care of the dead retains its meaning and worth in accord with the Judeo-Christian tradition. Having family and friends pray for the deceased and share the burden of sorrow through liturgical services is also a source of strength and support for bereaved people. Thus the legitimate customs of people at the time of death are not signs of superstition or blind fear; rather, they bespeak a noble belief about life, its purpose, and the enduring strength of human love.

In the Judeo-Christian tradition, respect for the dead was usually displayed through burial of the corpse in the ground or in a mausoleum. Cremation of the remains, although not a common part of this tradition, has never been considered a disrespectful treatment. For a long time, however, cremation was forbidden in the Catholic Church because anti-Christian groups in the eighteenth century advocated cremation as a means of denying symbolically the immortality of the human person and the Resurrection. Thus, not because it was immoral in itself, but rather because of what it might signify, cremation was not an acceptable form of caring for the remains of a person in the Catholic Church.

Because cremation is no longer associated with a denial of immortality today, although burying the dead is encouraged as the usual procedure, the discipline has changed, and according to the Revised Code of Canon Law (CIC 1983 [2000], c. 1176) the total remains of a person or an amputated member may be cremated if there is a serious reason (CDF 1963). For example, if a person or family determines that cremation is a suitable means of caring for the body, if the custom of the country favors cremation, if there is danger of spreading disease, or if suitable gravesites cannot be obtained at a reasonable cost, cremation is legitimate. If the request involves no certain sign of disrespect for Christian faith, cremation may be requested by a dying person or the next of kin. Those who direct that their bodies be cremated, then, may be given the sacraments of the Church, as well as liturgical rites of burial, provided that the latter are not performed in the actual place of cremation.

Autopsy

Autopsy is the examination of a cadaver performed to provide greater medical knowledge concerning the cause of death. Occasionally, the benefit of an autopsy will be to provide knowledge about a rare or contagious disease. In such cases, the good of the community would overrule the rights of the next of kin, and if the next of kin were not willing, the court could order that an autopsy be performed. In cases of violent death or unattended death in the United States, an autopsy is required by law, no matter what wishes are expressed by the next of kin.

Usually, however, the purpose of an autopsy is neither to trace the etiology of a rare disease nor to discover unknown or violent causes of death. More frequently, autopsies are performed to help health professionals achieve a higher level of efficiency in the care of the living (Haque 1996). The autopsy rate of a hospital is usually a good sign of concern for excellence and offers a gauge of professional integrity and interest in scientific advancement. Through autopsies, the diagnosis and treatment a person received can be evaluated and staff members encouraged to observe a high level of proficiency. For this reason, autopsies should be encouraged, and people should be encouraged to look on them as an ordinary part of the medical care process. Needless to say, the human remains of a person should always be treated with utmost respect during an autopsy.

In accord with the respect due to the remains of a human person, no organs should be removed from a corpse, nor should the body be dismembered in any way, unless a sufficient reason justifies such an action. Usually the next of kin or the person to whom the corpse is committed for care has the legal right to determine if organs may be removed from the body and if an autopsy may be performed (*Pierce v. Swan Point Cemetery*, 1872).

The right of the next of kin in regard to caring for the human body is not absolute. It may be superseded by statements made by the person while still alive, for example, through the Uniform Anatomical Gift Act (1968), or by the needs of society, for example, when an autopsy might help stave off a contagious disease. In the future, the need of organs for donation in society may change our assumptions in regard to family rights to donate organs of the deceased, and it will then be presumed that transplants are allowed if the person did not express opposition to such procedures when alive (English and Sommerville 2003). In Europe some countries have already made this presumption legal (Byk 1996).

The Uniform Anatomical Gift Act was "designed to facilitate the donation and use of human tissues and organs for transplantation and other medical purposes and provide a favorable legal environment for such activities" (Lehrman 1988; Sadler, Sadler, and Stason 1968). At present, all fifty states have enacted the Uniform Anatomical Gift Act, thus enabling persons who are of sound mind and eighteen years of age or older to give all or part of their bodies to persons or institutions authorized to practice or perform research medicine or to engage in tissue banking, with the gift to take effect at death. This law also recognizes the right of the next of kin to donate the body or any part for the same purpose, but in most states the law declares that if there is a conflict between the donor and the next of kin, the wishes of the donor have precedence. The person or institution to which the donation is made need not accept the gift. If the gift is accepted, the body, after removal of the part named, is transferred to the next of kin or other persons under obligation to dispose of the body. If the whole body is retained for research at a medical school, it will often be cremated upon completion of the research. If the person was Catholic there may not be a wake but a funeral service; a memorial mass, for example, is usually celebrated without the corpse being present if the person was Catholic.

Theoretically, the Uniform Anatomical Gift Act grants protection from civil and criminal proceedings that might result from the removal of organs or experimentation on the corpse to all persons concerned, including physicians, next of kin, funeral directors, and medical examiners. However, in practice, if the next of kin refuses the request for organ retrieval, even if the deceased person had signed an anatomical gift donation card, hospitals and physicians will usually follow the decision of the next of kin because they fear malpractice charges. Persons interested in donating a part or all of their body at death should inform their families of their desire so that possible conflicts will be avoided.

From a Christian point of view, the practice of donating organs and one's body for scientific research is ethical and even to be encouraged if a true need exists. Thus, as Pius XII (1956) and John Paul II (1995) advised, donating organs from a cadaver, if done from the motive of charity, does not seriously damage the integrity of the corpse.

Another ethical question, however, does not admit such an easy solution: Is it immoral to accept or solicit payment for the gift of certain organs? Although some defend such practices (de Castro 2003), other authors maintain that abuses could arise very quickly if cadaver organs were sold or contracted for money (Etzioni 2003). With this latter opinion we agree. If society is to live in a humane manner, generosity and charity rather than monetary gain and greed must serve as the basis for donation of human organs. The National Organ Transplant Act (McDonald 1988) prohibits the sale of human organs, although reasonable payments for expenses incurred by the health facility or donor are allowed.

6.6 SUICIDE, ASSISTED SUICIDE, AND EUTHANASIA

Suicide is the choice to destroy one's own bodily life, and "assisted" suicide is formal cooperation with the suicide of another. It is clear that it is unethical for a health care professional
to cooperate formally with suicide if suicide itself is unethical. A fortiori, if assisting suicide
is immoral, killing a person without their consent, even with the intention of relieving their
suffering, cannot be ethical. Hence we first discuss the morality of suicide, then of assisted
suicide, then of euthanasia (mercy killing).

Suicide

The Greeks and Romans both condemned and defended suicide, as did Eastern cultures
(Minois 1999; Cholbi 2004). The Epicureans, who considered pleasure and peace of mind
the highest of human goods, argued that it was better to kill oneself than to endure life if
it had become more painful than pleasurable or peaceful. The Stoics, who believed that
virtue or self-control was the highest good, argued that it was permissible to kill oneself if
suffering or torture might force one to lose self-control or act ignobly, or where a choice
had to be made to perish in a shameful way or "die with dignity." Dualists, such as some
Platonists, agnostics, and Manicheans, taught that the body in this life or in many re-
incarnations burdens the soul, which is the real person; thus suicide might be justified as
nothing more than a laying down of this burden.

The monotheistic religions of Judaism, Christianity, and Islam have always opposed suicide, however, because they regard life as God's gift, which his children are to use as faithful stewards. Moreover, these monotheistic religions, unlike others, hold that eternal life
is not the survival of a disembodied soul, nor endless reincarnation, but resurrected life
with God. Consequently, Christians cannot escape accounting to God for stewardship of
the life given them in their worldly existence, nor can they reject the body that will always be part of them. This view was already anticipated by the great Greek philosopher
Aristotle, who argued that suicide is against nature and an injustice to the community of
which the person is a part. In a very different way, another prominent philosopher, Kant,
argued that suicide is the greatest of crimes because it is a person's rejection of morality
itself, as a person must be his or her own moral lawgiver. To kill oneself is to treat oneself
as a thing (a means) rather than as a person.

Many of the modern experts on suicide seem to take it for granted that all suicides are
subjectively irrational and compulsive (Menninger 1938; Durkheim 1951); Pope John Paul
II (1995) indicated the same general evaluation of most suicides. Only when suicide is a
free and rational choice can we talk about its *subjective* morality. The Christian churches,
and especially the Catholic Church, have always condemned suicide as an offense against
the God who gave us life. As the Congregation for the Doctrine of the Faith (CDF 1980)
stated: "Intentionally causing one's own death, or suicide, is equally as wrong as murder;
such an action on the part of a person is to be considered as a rejection of God's sover-
eignty and loving plan. Furthermore, suicide is also often a refusal of love for self, the denial of the natural instinct to live, a flight from the duties of justice and charity owed to
one's neighbor, to various communities or to the whole of society" (II).

The Christian stand against suicide is again being questioned by philosophers and legal scholars (Philosophers' Brief 1997; Cohen-Almagor 2001). The Protestant moralist

Joseph Fletcher (1960, 141) stated, "The real issue is whether we can morally justify taking it into our own hands to hasten death for ourselves [suicide] or for others [mercy killing] out of reasons of compassion." Fletcher answers this in terms of his own situationism, according to which the only command of God is to "act lovingly" (see chapter 1, section 1.3). Hence any means is justified if it is effective for achieving loving ends because, "If we will the end, we will the means." Consequently, it appears to him that there are many situations in which persons can will their own death for the good of others (as a war prisoner who fears that torture may cause him to reveal the hiding place of others) or in which others may be put to death out of compassion for their sufferings, assuming that they would want this to be done for them. In the United States, the Hemlock Society and other organizations promulgate such views (Humphry 2002).

Physician-Assisted Suicide

Closely allied with the desire to accept suicide as a legal and ethical choice is the movement to approve physician-assisted suicide. Some of the proponents of this movement maintain that physicians have an ethical obligation to help their patients end their lives if they so desire, especially if they are experiencing physical or psychological pain (Quill 2000). In the United States, physician-assisted suicide is legal in the state of Oregon (Brumbaugh 2002), as it is in the European countries of The Netherlands and Belgium (Janssen 2002). Moreover, two federal circuit courts approved the practice in 1996, but the U.S. Supreme Court reversed the decisions of the lower courts and maintained that "there is no generalized right to commit suicide," also affirming that there is an important legal distinction between removing life support that is ineffective or burdensome, thus allowing the patient to die of a fatal pathology, and inducing the cause of death by means of lethal medications. The movement to accept and to legalize physician-assisted suicide has met with severe criticism on the part of philosophers, legal scholars, and physicians (Dyck 2002; Kass and Lund 1996; Foley and Hendin 2002). From the perspective of Catholic ethics, physician-assisted suicide is intrinsically evil because it involves active and formal cooperation on the part of the physician in an evil action. Even though the patient may take the lethal medication that in effect terminates life, the physician who prescribes such a medication cooperates formally with the person committing suicide. In recent years, there has been a great growth in the ability to control pain and offer palliative care to those who are suffering as death approaches (Byock 2003; Coberly 2003). Hence movement toward physician-assisted suicide has no foundation in good medicine or in a realistic person-centered ethics. As long as there is hope for a future, suicide is clearly unreasonable.

For Christians hope in God grounds the future. By God's providence even the most painful situations not only can be endured but also may be extremely important events in the completion of earthly life. In a secular humanist system in which ultimately no one cares for us except ourselves, this may not be true, but Christians ought to wait on the God who gave them life, because he knows best how to prepare them for the mystery of eternal life with him.

As for the argument that "If God shares with us a stewardship over life, why not over death?" it should be noted that our stewardship over life presupposes that we *preserve* our life, not destroy it. Suicide is a rejection of God's gift of life and therefore of God the giver, not a use of that life in the service of the purposes for which God gave it. Thus attempts to balance the various values of suicide lead back to the conclusion that suicide is intrinsically and always wrong, because in all circumstances it constitutes an abdication of one's responsibility to live out life in community with other persons and with God. Clearly, underlying all the modern arguments for suicide is the error of the absolute autonomy of the individual, that is, the notion that each of us ought to have total control of our own lives and therefore of our own deaths. In fact we do not create ourselves but are part of a human society and of a universe that has its origin in God. The Creator has made us partners in his wise governance of the world, and we must work in cooperation with him, not contradictory to his guidance. To reject his gift of life is to reject our relation to God and to humanity. The old saying holds that "while there is life, there is hope." Moreover, even beyond this life there is hope in God, if we have not rejected God here and now. Finally, Camus summed up the situation accurately: "There is but one philosophical problem and that is suicide. . . . Even if one does not believe in God, suicide is not legitimate" (1969, 1). Furthermore, "from the moment when life is accepted as good, it is good for all. . . . In a man's attachment to life, there is something stronger than all the ills in the world" (1956, 6).

Euthanasia

The word "euthanasia" is derived from two Greek words that mean "good death" or "happy death." For centuries, the term referred to an action by which a person was put to death painlessly, usually to avoid further suffering from an incurable disease or to end an irreversible comatose condition. *Webster's New International Dictionary* (6th ed.), for example, defines "euthanasia" as "a mode or act of inducing death painlessly as a relief from pain." Euthanasia in this sense is often called "mercy killing" or even "death with dignity."

The public discussion of this issue, however, is often confused by authors who speak of "passive" and "active" euthanasia; "passive euthanasia" means the withdrawal of life supports from patients even when such supports are no longer beneficial but harmful, a distinction that, as already stated, has been recognized by the U.S. Supreme Court. Hence it is better to avoid the term *passive euthanasia* and to follow the definition used by the Congregation for the Doctrine of the Faith in the "Declaration on Euthanasia": "By euthanasia is understood an action or omission of an action which of itself or by intention causes death in order that all suffering may be eliminated" (CDF 1980, II).

It is essential to note that according to this definition although euthanasia can be performed by either commission or omission, it is performed by omission only if the intention of the act of omission is to "cause death" and the intention of the agent is "in order that all suffering may be eliminated." When the intention of the act does not have this purpose, but is the result of a decision that treatment to sustain life is no longer beneficial to the patient or imposes an excessive burden and therefore is no longer obligatory, the action is not euthanasia, and its moral justification will be discussed later in this chapter. Confusion is also caused by the use of the term *death with dignity*, because this can beg the question "What is 'dignity' in death?" Certainly, if mercy killing is murder, to be murdered is not to die with dignity, but to have one's dignity as a human being denied in the most flagrant way.

In the traditional meaning of the term, euthanasia could be performed with or without the consent of the person to be put to death. In the Judeo-Christian tradition, euthanasia without the consent of the patient is equated with murder and with consent of the patient is both suicide and murder. Today, the proponents of euthanasia generally defend it in this latter form, where the patient's consent is given or at least presumed, so that it amounts to assisted suicide. Yet deciding to help with suicide in order to relieve suffering very quickly becomes a decision to relieve that suffering even when the patient does not or cannot consent. Evidence for this is supplied by the history of the medical profession in The Netherlands, a country otherwise known for its respect for human rights. In that country the government announced that while its laws forbade euthanasia, the mercy killing of patients with their consent would not be prosecuted provided physicians reported what they were doing (Janssen 2002). The result was that about half the deaths reported as euthanasia were performed *without the consent* of the patients.

In the United States the cause of euthanasia was dramatized by Dr. Jack Kevorkian, known as "Doctor Death," who was sentenced for second-degree murder in 1999 after carrying out some one hundred such mercy killings (Wikipedia 2005). If the motives of mercy killers are examined, their claim that they did it for the sake of the victim cannot be accepted easily. The real motive may well be that a relative or the health care professional did not want to accept the responsibility of helping the dying person to the end. Often the killer says, "I loved my mother, I couldn't bear to see her suffer!" It is true in such a case that the killer could not bear to see her suffer, but the quality of that love is not so certain. No doubt, however, sometimes mercy killers are themselves not free enough from tortured feelings to make a sane decision. Medical personnel hardly have such excuses. By consenting to help their patients die, they may simply be evading the painful and threatening task of adequate spiritual care for the dying, which is discussed in chapter 8.

Generally, the medical profession has rejected euthanasia absolutely (AMA 2000), as is evidenced by the Hippocratic oath as well as by more recent codes of medical ethics, such as the Geneva Declaration (WHO 1957) and the Helsinki Statement of the World Health Organization (1964). However, the tendency of the medical profession in the United States to prolong the act of dying even after it becomes evident that the patient does not benefit from life-prolonging therapy has caused many people to opt for euthanasia as a certain manner of ending life when medical therapy is no longer beneficial (Darley, Loeb, and Hunter 1999; Gillespie 2001). The fear of prolonged dying has also led to creation of the living will, and when the living will proved to be unsatisfactory, to creation of the durable power of attorney for incompetent people (Olick 2001). Although the living will and durable power of attorney are not unethical in themselves, and may even be helpful in some cases, they do not of themselves eliminate the decision-making problems that arise at the time of death (Guild of Catholic Doctors 1998).

Generally, the Christian churches have rejected euthanasia (Rice 1999). Repeating the consistent teaching of the Catholic Church, the "Declaration on Euthanasia" (CDF 1980, II) states:

> It is necessary to state firmly once more that nothing and no one can in any way permit the killing of an innocent human being, whether a fetus or an embryo, an infant or an old person, or one suffering from an incurable disease, or a person who is dying. Furthermore, no one is permitted to ask for this act of killing for himself or herself or for another person entrusted to his or her care, nor can he or she consent to it either explicitly or implicitly. Nor can any authority legitimately recommend or permit such an action. For it is a question of the violation of the divine law, an offense against the dignity of the human person, a crime against life, and an attack on humanity. (I)

Even more definitively, Pope John Paul II in the encyclical *The Gospel of Life* (1995, no. 65), stated: "In communion with the bishops of the Catholic Church I confirm that euthanasia is a grave violation of the law of God, since it is the deliberate and morally unacceptable killing of a human person. This doctrine is based upon the natural law and upon the written word of God, is transmitted by the church's tradition and taught by the ordinary and universal magisterium." This statement reaffirms that this teaching is for the Catholic conscience infallible and unchangeable moral truth.

6.7 ALLOWING TO DIE: WITHHOLDING OR WITHDRAWING LIFE SUPPORT

Under this title we consider many different topics in order to present clearly the distinctions that must be understood in order to make ethical decisions concerning the withholding or removal of life support: First, the distinction of allowing to die from suicide and euthanasia. Second, the distinction of basic or nursing care from medical therapy. Third, the distinction of the terms *ordinary* and *extraordinary* means of life support and how they coincide with the terms *proportionate* and *disproportionate* means of life support. Fourth, the distinction of the criteria that are used to determine whether life support is ordinary or proportionate, or extraordinary or disproportionate, and whether quality-of-life considerations may be used when evaluating these criteria. Fifth, the distinction of the timing of these decisions and by whom they should be made.

The Difference among Allowing to Die, Suicide, and Euthanasia

For Christians, and for many others as well, human life is considered to be a gift from the Creator, and the control of human life implies stewardship, not absolute autonomy. Human life may be compared to the talents given by the master to his servants, which he expects them to invest so that there will be a proper return (Mt 25:14–30). Hence this gift of life must be used wisely and prudently to strive for the purpose of life. As Thomas Aquinas stated, "Every man has it instilled in him by nature to love his own life and whatever is directed thereto; and to do so in due measure, that is, to love these things not as placing his end therein, but as things to be used for the sake of his last end" (*Summa Theologiae* I–II, q. 126, 1). For committed Christians, the last end, the purpose of life, is found in friendship with God and living with him forever (CCC 2000, 1, no. 356).

Yet the time may come in our lives when we realize that our death is inevitable and that prolonging life by additional medical treatment will not bring us closer to God. Family members or legal proxies may also be called upon to make a decision of this nature for patients who are unable to speak for themselves. In these circumstances one may decide that prolonging life is not the best investment of energy, time, or money that can be made in the time remaining. Seeking to prolong life in such a situation may not really benefit the patient and may interfere with the pursuit of other, more important goods or duties by the patient's caretakers. Hence, if further therapies to prolong life "do not offer a reasonable hope of benefit or entail an excessive burden," insofar as attaining the purpose of life is concerned, they may be refused (ERD 2001, D. 56 and 57). The intention inherent in an act of this nature does not constitute suicide or euthanasia. Rather, it is an act whose moral object may be accurately described as "allowing one to die for legitimate reasons." When a person chooses to have life support withheld or removed in such a case, or when the decision to do so is made by a proxy, the decision maker is not making a choice in favor of death. Rather, an *indirect* choice is made about when the patient will die, "taking into account the state of the sick person and his or her physical and moral resources" (CDF 1980, IV).

Suicide occurs when the intention inherent in the human act (the moral object, purpose, or *finis operis* of the act) is self-destruction. Euthanasia occurs when the intention inherent in the act is to end the life of another person, with or without the consent of that person, and the motive (or *finis operantis,* or intention of the agent) for the act is to alleviate or eliminate suffering. In both suicide and euthanasia the moral object of the act is to kill the patient, and the physical result of the act is the same, the person dies. In euthanasia, the act of killing may be accomplished by commission or omission, that is, by performing a lethal act or by withholding some life-prolonging therapy that should be utilized. The "Declaration on Euthanasia" defines such an act in the following manner: "By euthanasia is understood an action or an omission which of itself or by intention causes death, in order that all suffering may in this way be eliminated" (CDF 1980, II). The phrase "in order that" indicates the indirect intention or motive of the act (*finis operantis*).

Clearly, whether euthanasia has occurred cannot be discerned simply from the physical result of commission or omission of a medical act. Rather, the moral object of the act must be determined. To reject additional medical efforts that do not correspond to the actual circumstances of the patient (i.e., aggressive care) is not to reject life itself or the God who gave it, but is simply to reject efforts that will not help to complete the task of striving for the purpose of life. As Pope John Paul II (2004b) declared, "The refusal of aggressive treatment is neither a rejection of the patient nor of his or her life. Indeed, the object of the decision on whether to begin or to continue a treatment has nothing to do with the value of the patient's life, but rather with whether such medical intervention is beneficial for the patient." This act, which is contrary to euthanasia, is aptly described as "allowing to die for legitimate reasons." These legitimate reasons are either "no hope of benefit" or "excessive burden." Both euthanasia and allowing to die have the same physical result: death of the patient. But they have a radically different moral significance. Pope John Paul II explained the distinction between allowing to die and euthanasia in the following manner (1995, no. 65):

> Euthanasia must be distinguished from the decision to forgo so-called "aggressive medical treatment," in other words, medical procedures which no longer correspond to the real situation of the patient, either because they are now disproportionate to any expected results or because they impose an excessive burden on the patient and his family. . . . To forgo extraordinary or disproportionate means is not the equivalent of suicide or euthanasia; it rather expresses acceptance of the human condition in the face of death.

The Difference between Medical Therapy and Basic Health Care

Before discussing in detail the criteria for withholding or removing life support, for the sake of clarity let us distinguish those medical or surgical procedures that are employed to prolong life from those activities that furnish comfort care, sometimes called basic health care, normal care, or natural care (John Paul II 2004a). In the former category are all medical and surgical procedures designed to combat illness and disease and alleviate pain. Usually these procedures require the expertise of medical professionals in order to be utilized. In the latter category are those activities that may not improve the health of the patient but which demonstrate human compassion and respect for the person. For example, people who are suffering from illness or disease, no matter what their cognitive-affective function, should be bathed and kept clean and free from pain. Thirst and other effects of dehydration should be controlled insofar as possible. If they are in pain, analgesics should be administered even though health cannot be restored. When commenting upon the difference between medical procedures and comfort or natural care, some indicate that there is almost an absolute obligation to utilize natural care (Pontifical Council, 1995). But the criteria of benefit and burden must be applied to natural care as well as to medical care. Thus classical moral theology held that taking food and drink even in a normal manner ceases to be obligatory for a patient if its benefit no longer exceeds its burden. Whether normal care always includes the use of respirator or artificial hydration and nutrition when these are necessary to sustain life is a debated question that we will consider further in section 6.8.

Ordinary and Extraordinary Medical Means to Prolong Life

The phrase "ordinary and extraordinary means to prolong life" is familiar to many people inside and outside of the health care profession. From an ethical perspective, there is general agreement that ordinary means must be used to prolong life when fatal or terminal illness threatens, and extraordinary means may be forgone in the same circumstances. It sounds simple. Yet the application of these terms in clinical situations is never simple, either for people who will be making these ethical decisions or for health care professionals— the doctors, nurses, and pastoral care advisors—who will assist patients or their families in making these decisions. Theoretical, emotional, and ethical confusion often accompanies ethical decision making in these circumstances and beclouds the hearts and minds of decision makers.

Before the sixteenth century, in difficult circumstances people of faith often made decisions to forgo the medical or surgical means that might prolong human life, but their decisions were more the result of necessity than of theological analysis. A leader in the development of the theology of "death and dying" was Francisco de Vitoria, a Dominican theologian, called the "Father of International Law" (MacCulloch 2003), who taught at the Spanish University of Salamanca. When commenting upon the writing of St. Thomas Aquinas, especially in regard to homicide and abstinence, he formulated some theological principles that have endured to contemporary times (Ordanoz 1960; Doyle 1997). For example:

1. Human life is a great gift from God, a great good but not an absolute good, nor the ultimate good.
2. A person is not the master of life, but should use all fitting means to prolong life. If the means to prolong life are not fitting, that is, if they do not offer hope of benefit, or if they impose an excessive burden, they need not be utilized.
3. The ultimate human good is friendship with God. All human acts should be ordered toward this ultimate end.

4. God does not desire us to be interested in a long life; he wishes us to be interested in a good life.
5. It is one thing to kill oneself; it is a different thing to not prolong life.

Other theologians at Salamanca followed and developed the thought of de Vitoria concerning the duties in regard to prolonging life (Cronin 1989). It seems that Domingo Bañez, O.P., toward the end of the sixteenth century, coined the terms *ordinary* and *extraordinary means* to prolong life. In the ensuing centuries, the teaching of the Salamanca theologians was very important in developing moral teaching concerning the prolongation of life. The concepts mentioned above were applied to new methods in medicine and surgery, but later theologians never challenged the foundational principles (Cronin 1989). The consensus of theologians throughout the centuries in regard to use and removal of life support led to the first authentic papal teaching in this regard, by Pope Pius XII in 1957. This statement was followed by the "Declaration on Euthanasia" in 1980, issued by the CDF and approved by Pope John Paul II. Pope John Paul II also spoke about the removal of life support and the care of the dying, being careful to distinguish between the removal of unnecessary life support and euthanasia (John Paul II 1995, 65). Moreover, he considered the care of permanent vegetative state (PVS) patients and palliative care for the dying (2004a, 11, 12). Finally, the bishops of the United States have applied the teaching of the Church to issues involving Catholic hospitals and nursing homes in the ERD (2001).

Comparison of Terms

For centuries, the terms *ordinary* and *extraordinary means* were used for determining the use of life support. If the medical therapy was judged to be ordinary, there was a moral obligation to use it; if it was judged to be extraordinary, its use was optional. In 1980, the CDF suggested in the "Declaration on Euthanasia" that the terms *proportionate* and *disproportionate* might be more accurate descriptors of care than *ordinary* and *extraordinary*. In order to signify the meaning of both sets of terms, the declaration added: "In any case, it will be possible to make a correct judgment as to the means by studying the type of treatment to be used, its degree of complexity or risk, its cost and the possibilities of using it, and comparing these elements with the result that can be expected, taking into account the state of the sick person and his or her physical and moral resources" (sec. IV). It seems that the main reason for the suggested change in terminology arose from the tendency to interpret the terms *ordinary* and *extraordinary* in an abstract or generic manner; that is, the decision whether a medical means to prolong life was ordinary or extraordinary was often made without reference to the condition of a specific patient. Using the terms in an abstract or generic sense, only the cost, usual effectiveness, availability of a medical device, and potential pain inflicted would be considered when designating a medical or surgical procedure as ordinary or extraordinary. The overall condition of the patient was not considered until after the terms of ordinary or extraordinary care had been decided. This would often result in confusing terminology. The means in question might be considered ordinary in the abstract, but this designation would be changed to extraordinary once the condition of the patient had been considered. Thus a respirator or a feeding tube might be designated as an ordinary means to prolong life, but after consideration of the patient's condition, it might be considered extraordinary (Kelly 1950). The more accurate designation of moral responsibility in choosing or rejecting medical or surgical procedures rests on a diagnosis of pathology and prognosis of possible effects of medical care with regard to a specific patient.

Since the "Declaration on Euthanasia" was issued, Catholic theologians have used the terms *proportionate* and *disproportionate* as synonyms for *ordinary* and *extraordinary*, but they have not supplanted the original terms. Hence, before making a determination whether the means of medical care are ordinary or extraordinary, the condition of the patient and the potential effect upon the patient must be considered, insofar as possible.

The tendency to use the terms *ordinary* and *extraordinary* in an abstract manner can still be found in the writings of some physicians and other health care professionals, and very frequently in the conversations of people who must make decisions for loved ones concerning the use or removal of life support. Therapies that, in the abstract sense of the term, were at one time experimental or extraordinary and later became standard or ordinary care include, for example, blood transfusions and angioplasties (surgical reconstructions of blood vessels). But whether such a therapy should be utilized or may be withheld or withdrawn from a particular patient cannot be determined from the moral perspective until the condition of the patient is factored into the decision. Thus, in any oral or written discussion concerning life support, the meaning of the terms must be made clear at the beginning in order to avoid confusion later on.

The Criteria for Forgoing Life-Sustaining Interventions

The phrase "forgoing life-sustaining interventions" refers to withholding and withdrawing life support such as artificial hydration and nutrition or the respirator. The criteria for withholding life support are the same as those for withdrawing life support that is already being utilized. In the latter case, however, the ethical problem is often more difficult because the patient may die or will certainly die from their condition shortly after medical therapy is withdrawn. The specific criteria for distinguishing between ordinary and extraordinary or between proportionate and disproportionate medical therapy, as the ERD indicate (2001, DD. 56 and 57), are the hope of benefit that the therapy offers and the burden imposed by the therapy upon the patient, the family, and the community. Pope John Paul II expressed the same criteria in this way (2004b): "The possible decision either not to start or to halt a treatment will be deemed ethically correct if the treatment is ineffective or obviously disproportionate to the aims of sustaining life or recovering health."

Benefits.   In general, the benefits sought through medical care are the preservation or restoration of health and the alleviation of pain. In short, the goal of medicine is to promote optimal functioning, given the person's physical and mental capacities (Blum 1983). Medical therapy does not always result in a cure. It does not always improve or restore health or prolong life. Often it merely circumvents, abates, or alleviates the effects of an illness or disease, but does not eliminate it.

While medical care is directed primarily toward physiological or psychological functions, it often offers social or spiritual benefit indirectly. The benefit of medical care enables one to pursue the goods of life. These goods may be physical, psychological, social, or spiritual. These are proximate goods, explicitly or implicitly ordered toward the ultimate good of life, friendship with God. These proximate goods are often more prominent in the minds of persons as they evaluate hope of benefit associated with particular medical therapies. For example, when making serious medical decisions, people ponder what effects the therapies will have upon their health, their vocations, and their families. These goods are important insofar as achieving friendship with God is concerned, but this latter goal is not always prominent in the minds of people making decisions about health care.

Would this surgery improve my overall well-being and allow me a more pain-free life? Would this medicine enable me to cope with the stress of life more adequately? Will the medication or surgery enable me to return to work? Will this therapy enable my loved one, for whom I am the proxy, to regain consciousness, or will it simply prolong a comatose condition? How expensive will the medical procedure be? What other goods would the family have to forgo if we invest in this medical therapy? Thus, economic, psychic, and social goods more often are the immediate concern of decision makers. They are all included under the general category of hope of benefit. But these goods are at least implicitly ordered to a higher good. As Pope Pius XII stated in his famous "Declaration on Life Support" in 1957, "Life, health, all temporal activities are in fact subordinated to spiritual ends."

Burdens.   The burdens of medical care might also affect the pursuit of the goods that are significant in human life; thus the burdens might be economic, physiological, psychological, social, or spiritual. Since the sixteenth century, economic burdens, extreme pain, risk of losing life, and great subjective repugnance have been the principal burdens considered. In order to justify forgoing life support, the burden must be judged to be excessive. Determining an excessive burden is often a difficult process. All medical care is a burden in one sense. But an excessive burden makes striving for the continuation of life, or an important good of life, a moral impossibility—or at least very difficult (Cronin 1989). Certainly, some objective norms can be set for judging burden. Theologians seek to do this, presupposing a certain degree of courage (the virtue of fortitude). Thus direct killing of self or another, even to avoid suffering, is prohibited. But subjective disposition must also be considered.

At one time, some moral theologians suggested that a woman of tender conscience might find it an excessive burden to consult a male physician, and thus they thought that such a woman would be excused from consulting a physician. What seems to be an excessive burden by one person might be considered not an excessive burden by another person. As the "Declaration on Euthanasia" states: "In the final analysis, it pertains to the conscience either of the sick person, or of those qualified to speak in the sick person's name . . . to decide in the light of moral obligations and of the various aspects of the case" (IV). For this reason Catholic tradition has always insisted that the patient or the proxy has the right to make the final decision concerning the refusal of health care, as we shall see later.

Research on the burdens that people consider excessive indicates that many people in good health consider being paralyzed and being able to breathe only if assisted by a respirator an excessive burden (Jennett 2002, 73–86). Yet many people actually in this situation adjust to their situations very well and desire to prolong life by using life support. Thus, the ethical responsibility to consult the patient with regard to forgoing life support, and the need to afford these persons the proper counseling, cannot be emphasized too greatly. We shall have more to say about this factor when we consider personal and proxy decision making.

Future Burdens Considered.   When discussing burdens, theologians consider not only the present burden associated with a particular medication or medical procedure but also any future burden. As Connery says, "In assessing any particular means, it made no difference whether the burden to the patient was experienced before, during, or after the treatment" (1980). For example, the burden associated with respirator-assisted breathing is considered by most people to be a minimal burden, especially if intubation is necessary for only a short time. Nevertheless the length of time that this burden might endure must also be taken into consideration. For example, a young athlete fractured the C3 vertebra in a trampoline accident. Able to breathe only with a respirator, and now quadriplegic, he was informed two weeks after the accident that this condition would last for the rest of his life. Communicating with his family through eye contact, he convinced them to ask his physicians to remove the respirator because the prospect of living the rest of his life in this condition was an overwhelming burden. The family agreed with him. Having consulted with ethicists, the physicians brought in people who were living successfully with the same disability, but he and the family persisted in their request. After a time, the physicians ceded to their request. A less dramatic forgoing of life support often happens when a dialysis patient, experiencing severe and continual fatigue, realizes that she no longer benefits sufficiently from the treatment, determines to discontinue the treatment even though, if continued, it might prolong her life for the foreseeable future.

The financial burden resulting from prolonged medical therapy can be misconstrued. For example, the materials needed for tube feeding (i.e., assisted hydration and nutrition [AHN]) are inexpensive: a tube and some cans of Ensure. But inserting a gastrostomy tube or a tube into the vena cava (hyperalimentation) is a surgical procedure performed in a surgical suite, and long-term nursing care will be necessary for a person with these devices. These considerations are all part of the financial burden (Sulmasy 2006). What must be weighed is the burden not only to the patient but to the caretakers, and not only to the family of the patient and to the medical professionals and the health care facility but also to society at large. As John Paul II said, society has a duty to assist families in their palliative care of debilitated persons. In the United States, however, families often have to carry much of the burden. To set these considerations aside is unrealistic and an unjust imposition on the caretakers, who have other heavy responsibilities they cannot ethically neglect.

Two Criteria or One?   Are two criteria used when evaluating medical therapy, or are benefit and burden to be combined as one consideration? Connery expressed a preference for keeping them separate because they deal with different issues. "In practice, at least, the question of benefit seems limited largely to terminal cases; burden can be an issue even in cases which are not terminal" (1986). From a theoretical perspective, these are certainly two distinct criteria, and sometimes they are different in the practical situation. For instance, a patient suffering from cancer may determine that prolonging life for another ten days may not be beneficial, even though there is no serious pain or financial burden. Or drug therapy for patients with AIDS may offer hope of benefit, but some patients might deem it an excessive burden because of the expense involved.

More often, in an actual case, benefit and burden are compared to each other. The end result is a statement that the medical therapy in question is either a burden or a benefit. Some authors restrict their considerations to the benefit/burden terminology and seldom consider benefit and burden as separate criteria (Brock 1997, 360). In the ERD (2001),

Directives 56 and 57 distinguish between hope of benefit and excessive burden, but in Directive 58 the two are combined in the discussion on the use of AHN. Finally, it is important to consider benefit *before* burden, because, whatever the burden, it would be rigorism to hold that anyone is morally obliged to do something that is of no significant benefit to the recipient or society.

Quality-of-Life Considerations

The question is often asked whether quality-of-life considerations can be used as criteria for determining whether a medical procedure offers hope of benefit or imposes an excessive burden. But in any discussion of this nature it is necessary to realize that quality of life is an ambiguous term (Shannon and Walter 1990). In one sense, it refers to our relationship to God. In this sense, all persons have the same quality of life and dignity because God loves each person. But the term is also used in regard to measuring human function. People with impaired human function are said to have an impaired or lower quality of life. Some people have impaired human function as the result of a genetic or physical anomaly. If a person with a disability of this nature contracts a serious disease or pathology, it would be highly immoral to withhold care simply because of the genetic or physical disability. Consider, for example, a child with Down's syndrome who has a ruptured appendix. The parents' refusal of surgery or medication to treat the ruptured appendix would be a grave violation of the child's right to life.

There is, however, a third meaning to the term *quality of life*. Judgments of this nature "rely on the discernment of the patient" (Wildes 1996). Some people have impaired function resulting from illness or disease, and for these people the quality of life is fittingly considered when benefits and burdens are assessed, as the Pontifical Council *Cor Unum* affirmed in 1981 in a document cited with approval in the papal allocution of March 20, 2004, *On Care for PVS Patients* (John Paul II 2004a, no. 5). Let us suppose that one's mother has cancer, which has metastasized throughout her body, and her kidneys begin to fail. Should we consider her overall condition as we decide whether dialysis will be beneficial for her? In order to obviate the difficulties that arise from the use of the term *quality of life*, Fr. Thomas O'Donnell suggested in a private conversation that the term *quality of function* be used whenever a question arises about withdrawing life support from a person suffering impaired function from a serious illness or disease.

When Should the Decision to Forgo Life Support Be Made?

This is one of the more misunderstood questions in regard to forgoing life support. Because humans have a serious obligation to seek health in order to prolong life, they have a moral obligation to seek to overcome illness and disease, unless the means to accomplish this goal does not offer hope of benefit or imposes an excessive burden. When a less serious illness or disease is present, we often rely on the natural homeostasis of the body to resist it. For example, many people do not take medicines or antibiotics if they contract a minor case of influenza, relying instead on rest, liquids, and the natural resistance of the body to gradually restore health. However, when a more serious illness or disease threatens, one that might cause death if not eliminated or abated, the prudent person makes a decision to utilize medications or surgery to help the body overcome it, or at least to mitigate its effects.

Thus, the logical time to make decisions about utilizing the means to prolong life is when a person contracts a serious illness, that is, when a potentially lethal pathology is diagnosed. Usually the initial reaction to a serious illness will not involve a rejection of medical means due to lack of benefit or excessive burden. But in time, as the illness progresses, if the medical therapy is ineffective or becomes acutely onerous, a decision to reject medical means might be made for the reasons mentioned earlier. When decisions have to be made for persons unable to make decisions for themselves, proxy decision makers may decide to forgo life support for these reasons.

Often people believe that life support, either for oneself or for another who is incapable of making health care decisions, must be continued until it is no longer physically possible to keep the person alive. Thus, some physicians believe that life support cannot be removed until the disease can no longer be resisted and that death will occur within a short time *no matter what medications or medical procedures are utilized.* Physicians with this mentality often assert that life support cannot be removed because the patients are not suffering from terminal illness, that is, death is not imminent and inevitable. This seems to be the rationale underlying a recent statement of the World Federation of Catholic Medical Associations concerning patients in a "vegetative state" (VS; FIAMC 2004): "VS patients cannot in any way be considered terminal patients, since their condition can be stable and enduring."

O'Donnell states that "there is in the medical profession an ideal which demands the fighting off of pain and death until the last possible moment" (1957, 67). The assertion that life support cannot be removed unless death is imminent and inevitable is contrary to the consistent tradition in Catholic moral theology. When theologians of the sixteenth century considered questions concerning the duty to prolong life, they posited cases that did not presuppose the presence of terminal illness. Moreover, in the "Declaration on Euthanasia," the question is posed, "Is it necessary in all circumstances to have recourse to all possible remedies?" Section IV of the declaration indicates that several circumstances may prompt a decision to withdraw life support before a terminal illness is diagnosed. Guidance for withdrawing life support even before a so-called terminal illness is present is offered: "In any case, it will be possible to make a correct judgment as to the means by studying the type of treatment to be used, its degree of complexity or risk, its cost and the possibilities of using it, and comparing these elements with the result that can be expected, taking into account the state of the sick person and his or her physical and moral resources" (IV).

Furthermore, the notion that life support may be forgone only if the patient suffers from a terminal illness neglects the second criterion for forgoing life support: excessive burden. The lower courts in the famous Brophy, Conroy, and Cruzan cases thought that a terminal illness must be diagnosed before life support can be withdrawn. But these decisions were later reversed when the higher courts considered the matter more thoroughly and determined that the key issue was not whether a terminal illness was present but rather the effect of the therapy upon the patient. Some of the judges in the lower courts maintained that if death occurred after the removal of life support, the result was homicide. But the decision of the higher courts rightly inferred that if death occurred after the removal of life support, death was not the intention inherent in the action. Rather, the cause of death was the illness from which the patient suffered, not the removal of life support (O'Donnell 1987).

The notion that life support may be removed only if a terminal illness is present is expressed in that life support can be withdrawn only if death is "imminent and inevitable." This phrase is used in the encyclical *Evangelium vitae* (John Paul II 1995, no. 65), and it is also stated in a Vatican document seeking to summarize Church teaching on medical ethics (Pontifical Council for Pastoral Assistance to Health Care Workers 1995, no. 97). Of course, if death is imminent and inevitable, this diagnosis can be factored into the decision-making process. Indeed, it makes the decision whether or not to forgo life support easier. But the statement about "imminent and inevitable" death in the encyclical does not indicate that life support can be withdrawn *only* if death is imminent and inevitable. The encyclical quotes the "Declaration on Euthanasia" as the source of its teaching. As we have seen, this document envisions life support being removed even if death is not imminent and inevitable. Unfortunately, some people purporting to speak for the Church have recently focused upon this phrase and maintain that any removal of comfort care or life support that results in death is euthanasia, unless death is imminent and inevitable. This is contrary to five hundred years of theological analysis.

The Schiavo Case.   The recent case of Theresa Marie (Terri) Schiavo illustrates the inclination of many to maintain that life support cannot be withdrawn unless death is imminent and inevitable within a short time, no matter what medical intervention is employed (Furhman 2005, 219; Perry, Churchill, and Kirshner 2005). Schiavo was diagnosed by competent board certified neurologists as being in PVS, that is, as being permanently unresponsive due to injury to the cerebral cortex (Schiavo 2006, 200–213). There was moral certitude, later confirmed by an autopsy, that she would never recover cognitive-affective function and would not benefit from rehab therapy (345). Yet her mere physiological function could be sustained for the foreseeable future by means of AHN. Many vociferously maintained that because she was not in imminent danger of death, removing life support would be euthanasia. Some even maintained that she could recover limited cognitive-affective function if given the proper therapy. Others maintained that she suffered from a lethal pathology that was abated due to AHN and that no benefit would result from continued use of AHN. Still others maintained that there was "sufficient burden to outweigh the benefit" and thus in light of Directive 58, AHN could be removed (Eisenberg 2005, 55, 91). Cases of this nature are best decided by loved ones who act in the best interest of the patient. Unfortunately, because of disputes between her husband and her parents, the case was remanded to the courts in the state of Florida. The courts ruled that there was "clear and convincing evidence" that she had previously expressed a desire to have life support removed were she ever to be in a severely debilitated condition. AHN was removed on March 18, 2005, and she died on March 31.

Who Should Make the Decision?

Often, it is unclear which person has the right to determine whether the means to prolong life are ordinary or extraordinary. Clearly, the physician is deeply involved in the decision. He or she must present an opinion as to whether the means in question will cure, help significantly, or have no effect upon the ailing patient. In other words, the diagnosis and prognosis are primarily the responsibility of the physician. But other circumstances, in addition to medical effectiveness, must be considered. What about expense, pain, and inconvenience? What about the spiritual condition of the patient? Only the patient or the proxy can determine these factors accurately.

Insofar as this decision is concerned, the Catholic tradition does not rely upon the legal right of autonomy, as does the modern teaching of bioethics. Rather, the source of this personal responsibility is the "sacred and inviolable" character of the human person. Hence the radical right to make the ethical decision concerning means to prolong life belongs to the patient. Pope Pius XII (1957) spoke to this issue: "The rights and duties of the doctor are correlative to those of the patient. The doctor, in fact, has no separate or independent right where the patient is concerned. In general, he or she can take action only when the patient explicitly or implicitly, directly or indirectly, gives permission" (60). The ERD (2001, D. 26) also speaks to this issue:

> The free and informed consent of the person or the person's surrogate is required for medical treatments and procedures, except in an emergency situation when consent cannot be obtained and there is no indication that the patient would refuse consent to the treatment. Free and informed consent requires that the person or the person's surrogate receive all reasonable information about the essential nature of the proposed treatment and its benefits; its risks, side-effects, consequences, and cost; and any reasonable and morally legitimate alternatives, including no treatment at all.

The number of articles and books devoted to the topic of informed consent illustrates that the right of the patient to make health care decisions is prominent in the study of bioethics.

Proxy Consent.   The most difficult situation in regard to consent arises when the patient is incapable of decision making and another person must make decisions for the patient. If the patient is too young to indicate his or her wishes, or if the patient has failed to indicate the preferred therapy as death threatens, the proxy, usually a family member, acts *in the best interest of the patient.* That is, the proxy, acting with the advice of the attending physician, indicates the preferred therapy, or its forgoing, given the circumstances and using the criteria indicated earlier: hope of benefit and degree of burden. In the United States, the use of advance directives, in which the patient, when competent, names a proxy (not always a family member) to make health care decisions when he or she is not competent to do so, is recommended. The U.S. Bishops' Conference recognizes the advance directive as a legitimate means of preparing for future health care needs (ERD 2001, D. 25).

When acting under the guidance of an advance directive, the proxy should seek to offer *substitute judgment,* that is, to follow the previously expressed wishes of the patient insofar as possible if these wishes are in accord with the teaching of the Church. If, however, the circumstances are not the same as those envisioned by the patient, as often happens in crisis situations, the proxy may have to act in the best interest of the patient, always keeping in mind above all the patient's spiritual welfare.

Family Concerns.   While families are often called upon to offer substitute or best interest decisions when their loved ones are not able to make decisions for themselves, family decisions need not be totally altruistic. Often nursing a comatose patient imposes a serious burden upon those who have other obligations that they may not in conscience neglect. The ERD implies that family concerns should be recognized when decisions about life support are about to be made by a patient (2001, DD. 56 and 57). Connery stated, "A patient would be free to omit a means to preserve life even if he did so to remove a burden from the family" (1986). Moreover, Pius XII (1957) made two statements relevant to family decision making: "The rights and duties of the family depend in general upon the presumed will of the unconscious patient if he is of age and *sui juris*. Where the proper and independent duty of the family is concerned, they [the family] are usually bound only to the use of ordinary means." When discussing the removal of respirators, he added, "Consequently, if it appears that the attempt at resuscitation constitutes in reality such a burden for the family that one cannot in all conscience impose it upon them, they can lawfully insist that the doctor should discontinue these attempts, and the doctor can lawfully comply" (64). Finally, a statement of the U.S. Bishops' Committee for Pro-Life Activities in regard to family decisions about AHN should be kept in mind (NCCB 1992):

> We should not assume that all or most decisions to withhold or withdraw medically assisted nutrition and hydration are attempts to cause death. To be sure, any patient will die if all nutrition and hydration are withheld. But sometimes other causes may be at work—for example, the patient may be imminently dying, whether feeding takes place or not. At other times, although the shortening of the patient's life is one foreseeable result of an omission, the real purpose of the omission was to relieve the patient of a particular procedure that was of limited usefulness to the patient or unreasonably burdensome for the patient and the patient's family or caregivers. This kind of decision should not be equated with a decision to kill or with suicide. (707)

Of course, the family does not have a moral obligation to request withdrawal of life support if it seems to be extraordinary. The family may continue medical therapy if it does not violate the rights of other persons or facilities associated with caring for the patient. Thus the rights of doctors and hospitals to declare that life support should be withheld or withdrawn must be respected, even if the family does not wish to follow their advice. In these circumstances, economic burdens should not be assigned to the health care facilities.

Community Interest.   The community is also mentioned as a stakeholder when decisions about life support are necessary (DD. 56–57). People belong to small and large communities. In a small community, the expense and care that a particular therapy might impose could be a factor when decisions about life support are made, because if funds are not expended for one person, they may benefit another person. In religious communities, for example, there is usually a fund to finance health care. But this fund is not an insurance fund in the strict sense; the members of the community contribute to it. Thus, if a community member requires expensive therapy, others in the community may not have access to adequate therapy, or the contributions of individual members may have to be increased.

Some religious community members, not wanting to expend the funds of their community upon therapy that would have doubtful success, often refuse medical therapy, even though it would prolong their lives for a short time. At present, however, given the method of paying for health care in the United States, the larger community, the state, or the insurance company do not often become a significant factor in making decisions about forgoing life support. While the funding methods of state-sponsored health care and insurance companies are too complicated to discuss in this chapter, if care is withheld or removed from one person, there does not seem to be a direct benefit for another person, and the uninsured do not benefit from cost reduction for the insured. This situation could change if universal health care ever becomes a reality within the social policy in the United States.

6.8 CARE OF PERMANENTLY UNCONSCIOUS PATIENTS

In 1972, neurologists Fred Plum and Bryan Jennett distinguished the diagnosis of living (not brain-dead) patients who were unconscious, in a coma, that seldom lasted more than two or three weeks from those in a "persistent vegetative state" (PVS) that was irreversible and permanent because of serious brain damage (Jennett 2002). In 2002, however, the term "minimally conscious state" (MCS) came into use because certain patients diagnosed with PVS were found to slowly regain some low degree of consciousness; some patients eventually recovered full consciousness (Schiff and Fins 2003; Giacino et al. 2000). Some of these latter upon recovery reported that they had been in a "locked-in" state in which they could not communicate with others by any responsive acts, yet had some genuine self-consciousness and awareness of their environment. Dr. Joseph J. Fins, one of the first researchers to recognize this condition as distinct from PVS, summarizes the present state of research as follows: "It is now appreciated that a *persistent* vegetative state becomes *permanent* three months after an anoxic injury (from oxygen deprivation) and a year following traumatic injury. In the window between the persistent and permanent vegetative states, patients can progress to the *minimally conscious state*" (2005). Some estimates hold that some 100,000 Americans are in some state of partial consciousness in comparison to some 10,000 to 15,000 in a truly vegetative state.

In the 1997 edition of this book (Ashley and O'Rourke, 419–32) we proposed, in keeping with the principles already stated in this chapter and with the ERD, that the proxy of a person conservatively diagnosed to be in an irreversible, permanent state of unconsciousness can prudentially judge that, because such a person can no longer perform acts that will serve the ultimate end of human life, union with God, the benefit of any treatment or care beyond that required to show respect for the person can be withdrawn. The theory that human physical life is an "incommensurate good," that is, without any exception a benefit outweighing any burden, was also considered but not accepted in the 1997 edition. Also it was noted how inconsistent it is to hold, as do some adherents to this theory, that the respirator can be withdrawn when it is no longer beneficial for the patient, but not hydration and nutrition by intubation.

Pope John Paul II (1998a), in his "Address to the Bishops of the Episcopal Conference of the United States of America (California, Nevada, and Hawaii)," said:

> As ecumenical witness in defense of life develops, a great teaching effort is needed to clarify the substantive moral difference between discontinuing medical procedures that may be burdensome, dangerous or disproportionate to the expected outcome—what the *Catechism* calls "the refusal of 'over-zealous' treatment" (no. 2278; cf. *Gospel of Life*, 1995, 65)—and taking away the ordinary means of preserving life, such as feeding, hydration and normal medical care. The statement of the United States Bishops' Pro-Life Committee, *Nutrition and Hydration: Moral and Pastoral Considerations*, rightly emphasizes that the omission of nutrition and hydration intended to cause a patient's death must be rejected and that, while giving careful

consideration to all the factors involved, the presumption should be in favor of providing medically assisted nutrition and hydration to all patients who need them. (John Paul II 1998a)

This statement, while urging caution when it says, "giving careful consideration to all the factors involved, the presumption should be in favor of providing medically assisted nutrition and hydration to all patients who need them," also clearly reaffirms the principles explained in this chapter. The Pope repeated this in what seems to have been his final teaching on the subject, his "Allocution to the Participants in the 19th International Conference of the Pontifical Council for Health Pastoral Care," (2004b, no. 4):

True compassion, on the contrary, encourages every reasonable effort for the patient's recovery. At the same time, it helps draw the line when it is clear that no further treatment will serve this purpose. The refusal of *aggressive treatment* is neither a rejection of the patient nor of his or her life. Indeed, the object of the decision on whether to begin or to continue a treatment has nothing to do with the value of the patient's life but rather with whether such medical intervention is beneficial to the patient.

The possible decision either not to start or to halt treatment will be deemed ethically correct if the treatment is ineffective or obviously disproportionate to the aims of sustaining life or recovering health. Consequently, the decision to forego aggressive treatment is an expression of the respect due to the patient at every moment.

Controversy has arisen, however, with regard to Pope John Paul II's previous address of that year (2004a), "To the Participants in the International Congress on 'Life-Sustaining Treatments and Vegetative State': Scientific Advances and Ethical Dilemmas," which, after deploring the use of the term PVS as leading to a denial of the personhood of such victims, went on to say (no. 4),

The sick person in a vegetative state, awaiting recovery or a natural end, still has the right to basic health care (nutrition, hydration, cleanliness, warmth, etc), and to the prevention of complications related to his confinement to bed. He also has the right to appropriate rehabilitative care and to be monitored for clinical signs of eventual recovery. I should like particularly, to underline how the administration of water and food, even when provided by artificial means, always represents a natural means of preserving life, not a medical act. Its use, furthermore, should be considered, in principle, ordinary and proportionate, and as such morally obligatory, insofar as and until it is seen to have attained its proper finality, which in the present case consists in providing nourishment to the patient and alleviation of his suffering. The obligation to provide the "normal care due to the sick in such cases . . . includes, in fact, the use of nutrition and hydration."

The question in this statement is not about the difference between medical treatment and comfort or basic care, as some commentators have supposed, because the principle of burden and benefit, as we have seen, applies to both natural or normal care and to medical treatment (section 6.7). If either treatment or care is withdrawn with the intention of causing death, the withdrawal is euthanasia as the Pope has stated, but if the intention of the act (*finis operis*) is simply "letting die," it is not euthanasia, as the Pope stated in the previously quoted address (2004b). What is new, however, is that in the address in March (2004a) he did not speak of "presumption," but seems to accept the medical view that was formulated by the medical participants in this Congress (FIAMC 2004, 579) in their concluding summary about VS.

5) VS diagnosis is still clinical in nature and requires careful and prolonged observation, carried out by specialized and experienced personnel using specific assessment standardized for VS patients in an optimum-controlled environment. Medical literature, in fact, shows diagnostic errors in a substantially high proportion of cases. For this reason, when needed, all available modern technologies should be used to substantiate the diagnosis.

6) Modern neuroimaging techniques have demonstrated the persistence of cortical activity and response to certain kinds of stimuli, including painful stimuli, in VS patients. Although it is not possible to determine the subjective quality of such perceptions, some elementary discriminatory processes between meaningful and neutral stimuli seem to be nevertheless possible.

7) No single investigation method available today allows us to predict, in individual cases, who will recover and who will not among VS patients.

8) Until today, statistical prognostic indexes regarding VS have been obtained from studies quite limited as to number of cases considered and duration of observation. Therefore, the use of misleading terms like "permanent" referred to VS should be discouraged, by indicating only the cause and duration of VS. (579)

Thus when John Paul II (2004a, no. 4) said, "The evaluation of probabilities, founded on waning hopes for recovery when the vegetative state is prolonged beyond a year, cannot ethically justify the cessation or interruption of minimal care for the patient including nutrition and hydration," he left open whether in this so-called vegetative state there is a reasonable hope of recovery, although he leans in the direction adopted by the medical statement of the conference (FIAMC 2004) that "no single investigation method available today allows us to predict, in individual cases, who will recover and who will not among VS patients." Yet even their statement, although it "discourages" the term *permanent*, does not deny that it can be permanent. Thus it is forcing the papal statement to claim that we do not still have to consider the benefit-burden principle in deciding how long the continuation of hydration and nutrition is ethically obligatory. Catholic moral theology has never imposed moral obligations on persons, especially if they were burdensome, except in cases of moral certitude. Moral certitude, however, is prudentially, not factually, certain, and this factual probability is sufficient if it is the best information available to us. In the case of medical diagnosis, this prudential certitude is all that is usually possible, even in declaring brain death. Therefore to conclude that it is morally obligatory to keep all PVS patients alive as long as possible, including the use of artificial respiration and nutrition and hydration, is excessive.

"In Principle" Admits of Exceptions

As a number of commentators have pointed out, John Paul II in the previously cited address (2004a), qualified his remarks by saying, "in principle," which the French translation most clearly renders as *en règle générale*, "as a general rule," thus leaving room for exceptions, as he had done previously by the term *presumption*. It follows that while, as already noted, suicide and euthanasia are intrinsically immoral and admit of no exceptions, this is a question of "allowing to die." Thus, in principle, the obligation of hydration and nutrition as comfort or basic care does admit of exceptions when the medical diagnosis of irreversible and permanent unconsciousness has been conservatively made on the basis of current knowledge and when it can be prudently judged that its burden to patient and to the caregivers exceeds its benefit to the patient.

Our understanding of the papal teaching, however, is not accepted by all, either because they support the theory of "incommensurable goods" that makes physical life always a benefit except when the person is actually dying or because they understand John Paul II to have magisterially ruled out any possibility of a morally certain diagnosis of permanent unconsciousness (Shannon and Walter 2004; Doerflinger 2004). It is, however, supported by others who like ourselves seek to be faithful to magisterial teaching. Thus the National Catholic Bioethics Center (NCBC 2004) in their statement following the Pope's March 10 (2004a) statement concluded that, "In general the provision of nutrition and hydration to the patient in the vegetative state is proportionate and morally obligatory, but that in a particular case nutrition and hydration may be extraordinary and disproportionate, and, therefore, morally optional." The Catholic Health Association (CHA) very cautiously answers questions of its members in much the same sense.

A group of philosophers, theologians, and pastoral care and clinical personnel, meeting in Canada in June 2004, stated that the Allocution of the previous March must be interpreted in accord with the traditional teaching of the Church (CCBI 2004). For this reason, the phrase "in principle" does not mean "absolute in the sense of exceptionless," but allows the consideration of other duties that might apply. These considerations would include cost and other burdens. In September 2004 the Australian Bishops' Conference affirmed the teaching of the papal address of the previous March on this point, but also stated, "In particular cases, however, the provision of nutrition and hydration may cease to be obligatory, e.g. if the patient is unable to assimilate the material provided or if the manner of the provision itself causes undue suffering to the patient, or involves an undue burden to others." Others, however, for example Richard M. Doerflinger, of the pro-life committee of the NCCB, have read John Paul II's address of March 20 as forbidding the withdrawing of hydration and nutrition as normal care until the patient is actually dying (2004). What, therefore, are our Catholic health care facilities and families to do when they are faced with this situation? In practice it seems that, unless the Holy See further clarifies the issue and teaches that it is always wrong to withhold artificial respiration or hydration and nutrition until the patient is dying, Directive 58 of the ERD (2001) (for its history, see Kopfensteiner 2005) still covers the care of PVS patients: "There should be presumption in favor of providing nutrition and hydration to all patients, including patients who require medically assisted nutrition and hydration, as long as this is of sufficient benefit to outweigh the burdens involved to the patient." When applying this directive, the burdens of the family and the community may be considered, as indicated in Directives 56 and 57 and the traditional teaching of the Church whose teaching on such subjects is open to development in light of the progress of medicine. Ultimately, when medical opinion becomes more uniform, the Holy See will probably further clarify the ethical question, and its guidance should be followed by Catholics as having authority superior to theological opinion, including, of course, of this present book.

6.9 TREATMENT OF PAIN

Patients recovering from surgery, undergoing therapy for serious pathologies, or in proximate stages of dying often experience severe pain and suffering (Fine 2002). Three principles should govern pain control.

First, alleviating pain by means of medication or narcotics does not constitute euthanasia, even if the suffering person's life might be shortened as a result of the medication (John Paul II, 1995). As indicated earlier, the intention inherent in the act of euthanasia (*finis operis*) is ending the life of the person in question. The intention inherent in the act of pain control is to moderate the pain of the patient, even though it is possible that this may result in the patient dying sooner. The ERD declares (2001, D. 61):

> Patients should be kept as free of pain as possible so that they may die comfortable and with dignity, and in the place where they wish to die. Since a person has the right to prepare for his or her death while fully conscious, he or she should not be deprived of consciousness without a compelling reason. Medicines capable of alleviating or suppressing pain may be given to a dying person, even if this therapy may indirectly shorten the person's life, as long as the intent is not to hasten death. Patients experiencing suffering that cannot be alleviated should be helped to appreciate the understanding of redemptive suffering.

Second, pain is not an absolute human evil. Although suffering is to be alleviated whenever possible, it is not in itself a moral evil nor without supernatural benefits if rightly used. The Christian tradition holds that great spiritual good can come out of suffering when it is joined to the sufferings of Jesus. St. Paul said, "Now I rejoice in my sufferings for your sake, and in my flesh I am filling up what is lacking in the afflictions of Christ on behalf of his body, which is the church" (Col 1:24). Christian teaching in this regard does not imply a masochistic desire for pain, nor does it stand in the way of medical progress. As one group of Christians maintained (Church of England 1975), "A terminal illness can be transformed into a time for which everyone concerned is grateful." The opportunity to use suffering as a means of spiritual growth is not destroyed if pain-killing drugs are used. Rather, the individual and those who care for him or her have the right to use such drugs in a way that will permit the best use of the patient's remaining energies and time of consciousness, so that the patient can complete life with maximal composure.

Third, in recent years, medical and psychological breakthroughs have occurred in regard to pain (Carr and Goudas 1999). Pharmaceutical and surgical procedures make it possible to control and alleviate pain in the hospital and at home. Severe and excruciating pain, then, is hardly a realistic excuse for direct euthanasia or suicide (Foley and Hendin 2002). Moreover, people in the hospice movement have made an even more startling discovery in the psychological control of pain. Case studies demonstrate that pain is alleviated and controlled when human concern and care are given to the elderly. The ultimate human pain seems to be the fear and the loneliness of dying alone. If these feelings are overcome, it seems that pain is not so unbearable, even for those who are dying of debilitating disease (Cassem 2003).

6.10 CONCLUSION

In summary, the following pastoral norms for decision making in regard to allowing to die can be formulated thus:

1. A physician may admit that a patient is incurable and cease trying to effect a cure; however, physicians should not cease trying to find a remedy for disease itself.

2. As long as there is a slight hope for curing patients or checking the progress of their illness, the physician should use the available remedies at hand, if this is the desire of the patient or proxy. However, the patient or proxy may refuse treatment if the patient or proxy considers it to be ineffective or constitutes a serious burden to the patient. The burden may be psychic, social, or spiritual, as well as physiological.

3. The patient, considering his or her medical prognosis as well as other spiritual and temporal circumstances of life, should determine in consultation with the physician whether a particular means is ordinary or extraordinary from an ethical point of view.

4. If the means are ordinary, they must be used; if the means are extraordinary, they may be used but need not be. Minimal means of maintaining the patient's comfort and well-being are always considered ordinary means (CDF 1980).

5. If the patient is unable to make the pertinent decisions, family members, in consultation with the physician, have the right and obligation to determine whether the means in question are ordinary or extraordinary and whether extraordinary means will be used. In making this decision, the family should decide in the best interest of the patient, not solely for the benefit of the family.

6. Documents such as Advance Directives may be used by patients as a means of informing family and physician and as help in preparing for death (ERD 2001, D. 25). We do not, however, favor that such documents be given legal status. Although such documents are not in themselves wrong, they do not always solve the problems of decision making.

7. In accordance with the advice of St. Paul (1 Cor 6:1–6), "How can any one of you with a case against another dare to bring it to the unjust for judgment instead of to the holy ones?" When Catholic families cannot agree about what to do in the care of such persons they should ask the advice of their bishop rather than sue each other in the secular courts.

Part III

SOCIAL AND PASTORAL RESPONSIBILITIES

Chapter Seven

SOCIAL RESPONSIBILITY

OVERVIEW

ALTHOUGH INDIVIDUALS HAVE PRIMARY RESPONSIBILITY TO care for their own physiological health as well as for the psychological, ethical, and spiritual aspects of their personal development, such development can be achieved only with the help of other members of the community. People belong to many different communities: their family, various social organizations, business organizations, and various civic entities. Many of these communities have a direct or indirect relationship to a person's health or health care. In advanced communities, such help is furnished by persons who have committed themselves to this vocation and been educated for the special social roles called the health care professions and also by society, that is, by government funding. This chapter considers the chief ethical responsibilities of these various social entities. Because the health care profession is one among several professions basic to the culture of any advanced community, we consider the nature of professions in general, then specific characteristics of the health care profession. Because the health care profession is founded upon trust, we focus upon the activities in the physician-patient relationship that foster trust, counseling, and communication and confidentiality. When considering the responsibilities of the civic society, an analysis of the task of local communities is beyond the scope of our concern. We focus instead on the federal level and begin by examining the politics in the United States in regard to health care, the principles that should inform health care policy, and the efforts of society to formulate ethical public policy for health care. Finally, we consider the responsibility of Catholic institutions as they contribute to provision of health care in the United States.

7.1 PROFESSIONS: DEPERSONALIZING TRENDS

The traditional professions are divinity (theology), physic (medicine), law, and teaching. They are "person professions" centered on a counselor-client relation (Pellegrino 2002). They do not produce goods for sale or works of art for enjoyment, but seek to heal, guide, or protect some person in a life crisis. Industrial society has greatly fostered the professions, but it has also depersonalized them. No longer are they centered on the relationship of persons (Engelhardt and Cherry 2002), but on the productivity of an impersonal system. They no longer deal with better interpersonal communication, but with more efficient exchange of energy (Brint 1994).

This slow depersonalizing transformation of the professions is reaching its completion today, just as industrial society itself seems about to yield to a new postindustrial society. Neither progressive capitalism nor revolutionary Marxism has been able to fulfill the promises of scientific technology to produce a society of abundance and freedom. Even this promise begins to seem illusory in view of the ecological doomsday predicted by some authorities.

In postindustrial society, the source of power will no longer be economic ownership (whether capitalist or socialist), but rather *knowledge and its communication.* Such power means a still greater role for the professions (Callahan 1988). This knowledge can be used to bring about greater social conformism and dependency on professionals, or it can be used to open the system to wider and more genuine social participation by all. In either case, the professions, especially the profession of medicine, will be significant cultural factors.

Will professionals become technocrats whose technological mastery must extend itself to behavior control? Or will they become the persons who help others to transcend the depersonalization of technological systems by "putting the good of the weaker party over one's own interests" (Moline 1986)? If professionals choose the latter alternative, the professions must again be personalized. They must be reconstructed so as to eliminate the threefold depersonalization that the professions have suffered in the epoch of industrial society.

In medical practice, depersonalization is increasingly evident (Williams 2001). First, *patients* have been depersonalized by the proliferation of specialization. Often, they are no longer thought of as organisms, but as collections of organs (Isaacs and Knickman 2002). The parts are healed, not the person, such that the very meaning of *healing*—that is, "to make *whole*"—has been lost. Even the efforts of interdisciplinary healing teams never quite seem to succeed in getting it all together again. In this book we have tried to avoid the term *patient* as much as possible, too, because it tends to depersonalize the sick as if they were merely passive recipients of healing rather than persons who are themselves striving to recover health.

Second, *professionals themselves* have been depersonalized by a loss of clear identity. This loss is notoriously true for the ordained ministry (Cozzens 2000) and is now evident in law, teaching, and medicine (Beck and Young 2005). Psychiatrists, psychoanalysts, and psychiatric social workers all perform similar tasks but are considered members of three different professions. Even more confusing, many ordained ministers, lawyers, and physicians counsel clients in ways not easily distinguishable from those used by psychotherapists.

Contributing to this confusion of identity today is the tension within the profession between the goals of research and the goals of practice (Katz 2002). In addition, many areas of professional practice may soon be handed over to computers (Mitchell 1997). How, then, can a professional make that type of personal commitment always regarded as a mark of a profession if it is not clear to what he or she is professed?

Third, the *validity of the professional-client relationship* is being questioned. Professionalism seems to imply an elitism that is ultimately socially destructive. Ivan Illich (1972; Illich, Zola, and McKnight 1978) masterfully studied the problems of underdeveloped countries and launched an all-out attack on schooling and the concept of the teaching profession and extends the same criticism to medicine. He contends that the industrial model for organizing the professions has progressively restricted access to knowledge and skill, placing them in the hands of elites on whom the public is more and more dependent, but from whom the public receives less and less adequate service. The result is that service institutions have become "production funnels" that proliferate subordinate professions and para-professions, and he indicates that developing nations are desperately striving to make the same mistake.

Fourth, the contemporary practice of health maintenance organizations (HMOs) or other managed care corporations to contract with physicians in the practice of medicine disposes physicians to be more interested in practicing within economic guidelines than in serving patient well-being (Bennet 2001).

These four sources of depersonalization are most easily illustrated in the case of the medical profession (Stevens 2001), but they also occur in the most unlikely profession—the religious ministry, which has always claimed to be concerned with and for the whole person. In recent years, many priests, ministers, and rabbis have deserted their calling to serve. The clergy have accepted elitist status and are neither sure of their own role nor competent to give interdisciplinary guidance to other professionals in the service of persons (O'Meara 2000).

A Person-Centered Concept of a Profession

Today the term *profession* is used for almost any prestigious occupation because it has the aura of an ideal. It is a symbol rather than a reality. The distinguished sociologist Howard Becker (1960) wrote,

> The symbol systematically ignores such facts as the failure of the professions to monopolize their area of knowledge, the lack of homogeneity within professions, the frequent failure of clients to accept professional judgment, the chronic presence of unethical practitioners as an integrated segment of the professional structure, and the organizational constraints on professional autonomy. A symbol which ignores so many features of occupational life cannot provide an adequate guide for professional activity. (46)

Nevertheless, sociologists have devoted much time to developing a good empirical definition of a profession. Merton (1960) explained the social value of a profession very succinctly: "First, the value placed upon systematic knowledge and intellect: *knowing*. Second, the value placed upon technical skill and trained capacity: *doing*. And third, the value placed upon putting this conjoint knowledge and skill to work in the service of others: *helping*" (9). Today, engineering, accounting, architecture and the other arts, and business are considered professions because they also involve knowing, doing, and helping. Their immediate objective, however, is not personal but productive; they do not have direct contact with persons, or with their development as persons. This obliteration of the distinction between the person professions and productive occupations is characteristic of industrial society and its depersonalization of the professions. A true profession, therefore, is rooted in theory but aimed at practice—a practice that does not produce things external to persons, but a service directly to persons themselves. Furthermore, this service is not applied to persons who receive it passively, but facilitates those persons' own activity. It aims at healing them, at making them whole, at freeing them to act on their own. Counselors should not act on clients nor dominate them, but should enable them to become fully, autonomously themselves. Thus a profession cannot properly be elitist. It communicates power rather than enforces dependency.

To call the technologies and the arts (engineering, business, and fine arts) professions is confusing and dangerous because this designation disguises the fact that they produce *things* and do not directly help persons. Certainly the technologies should educate their practitioners to be more sensitive to the human uses to which their products will be put. This humanization of technology, however, will be hindered if industrial society continues the previous tendency of lumping the technologies and the person professions together under one name and judging them all in terms of productivity. Finally, professional help in the full sense is concerned precisely with those problems that are deeply personal, that are matters of life and death. Therefore such help engages both counselor and client in a profound responsibility both to each other and to the community. This person-centered concept of a profession can reconstruct the professions and professional education for the future.

7.2 CHARACTERISTICS OF MEDICINE AS A PROFESSION

To make sure that the personalistic concept of the medical profession is not mere theory requires a brief look at the ideals of medicine as a profession as developed through its history.

The standard histories of medicine (Garrison 1960; Sigerist 1951) usually divide this history into the prescientific period and the scientific period, which begins in the seventeenth century after Vesalius and Harvey. Michael Foucault, in his fascinating book *The Birth of the Clinic* (1973), shows that a crucial step was taken as a result of the efforts of the radical wing of the French Revolution to abolish all professions, including the medical profession, as a means to establishing a classless society. The resulting chaos in health care then led to the reestablishment of the medical profession and its hospitals on a new basis under the domination of the scientific ideals of the Enlightenment.

Freymann (1974) has also shown that from 1700 to 1850 health care was fragmented, and the profession was at a low ebb until the age of Pasteur, with its emphasis on the scientific education of physicians to fight acute diseases. Thus medicine as an effective scientific technology is a very recent development in human history.

On closer examination, however, it becomes evident that this sharp division into prescientific and scientific periods is somewhat misleading because it is only a manifestation of two aspects of medical tradition that have always coexisted. Today, along with orthodox scientific medicine, a vast field of heretical medicine exists, ranging from naturopathy, faith healing, homeopathy, and chiropractic to osteopathy, acupuncture, and "holistic" medicine, not to mention countless forms of pure quackery (Callahan 1993). These therapies evidently complement orthodox medicine because they seem to meet health needs that orthodox medicine does not. Also, it is no secret that even within orthodox medicine the field of psychotherapy is a borderline area that many medical physicians consider unscientific.

This duality, on closer examination, reflects the mind–body or psychosomatic duality of the human being who is sick. In early times the learned professions all originated from the one rather confused profession of priest (or perhaps priest-king). Priests were looked on as custodians of sacred wisdom and power over the forces of nature, a gift from the gods, who alone possessed cosmic secrets.

In Greece (whence modern Western medicine is directly descended) the first father of medicine was Asclepius, who was so kind and known as the "mild god" that he was to prove a great rival of Christ as Christianity spread throughout the pagan world (Edelstein 1967). Asclepius's priests presided over shrines (the first clinics) where the sick came to worship, sleep, and have their dreams interpreted. The symbol of the medical profession today is still a staff with entwined serpents because the serpent, symbol of wisdom and the healing power of mother earth (i.e., nature), was the cult animal at these shrines. To-day in the city of Rome, the Hospital of the Benefratelli of medieval origin is built on an island in the River Tiber over remains of a shrine of Asclepius transferred from Greece in classical times. A great snake is still to be seen carved on the ancient ruins.

This myth manifests a basic truth about the medical profession: the physician to this day retains something of a priestly ministry in the service of the healing forces of nature. Something similar is true of every profession, as all professions deal with the sacred dignity of the human person and rest on the sacred covenant of trust between client and professional. This priestly ministry is especially true of the medical profession because its direct relation to life and death gives it a fundamental, primitive character (Ross 1994). A person's trust in the physician is almost the same as trust in one's mother; it is a primordial confidence in life support.

No wonder, then, that even today the physician is a charismatic figure, surrounded by a priestly atmosphere (witness the myths of television doctor shows). Although this trust can be abused and exploited, it is valuable when it is authentic. No one can be healed without trust. Thus the most significant distinction in understanding the history of medicine is not between scientific and nonscientific medicine, but between *authentic* medicine and quackery. Thus authentic medicine has both priestly and scientific dimensions.

Why did it take until the seventeenth and even the nineteenth century for the rapid development of this scientific side of medicine to begin? The empirical rational method was already well understood in the time of Hippocrates, about 400 BC. Hippocrates rejected the designation of epilepsy and other ailments as sacred diseases and attempted to explain them biologically. In the next century, Aristotle (himself a son of an Asclepian doctor who was the physician of Alexander the Great), in *De Somniis,* demythologized the notion of dreams, often used to diagnose diseases, by giving such psychic phenomena a physiological explanation. This tradition of scientific medicine was further developed by Hellenistic physicians such as Galen and by medieval Arabian, Jewish, and Christian physicians. Before Harvey (d. 1657) described the circulation of blood, however, the practical fruits of this scientific approach were sparse.

Why Did Medicine Develop So Slowly?

Why did it take so long for medicine to develop its scientific side? One explanation is that the scientific aspect of medicine was held back by its priestly aspect (White 1896). It is not inevitable, however, that these two aspects should hinder rather than complement each other. Others have pointed out that scientific medicine could not get far until the development of chemistry and biology. But why were these sciences also so slow to develop? Perhaps the better explanation is given by some Marxist sociologists and other authorities. Greek thinkers clearly recognized the method and value of empirical science, but they practiced in medicine in a social system based on the sharp division between the liberally educated freemen who despised manual work and the slaves or serfs. This barrier between theory and practice, between attention to the spiritual care of sick and dying persons and attention to the care of their material bodies, was the major obstacle to the development of science and scientific medicine.

Elevation of the physician to the status of a learned professional increasingly separated from the suffering patient was intensified by the university education that emerged in the Middle Ages. Nevertheless, the Christian concern for the poor began to break through this Greek contempt for practical involvement. Christianity, particularly in its Roman Catholic form, has been the religion most concerned with organized health care because of its belief in personal charity and the integral relation of the body to the human person. Despite practical efforts to realize this Christian ideal, however, the state of scientific knowledge and the level of social organization were so low that, until the end of the Middle Ages, the chief efforts were directed to caring for sick and dying persons rather than to healing them.

Practical and material concerns were clearly seen to have religious and ethical values only with the Renaissance and the development of Christian humanism in Catholic Europe and Calvinist emphasis on work as a vocation in Protestant Europe. Thus the groundwork for the rapid rise of empirical science and modern medical technology was finally laid. Undoubtedly the secular humanism of the Enlightenment built well on this basis, but it did not lay its foundation. The role of the French Revolution was essentially negative. It broke down the old, fixed patterns of the medical profession so that the new model might develop fully (Foucault 1973).

Does the previous tension between the liberal and the service aspects of medicine exist today? At first glance such a suspicion seems absurd. The modern physician is above all interested in practice, and no class of physicians has greater prestige and remuneration than surgeons, who certainly get their hands dirty. A closer look, however, reveals that the emphasis on the specialist, as opposed to the general practitioner, and the building up of a pyramid of paramedical professionals in the service of the physician, who mediate between the physician and patient, is the modern version of this class distinction (Pew Commission 1993; Institute of Medicine 1996).

The Twenty-First-Century Physician

Alternatively, the rise of psychiatry and psychosomatic medicine in the twentieth century has strengthened and developed the other, priestly aspect of medicine in which the physician as counselor becomes less the scientific technologist and more the artist in direct contact with the patient. The current debates about the humanization of medicine reflect the resurgence of this other aspect of the medical tradition, which has never died and will always be part of medicine (Brennan 1994). Many of the real needs of the sick that nineteenth-century medicine tended to abandon to the medical heretics are now being recovered as legitimate concerns of the orthodox medical profession (Moyers 1993). These debates, however, continue. The problem of the personalization of health care is far from solved, but the emphasis on patient needs speaks well for a re-personalization of medicine (Pew Commission 1995). Therefore the charismatic character of the physician, which arises from the priestly side of medicine but is also enhanced by the astounding power of scientific technology, should be respected. In all professions the charismatic atmosphere is an important element of the professional relation and is essential to the healing process. This atmosphere makes it possible for the patient, often skeptical or distrustful, to place the necessary trust in professional help. It also gives medical professionals a sense of personal dignity, dedication, and responsibility that immeasurably contributes to their satisfaction and persistence in a difficult vocation.

This charismatic aspect is also a guard of other ethical values, because nothing is so likely to keep medical professionals from abusing their position for financial or other gains as this sense of self-respect. It would be disastrous if the increasing mechanization of medicine or the reduction of the medical professional to an anonymous functionary in a government bureaucracy would destroy the priestly charisma of the profession (Pellegrino 1987; Crawshaw et al. 1996).

On the negative side, however, as with the clergyman, overemphasis on the special status of the physician is open to great abuses (Martin, Lloyd, and Sough 2002). The physician can become an unquestioned, dogmatic authority in medicine and in all other matters as well. The medical profession often jealously defends its authority and its prerogatives, refuses to discipline members of the profession, and claims the right to settle ethical and social questions that affect the profession on the grounds that laypersons have no right to opinions in such matters.

Therefore the physician who wants to develop a sound ethical judgment must have (1) a profound respect for the medical profession as a vocation that has both scientific and priestly aspects, (2) a clear understanding of the limits of this profession, and (3) a sense of personal responsibility to develop the attitudes and skills that enable one to personalize the profession (O'Rourke 1988).

The Christian Physician

Christian health care professionals are called by their faith to understand this vocation in a special way, just as professionals of other religions or philosophies of life are called by theirs. Christians think of life as a gift from God and the body as a marvelous work of divine creation to be reverenced as a temple of God (1 Cor 6:19, 2 Cor 6:16). They also think of the human person not only as a living body but also as a body living with spiritual life open to a share in the eternal life of God. Even when sickness cannot be overcome, the struggle against it can be lived through as an experience that can further moral and spiritual growth. Thus the Christian physician or nurse is truly a minister of God, cooperating with him in helping human beings overcome their suffering to live more fully.

The Christian medical professional finds a model in Jesus Christ, the healer. Although physicians do not have supernatural or miraculous powers, they do have medical skill, which is also a gift from God. They can imitate Jesus's compassion for the patient and his reaching out to the most neglected, even the lepers. This Christian attitude cannot be a matter of mere pious words; rather, it is a profound dependence on God, who gives the physician and nurse the inspiration, insight, and courage to carry out their work as professionally and as skillfully as possible.

Moreover, one should not make the mistake of thinking that the ethical aspect of medicine pertains only to its personal, priestly side. It also penetrates the scientific aspect. A scientific approach to disease is built on devotion to objective truth and the courageous, persevering effort to advance this truth through research and criticism. Though there are some examples of scientists being interested in their own reputations at the expense of truth, on the whole, the scientific approach, with its insistence on objective evidence and critical review by peers, has a splendid record. Scientific integrity has been very effective in limiting excessive charismatic pretensions and ambitions.

On the negative side, however, the scientific method, as now understood and practiced, often tends to reductionism, that is, the assertion that the scientific method is the exclusive road to truth. Because the scientific method deals only with the limited aspects of reality that can be measured and experimented on, such a reductionist attitude can compel physicians to ignore and deny facts and experiences outside those rather narrow limits. When reductionism is rigidly applied, the patient is treated as a soulless machine. In the history of medicine, this mechanistic approach has been profitable to the degree that it has used the scientific method intensively, but it has ultimately limited the advance of medicine. Biologists and physicians sensitive to the holistic character of living organisms and the human person have revolted repeatedly against reductionism and opened new, broader, and more fruitful lines of research (Kass 1985).

Thus sound ethical judgment must completely respect scientifically established medical facts, but it cannot rest on these facts alone. It must be open to all humanistic approaches to understanding and evaluating the human condition.

7.3 HEALTH CARE COUNSELING

In order to serve clients well, every professional must be an adept counselor. Originally the term *counseling* pertained to rational, moral, and ethical functioning, and in particular to the legal profession, as the British use of the term *counselor* indicates (Gladding 2004). Counseling also found a place in the religious ministry; the rabbi was a type of religious lawyer, and this role was passed on to Christian priests. The specific type of counseling proper to the ministerial profession is deeper than the legal profession and pertains to the spiritual dimension of the human person. One can argue that the teaching profession, in arousing the creativity of the student, also reaches this level of intuitive life.

The medical professional often performs one or the other of these types of counseling proper to the other professions. A physician may have to discuss with an ailing person certain ethical and legal issues, such as those involved in an abortion decision. Sometimes a physician is involved in a sick person's spiritual struggles about death and the meaning of life. Often physicians must play the role of teacher, helping persons understand their bodies and their feelings about them. All these involvements, however, are incidental and substitutional. A prudent physician is quick to refer the patient to experts in other professions when the issues are ethical and spiritual rather than medical.

The proper task of the medical professional is to deal with problems at the biological and psychological levels of human functioning (Pellegrino and Thomasma 1981, 1988). At the psychological level, counseling of a certain type plays a major therapeutic role. At the biological level, however, it is not so obvious that the physician's role is still primarily that of a counselor.

However, all persons have primary responsibility for their own health; thus the physician's primary responsibility is to help patients make good health decisions, which requires a counseling process. People cannot make good decisions about how to care for their health unless they have the required information. In more complicated cases, this information can be obtained only by consulting a physician. To some extent the physician is playing the role of a teacher in giving this information. More is involved than this, however, as the information required is not abstract biological truth but a concrete assessment of personal health and the possible ways of dealing with the problems this assessment presents. This form of guidance is required of a physician, and it engages the physician in a special type of counseling.

This basic counseling relation on which the whole medical profession is built is *trusteeship*. Ramsey (1970) describes this relationship as *a covenant* similar to the pact between Yahweh and his people described in the Jewish scriptures. Technological progress in medicine has temporarily obscured the importance of trusteeship, making it appear that the physician is a scientist-technician rather than a counselor, but this same technological progress will eventually expose what it covers up (Campbell 1994).

Nursing is truly a profession because it shares in this counseling task of the physician (Johnstone 2004). Today the role of the nurse has become very ambiguous (Crissman and Betz 1987; Jecker and Self 1991). Health care has always had the double dimension of cure and care. Thus medicine often requires a distinction between the curing task of the physician and the caring task of the nurse. What is common to both cure and care is that the patient must consent to both and cooperate actively with both, so that both physician and nurse must enter into the trustee relationship with the patient.

Also, this basic relationship will not be eliminated as patients in managed care plans relate more and more to a health team rather than one-to-one with a personal physician. Group psychotherapy has proved that personalism need not be eliminated just because the one-to-one relationship with a therapist is expanded into a more complex social relationship.

In the medical model, the professional goal is to treat a physical pathology so as to restore normal physiological function insofar as possible. The physician first seeks to diagnose the disease then to prescribe a course of treatment through medicine, surgery, nursing, and change of regimen. The physician must also offer a prognosis and, if possible, give the patient hope. At the first stages of medical counseling, the patient is not overly active; but more activity is required in the recovery or rehabilitative stage of the relationship. At the foundation of the medical relationship of counseling are concern, knowledge, and skill.

Concern

Fundamental to the counseling relationship is the physician's concern for the client's well-being. Trust will never exist if the client believes that the physician is only interested in her or him as a specimen of some pathology, performing a routine in a mechanistic manner, or as a bureaucratic employee. The physician must communicate interest in the patient as a person, not as a kidney or a transplant donor. In the concept of "covenant," God makes a pact with the chosen people not because of their worthiness but because of his generous love for them. The professional contract is analogous to such a promise in the sense that the professional undertakes to help the sick person not because that person is ethically worthy of help, or even because he or she is able to pay for the service, but primarily because of human need.

This concept of covenant should not be exaggerated. God himself insisted on the responsibility of his chosen people to respond to their obligations. Thus the physician also has the right to demand cooperation from the patient. Moreover, the physician's responsibility is related to his or her own competency and should refer the patient to another medical or nonmedical counselor if the problem requires such referral. Health care professionals have the fundamental responsibility to be expert in regard to the theory and art of medicine within the realm of their specialties. The field of medicine is characterized by research and new knowledge, and keeping abreast of the new knowledge is a daunting task. The physician who does not consider herself or himself engaged in a lifelong learning process will mistreat clients and become personally dissatisfied. Thus there is no substitute for assiduous continuing education on the part of physicians. Personal warmth does not substitute for medical expertise. Humanistic concern must be based upon scientific competency.

7.4 PROFESSIONAL COMMUNICATION AND CONFIDENTIALITY

In health care, as in all professional relationships, adequate communication between professional and client is a fundamental ethical requirement. In medical counseling the opportunity for communication may be limited by an inability on the part of the patient to understand scientific terminology. This is especially difficult if the client is not familiar with the language of the professional. Yet some effort must be made, perhaps by a translator, to help the client comprehend the situation and make reasonable choices of treatment. A commission appointed in the early days of concern focusing on malpractice litigation found that a major cause of the problem was poor communication on the part of health care professionals (GAO 1987). This problem exists today as well and should be a continuing concern of all health care professionals.

The first requirement for good communication on the part of the health care professional is to listen carefully to the patient. Pathologies are often disguised by clients; thus the professional must sift through the statements and evasions of the client in order to discern the "real problem" (Reiser 1993). Somehow professionals must cut through the noise and get at the real message, remembering that "the medium is the message," that is, the way clients are or are not communicating may be the most significant symptom.

Therefore no matter how busy they might be, health care professionals must not rush through interviews or simply rely on lab test results. They have a responsibility to acquire the art of medical dialogue, by which they can help clients say what has to be said. The first rule of this art is for the professional to repeat back to the client what seems to the professional to have been significant and to ask the client if that is what he or she meant.

This form of feedback not only reassures the client but also can train the client to give relevant information. A second rule is to obtain the client's cooperation by explaining the purpose of the questions, because unexpected questions are threatening to some clients. Physicians my find it necessary to work with other persons, for example nurses, in order to achieve better communication skills.

Professionals have the right to require honesty and frankness from clients. When professionals suspect deliberate deceit, they should deal with the situation explicitly and directly. In some illnesses, however, psychological factors may cause communication to be distorted by unconscious elements of self-deceit, denial, confusion, or panic. Psychotherapists have to deal with this type of situation more often than other medical professionals experience this form of ambiguity. Even in these situations, the patient has the right to the truth, however difficult it may be for them to face it (Thomasma 1994).

Confidentiality

Clients have a right to the truth about their health because they have the primary responsibility for their health. They also have the right to privacy about those aspects of their life that do not directly affect others. Federal legislation has offered greater protection for personal privacy (Annas 2002). Thus health care professionals have a serious obligation to maintain such confidences that protect the client's right of privacy.

How is a professional to act when questioned by others about a patient's condition? Can confidentiality be protected by lying? All Catholic moralists agree that it is wrong to lie, even to protect privacy, but not all agree on the definition of *lying*. Some distinguish between a *false statement* and a *lie*, which is a false statement made to a person who has the right to a true answer. Thus, as Knauer stated when this issue was discussed a few decades ago (1967), the meaning of any human statement must be determined from the context in which the statement occurs. Therefore, when persons ask questions that they have no right to ask, the context renders any answer given essentially meaningless. Thus health care professionals who are questioned about confidential matters, without lying, give an ambiguous or irrelevant answer. This distinction between a falsehood and lying has been challenged (Fisher 1996), but still seems to have validity. Of course, this distinction would never excuse a physician from answering the questions of clients or their guardians, because these persons have a right to know (Capron 1993). If there is need to discuss a client's condition with another physician or member of a health care team, the physician responsible for care should obtain informed consent from the client before sharing information that might be demeaning with others. Researchers who search medical records also must be aware of the need to protect confidentiality of patients (Annas 2002).

Nevertheless, the right of privacy, even though important, is limited by other persons' rights and the right to the help of others that persons have. Sick persons may behave in ways that injure themselves or others. For example, patients may threaten suicide, seek ways to continue chemical addiction, or spread contagious diseases. In the well-known case of *Tarasoff v. Regents of University of California*, the court decreed that a therapist is responsible for not warning third parties that his client might be dangerous (Goldstein 1993). In all cases, the professional, acting as a representative of society, has the responsibility to prevent harm to clients and other members of the community. Thus, in general, when information is given in confidence that might endanger patients or other people, professionals have the obligation to communicate this knowledge to those who would be able to prevent the harm anticipated. When a client reveals that he or she might commit suicide or commit a crime against others, the professional has the right and responsibility to communicate such knowledge that would prevent the adverse event.

In recent years the spread of acquired immunodeficiency syndrome (AIDS) has reminded health care workers of the serious responsibility of confidentiality (Boyd 1992). Mainly because of the way in which AIDS is often transmitted (through homosexual acts or intravenous drug use) severe discrimination is often exercised against AIDS victims. People seem to forget that this pathology may be acquired through blood transfusions or by means of licit sexual activity. Moreover, Christian compassion demands that respect be shown to all AIDS sufferers, even those who acquired the disease through aberrant behavior. Jesus never asked those he healed how they became ill. Health care workers therefore have a serious obligation to maintain confidentiality in regard to AIDS sufferers. They must be careful about gossip and casual conversation. However, those who counsel AIDS patients must insist that they reveal their condition to their sexual partners. If they refuse to reveal this information, the health care professional might be held in justice and charity to reveal this information (Solomon et al. 1999).

A New Paradigm for Health Care

Even people who are more or less bystanders realize that the profession of health care is changing. Theorists interpret these changes in terms of paradigms; that is, they maintain that the fundamental model, blueprint, or archetype for the profession of health care is changing. For years the paradigm revolved around highly trained physicians and well-equipped acute care facilities. The paradigm could have been phrased in this manner: "Good health depends on highly trained physicians and acute care hospitals with state-of-the-art technology." Guided by this paradigm, specialists outnumbered primary care physicians; physicians' medical decisions usually were not subject to objective accountability; there was no effort to limit the number of physicians; cost was not a factor in evaluating quality of care; and performing high-tech surgical procedures such as transplantation or cardiac angioplasty, which benefit a comparative few, became the standard for excellence when evaluating acute care hospitals. But this paradigm did not respond to the needs of the American public. It resulted in a continual spiral of expenses, and it neglected health needs of several segments of the public such as the poor and elderly.

What is the new paradigm for health care? It seems that two paradigms are vying with each other for acceptance. The first paradigm might be expressed as follows: "Health care is a business, and everything should be structured with a view to making the greatest profit." Those who accept this paradigm bargain with health care professionals, whether physicians or acute care hospital administrations, to accept less remuneration for their efforts. In other words, cutting the cost of health care and making a profit for stockholders receives top priority, even though quality care and client satisfaction are also mentioned as secondary objectives.

Fortunately, there is another paradigm developing (O'Rourke 1996). This new paradigm also features a more cost-conscious offering of health care, but its main perspective is to continue not-for-profit health care facilities and care for personal needs in a holistic manner. Hopefully, the renewed emphasis on clients' needs will lead health care professionals to stimulate society toward a greater effort to make access to health care a reality for all.

The effects of the second new paradigm in health care professions will occur in five areas of health care. To wit:

1. *Client participation:* The emphasis shifts from patient compliance to client participation. People increasingly expect to know not only their diagnosis, but also details of patho-physiology, treatment options, and prognosis.
2. *Medical decision making:* Individuals differ with respect to the amount of detail regarding their health they wish to know and the degree to which they wish to participate in decision making. Consequently, the art of person-centered care involves determining the appropriate amount of information and participation from the individual patient's perspective.
3. *Medical law:* The Quinlan, Cruzan, and Schiavo cases ignited public interest in advance directives. The mere enactment of state laws recognizing this legal device demonstrates that medical law now bends over backward in order to support person-centered decision making.
4. *Medical education:* The person-centered paradigm will demand a change in emphasis and content in the medical school curriculum. Curriculum revision in medical schools has been devoted to utilizing new learning methods. Little attention has been given to preparing young people for a new vision of health care.
5. *Medical research:* Hard biomedical outcomes have long been the currency of medical research. Over recent years, however, there has been increasing realization that other "softer" outcomes such as functional states, quality of life, and client satisfaction may be at least as relevant. The primary difference between traditional outcomes and newer outcomes is that the latter requires person-centered perspectives.

If health care as a business becomes the dominant paradigm for the provision of health care, then a noble profession will be destroyed. Moreover, the quality of health care for all people in the country will be diminished. One does not need a host of empirical studies to prove these conclusions. When profit becomes the principle goal of any enterprise, all other partial goals, no matter how noble, are sooner or later sacrificed. Conversely, if the person-centered paradigm becomes predominant, then we can retain the best qualities from the past, develop a health care system that fulfills our personal and social needs, and hopefully extends access to health care to all in need of it.

7.5 THE POLITICAL SITUATION OF HEALTH CARE TODAY

In the early 1990s most Americans realized that the health care system in this country was deeply flawed, if not altogether broken. It consisted of a rather random collection of players—providers, payers, and consumers—who more often than not were seeking disparate goals for a variety of reasons, some laudatory and some less than honorable. Moreover, millions of citizens were without access to even basic care. While there was little that people could agree on with regard to American health care, everyone was certain of one thing: the costs related to health care were escalating out of control. This was having very harmful effects on all parties, from local and state governments to employers and employees, from health care workers to patients. And the upward spiral of costs only threatened to worsen.

Pledging to reform American health care in a comprehensive and inclusive manner, then presidential candidate Bill Clinton promised in 1992 that, if elected, he would tackle the issue of fundamental health care reform that presidents before him had evaded for many decades. After capturing the presidency, Clinton proposed a system that would rein in the costs of the health care industry while offering simplicity, savings, choice, and quality health care to every American. However, when the Clinton plan saw the light of day it appeared as an overly complex, highly bureaucratic, and excessively regulated system that would scrupulously oversee every detail of the delivery and the financing of health care services. For a variety of reasons, the plan never made it to a vote in Congress. Among the more significant reasons for its failure seems to be that Clinton underestimated the depth of anti-government sentiment triggered by the Reagan era budget deficits that preceded him (Skocpol 1996). The Clinton proposal had governmental control written all over it and was rejected outright as big government intervention. More important, the Clinton proposal failed because many Americans were convinced by a clever media campaign featuring a middle-class couple, Harry and Louise, who fretted over all the health benefits they would lose should universal coverage become a reality.

We will talk more later about the principle of the common good. But it is worth mentioning here that appeals to this principle during the debate over the Clinton plan fell quickly to the deeply rooted individualism that was so well articulated by Ronald Reagan and that has been documented by scholars such as Robert Bellah (1986, 1991) and Mary Ann Glendon (1991).

In the wake of the failure of the 1993 Health Security Act, managed care schemes gained greater appeal. Although managed care plans had been around for many decades, the 1990s witnessed their zenith. In general, managed care was an attempt by insurers, employers, and some physicians to rein in costs by using approaches such as gatekeeping, utilization review, restricted physician panels, and capitation. And while the economic outcomes of managed care were positive, the backlash created by its essential features proved to be its undoing (Stone 1999; Vladeck 1999). The reasons for this are many and complex. At least four are worth mentioning here. First, the mechanisms that managed care organizations used to contain costs raised questions in the minds of consumers about the physicians' motives for providing care. People long accustomed to doctors "doing every test in the book" when presented with a person's health care complaint under the "fee for service" approach were worried that physicians were being incentivized to undertreat so as to conserve resources in a capitated environment. Second, persons enrolled in managed care plans, whether by their own choice or by the choice of their employer, found that they were no longer free, as they were in the past, to choose any physician they wanted but were limited to a preselected group of providers. This limitation of choice of provider was a particularly troublesome aspect of managed care (Swartz 1999). Finally, the effects of managed care plans on relationships in the workplace between employer and employee were less than positive. When employers found that they could contain some of the rising costs they paid for health insurance for their employees by enrolling employees in managed care plans, they did just that. Employees found, in many instances, that the new plans both restricted benefits and cost them more out-of-pocket expenses as well. This in turn has contributed to an increasing number of employers that do not provide health insurance coverage for employees as well as a growing number of employees that decline employment-based coverage when offered because of the high co-pays involved (Robinson 2001).

Failure of Managed Care

Ultimately, the American public came to believe that managed care could not deliver on its fundamental promises to contain costs and improve quality (Robinson 2001). In fact, in the minds of many, managed care did just the opposite. While it is clear that the cost containment promises made by proponents of managed care failed to be realized, the impact of managed care on quality is not so clear (Shaller, Sharpe, and Rubin 1998). But perception is often reality. When people had to wait for appointments and/or procedures, when their choice of physician was limited to a predetermined list, or when they were denied access to drugs or medical interventions by a distant third party, they came to believe that quality was diminishing. In fact, a 1998 report issued by the National Roundtable on Health Care Quality, a group convened by the Institute of Medicine, warned that serious problems of underuse, overuse, and misuse of health care harmed many Americans and existed equally in fee-for-service and managed care (Chassin and Glavin 1998). By the end of the decade—and the century—it was clear that managed care and its advocates had failed to convince the American people that employers, insurers, and physicians, working together, could effectively establish priorities and make decisions about who gets what from the health care system. As the resentment against managed care plans heightened, managed care companies began to loosen their restrictions, open physician panels, and move away from capitation (Robinson 2001). At the same time, the American consumer was becoming more convinced that allowing others, no matter how well intentioned or qualified, to make health care decisions for him or her was a mistake. Many things have fueled the growing confidence of the contemporary health care consumer. For example, the Internet has expanded to the point that information on health, health care, diagnoses, pharmaceuticals, treatment regimens, and so on is ubiquitous. This gives many people the impression, perhaps more appropriately the illusion, that by accessing that information they will be well equipped to make complex health-related decisions unencumbered as they were in the past by plan restrictions, utilization review, and the like. While some people will be able to navigate the system and get the care they need on their own, armed only with a computer and a web browser, many others will not. Moreover, as pieces of the managed care apparatus are modified or dismantled, for example, allowing out-of-plan point-of-service options for those who can afford them, people with limited means will be restricted in their choices while people with money will not be—a situation only exacerbating the access issue.

By the end of the century more than 44 million Americans, 16 percent of the total population, were without health care insurance, and in the first five years of the new millennium that number grew by 4 million and is projected to continue to increase well into the future (Families USA 2005). After decades of failed efforts to reform American health care, the system appears to be in crisis. Even though the negative effects of this crisis are being felt by providers, employers, and consumers alike, there appears to be no reasonable hope of alleviating it in the near or even distant future (Lofton 2005). Underlying the persistent problems at the heart of this long-standing predicament is the widely held conviction that health care is a commodity rather than a public or social good (Chollet

2005). This notion is supported and furthered by the predominance of the market ethos that drives both for-profit and not-for-profit health care providers and drowns out any claim that health care is a basic human right. Sooner or later, however, the costs of caring for the growing number of uninsured will be felt by every insured person in this country (Families USA 2005). Perhaps then we will consider seriously the need to fundamentally reform American health care and ensure that every person has access to needed care. What values and principles can be derived from Catholic social teaching to guide this process?

7.6 PRINCIPLES OF HEALTH CARE POLICY

Given the economic difficulties with the present health care system, just as in previous chapters we urged a new paradigm of person-centered health care, so we must now consider a new model for its economic structure. Whether this new model should provide coverage for all persons by means of private or public financing is open to debate (Chollet 2005). But whatever model is adopted, certain principles should be reflected in both the development of the model as well as in its application.

The Principle of the Common Good

The first step in formulating a better approach to providing health care services in the United States must be to back away from our tendency as Americans to analyze every social issue solely in terms of individual freedoms and rights. As noted earlier, this tendency has deep roots in the American psyche and leads too often to a neglect or outright denial of our social nature as persons and of the shared obligations of all that derive from that nature (Glendon 1991).

The authentic social teaching of the Catholic Church has been formulated since Leo XIII's great encyclical *Rights and Duties of Capital and Labor* (1891), in many papal encyclicals and documents, by the Second Vatican Council in *The Church in the Modern World* (Vatican Council II 1966), and most recently in the encyclicals of Pope John Paul II, *On Social Development* (1987) and *The 100th Year* (1991). This teaching contains some strong criticisms of socialism, chiefly on three grounds: (1) its materialism, (2) its denial of the right of private property, and (3) its tendency to promote totalitarian government. Yet it approves its concern for distributive justice as against exploitation of poor workers by the rich. This teaching also contains a vigorous criticism of capitalism on three grounds: (1) its deterministic reliance on economic laws, (2) its advocacy of unregulated competition and the profit motive, and (3) its neglect of the Christian advocacy of the poor. Yet it approves capitalism's proven ability to increase productivity through private initiatives and its support of private property.

Moreover, recent papal documents (e.g., John XXIII's *Christianity and Social Progress* [1961], Paul VI's *The Development of Peoples* [1967], and John Paul II's *On Social Development* [1987]) have pointed out that capitalism and socialism alike have become colonializing powers either politically or economically and are thus largely responsible for the wars and poverty that oppress the great majority of humankind (Curran and McCormick 1986). Christian health care professionals, therefore, should base their thinking about the social organization of health care on the principles of the Gospel, not on a one-sided choice of either socialism or capitalism (USCCB 1998).

Apart from ideological bias, no one economic system any more than one political system is simply natural, right, or Christian. Such systems are human inventions, each with some advantages and some disadvantages, to be selected and balanced against each other according to particular historical circumstances and for the common good of all. These merits need to be evaluated both from a theoretical point of view and from a practical, experiential point of view. In judging them ethically, both their congruity with fundamental moral and Gospel principles and their pragmatic results in a given situation must be considered. A theoretically correct system in some circumstances may result in ethical disaster, whereas it is sometimes necessary to tolerate theoretically wrong institutions because they are the best that can be hoped for at the moment. In the long run, however, bad principles will have bad consequences. Christians must constantly strive to test their understanding of principles by experience and to bring the real situation into line with these principles once they are refined.

Catholic health care professionals thus have the responsibility at present to study all proposals for a plan for health care and attempt to judge them in terms of theoretical principles and practical experience. Such a study is beyond the scope of this book, but it may be useful to indicate the first steps in such an ethical inquiry seeking a solution to the problem of providing access to health care for all. To face this fundamental dilemma requires radical thinking, and it is here that Catholic social thought can make an important contribution to finding a new solution. This solution must rest on three propositions that have been previously expounded in this book: (1) every human being does have a fundamental right to health, as acknowledged in the *Universal Declaration of Human Rights* (United Nations, 1948, Article 25), because human rights are based on essential human needs; (2) individual persons have the primary responsibility to promote their own health; and (3) as social beings, however, people also have the right to seek the help of others when necessary to fulfill this responsibility and reciprocally have the duty to give the same help to others as much as they are able.

Subsidiarity

The papal encyclicals and the Second Vatican Council have repeatedly proposed a universal social principle (of which the second proposition discussed in this book is only an application to health care) that is called the *principle of subsidiarity* (from the Latin equivalent of "supplementarity") or, more comprehensively, the *principle of participation*. This principle follows from the need of the person in the community, which is to be realized in communal sharing or in the common good, one citizen supplementing the efforts of another. Each individual, therefore, in order to fulfill human need, has a moral obligation to contribute to the common good and a consequent right to share in it.

Most social evils and injustices are the result of exclusion of some persons from the common good in which they have a right to share (Williams and Houck 1987). The ancient evil of slavery was precisely such an unjust institution. The slaves contributed to the common good but were not permitted to share fully in it, not only in regard to economic goods but also in regard to spiritual goods such as education, freedom, political participation, respect, and even the right to worship the "gods of the city." Thus the distribution of the common good is a fundamental demand of social justice.

Jesus, moreover, taught an ethics that clearly went beyond even this demand for distributive justice based on merit. Jesus proclaimed the coming of the kingdom of God (Mk 1:15), which was not merely a heavenly kingdom but also the fulfillment of the Old Testament prophecies of the reign of God on Earth (Viviano 1988). When Jesus said to Pilate, "My kingship is not of this world" (Jn 18:36), he did not mean by "world" the Earth, but the present sinful order of power struggle. He was saying to Pilate, "I am not competing with you power brokers. I am building a kingdom built on a different principle: on service, not on dominion." He taught his followers to pray, "Your Kingdom come, your will be done, on earth as it is in heaven" (Mt 6:10). According to the exegete Jacques Dupont (1969), the Beatitudes (Lk 6:20–22; Mt 5:3–11), in their original Lucan form, were the joyful announcement to the poor (i.e., those excluded from the common good) that at last they were to be included in that common good, not only economically but spiritually ("The poor have the good news preached to them"; Lk 7:22). Consequently, the principle of the early church was "from each according to his ability, to each according to his needs," a principle that Marx borrowed from the Acts of the Apostles (4:32–35). Thus the principle of the common good requires love and mercy and the distribution of the common good not according to merit but according to need. Thus the mark of all Jesus's work was his concern for the neglected, the outcast, the leper, the prostitute, the Samaritan heretic, and the pagan unbeliever.

A Christian ethics of health care distribution must be based not on merit, and certainly not on the ability to pay, *but on need,* because the needy are the most neglected. Those who can care for themselves do not need social help. Moreover, social oppression of the needy is the major cause of their illness, an oppression from which the more affluent members of society profit. Thus those who are helpless by reason of poverty, disease, defect, or age (the unborn or the senile) should be the first consideration of any health plan.

However, all persons should contribute to the plan according to their *ability.* Thus the social responsibility for health care falls first on those who have the ability to heal, the health care professionals, and second on those who have the ability to pay, that is, those who have financially profited the most from society. For such affluent individuals to claim that they have made their wealth simply by their own efforts is an absurdity. They may have worked hard, but their wealth would not have been possible exclusive of the society of which they are a part. Consequently, their debt to the common good is in proportion to the wealth they have received from it.

From this notion of the common good, the idea of subsidiarity follows logically. *Subsidiarity* implies that the first responsibility in meeting human needs rests with the free and competent individual, then with the local group. Higher and higher levels of the community must assume this responsibility when the lower unit cannot assume it and when the lower unit refuses to assume it.

Although all persons are primarily responsible for their own health, when, because they are too young, too old, too poor, too uneducated, or possessed of any other handicap, they cannot assume this responsibility, the community at higher levels must come to their aid. If a lower level neglects to fulfill the responsibility, a higher level must correct the oversight by punishment or other remedies. The higher level should never be content merely to take over responsibility, however; it must work to return responsibility to a lower level. Thus people should be educated about personal health care, helped to pay for such care, and held responsible for neglecting it. *The main objection to many social reforms has been that they have not provided for this progressive decentralization.* For example, the welfare system in the Untied States has perpetuated poverty rather than helped the dependent to become independent.

The growing criticism of liberalism and the excesses of government bureaucracy, however, should not lead to identifying Catholic social thought with the conservative movement, which has grown more and more powerful in the United States since World War II. As Nash (1976) has shown in *The Conservative Intellectual Movement in America since 1945,* American conservatism is of three varieties: (1) libertarianism, which advocates a laissez faire government; (2) traditionalism, which deplores the loss of Western cultural heritage through overrapid social change; and (3) nationalistic anticommunism. Catholic social doctrine has always opposed laissez faire capitalism, which the papal encyclicals label "liberalism," in the original sense the term had in the economic thought of Adam Smith and the political thought of the French Revolution, because it is based on economic determinism rather than prudence and justice. Although Catholicism has conserved the Western cultural heritage, the Gospel message, as Vatican II made very clear, is to build the kingdom of God on Earth by a radical reform of society according to the demands of peace and justice. Likewise, Catholicism opposes communism because it denies the right of private property and tends either to totalitarianism or to anarchism. Thus Catholic thinking in social matters must remain independent of both the liberal and the conservative tendencies, both of which arise from the basic assumption of humanism (USCC 1995).

Therefore the type of health care program that Catholics can consistently support must be economically sound yet aim at preventive medicine, at achieving a healthier people who can care for themselves, rather than an ever-increasing dependence on technical medical care and professional help. As Plato observed, "A society that is always going to the doctor is a sick society" (*Republic* III 405A).

Functionalism

The popes have also stressed that one of the evils of historical capitalism and socialism alike has been the tendency of both systems to concentrate all the power of decision making in the state. Before secular humanism became the dominant philosophy of modern society, Christian thinking was able to advance the notion that a society is not simply a two-level structure of government and citizenry, but an organic community containing many *functions* that are mutually interdependent.

This concept of the mutual interdependence or solidarity of a community was enunciated by St. Paul in 1 Corinthians 12–13 and linked by him with Jesus's teaching that the greatest should become the servants of the least in the kingdom of God. Thus the power to make social decisions ought to be kept as close as possible to those who experience those problems and are most strongly affected by the decisions concerning them. Only in this way can the dignity of the least members of a community be acknowledged and their interests effectively served by the greater. A paternalism that decides everything for those it claims to serve is really nothing but a form of domination and tends to become self-serving. Thus St. Paul, without directly attacking slavery, admonished the master that he should treat his slave not as a child but as a "most dear brother" (Phil v. 16), that is, as an equal by reason of their mutual interdependence in Christ.

The principle of subsidiarity therefore requires us to share decision-making power not only at various vertical levels of local, state, and federal government but also among horizontal sectors representing various functional bodies. Thus education, as a basic function of society, forms a body of persons, some with expertise (the educators) and others (the students) who are trying to educate themselves through the services of the experts. Decisions about education pertain first not to government but to bodies of cooperating teachers and students mutually dependent on each other. The same holds true for other basic social functions—especially for the economy, with its interdependence of management, workers, and consumers—as well as for the social organization of health care, with its mutual interdependence of professional healers and health seekers. Each person in a society is related to as many such functional bodies as he or she has basic needs. The role of government is to coordinate and encourage the full development of these different organs of society, not to deprive them of their decision-making capacity.

This application of subsidiarity to the organization of society on the basis of social functions, rather than on the basis of a struggle between isolated individuals defending their rights and a centralized government having all the powers of social decision, is usually referred to as *corporatism* in Catholic documents. This term somewhat misleads Americans, who usually view corporations as purely economic organizations. The term has also been discredited because it was used by fascist political parties in Europe to win Catholic support for its exact opposite, namely, totalitarianism or total state power. The following discussion will use the term *functionalism* instead.

Functionalism is opposed, on the one hand, to communism and national socialism because they are totalitarian, concentrating all decision-making power in the hands of the state and the military. On the other hand, it is opposed to the competitive individualism of unregulated capitalism or free enterprise, with its hidden tendency toward monopolism, resulting in concentration of decision-making power in the hands of an interlocking power elite or the industrial-military complex. Functionalism is not a mere theory, because it has a powerful influence, through Catholic leaders, on the formation of the European Common Market and of codetermination by management and labor in Germany, Japan, and other countries. Some of its implications are also evident in Latin America in the efforts of Catholic theologians and political leaders to develop a theology of liberation that is not capitalist, fascist, or Marxist (Boff 1987, 1992).

Politically, it might seem that functionalism would have little chance in the United States. Certain features of some institutions, however, are in fact functionalist. For example, higher education in the United States, in contrast to the statism of the lower school system, remains largely functionalist. Decisions about educational policies in our colleges and universities are made independently of government by faculties and accrediting agencies and by the right of students to choose their own schools. The student revolt of the 1960s, however, seemed to show that schools needed to allow students greater participation in policymaking, and to a certain extent this has taken place, rendering the system still more functionalist. In contrast, the increasing control of the government over schools by reason of their economic dependency is working strongly to destroy their functionalist character.

Similarly, after the Great Depression the growth of labor unions in the United States, to a considerable degree under the influence of Catholic social thought (Cronin 1950), portended the eventual development of functionalism in the economic sphere. Unfortunately, the unions have largely neglected the social aspects of their original purpose and have been co-opted by the capitalist market system, in which they tended to become just another monopoly. The result has been the recent marked decline of the labor unions' influences in American life. Renewed Catholic leadership in unions, including hospital unions, could remedy this neglect. Fortunately, this trend toward monopoly shows some signs of a reversal in the growth of consumer activism, participatory democracy, and social ecology, as well as in the increasing dissatisfaction with resulting liberal reforms, so many of which have served only to enlarge the power of government bureaucracy. Catholics need to take advantage of this growing criticism of the so-called American way of life to propose a more personalistic and functionalist conception of society.

In health care, these general ethical principles of subsidiarity and functionalism have to be applied to the concrete historical situation of American medical institutions. The medical profession, as it has operated in the United States, has been influenced by three somewhat inconsistent principles: (1) the ancient ideal of a profession as service, which was formulated in the Hippocratic oath and reinforced by Christian ethics; (2) the philosophy of secular humanism, with its strong emphasis on human rights and the duty of man to use scientific knowledge to solve human problems; and (3) the ideology of capitalism, which has been fostered by secular humanism. Many liberal secularists recognize that this capitalist ideology is at odds with their concern for human rights and the full application of the social sciences to the planning of economic and political life. Conservatives, however, have defended this capitalist ideology out of fear of socialism.

In view of Christian goals, a Catholic should be particularly aware of the lessons learned in the United States. The first of these is that our existing health care system has not adequately cared for the poor or emphasized preventive medicine (AHA 1986a; Aday 1993). Rather, it has tended to foster an exaggerated professional elitism, to place strong emphasis on monopolization and the profit motive, and has produced a system of medical education lacking in humanistic breadth and depth. Alternatively, the existing system should be credited with promoting very rapid technological and scientific progress and with developing many health care facilities equipped to give acute care. It must be noted, however, that this progress has led to greater expenditure of resources on the sophisticated treatment of relatively rare ailments rather than to better care for the health of the majority (Fox and Swazy 1992).

Single-Payer System

Many today favor a centralized single-payer system aimed at correcting some of these defects, as we will see in the next session. Yet there is also danger that such a system, if adopted, will greatly increase bureaucratization, which, as evidenced by our experience with a welfare system, can cost a great deal and accomplish very little. A centralized system will provide more health care, but there is no certainty that it will promote better health. A bureaucracy also is not likely to personalize the health care it gives. Even if this system makes a sincere effort to humanize medicine, such an effort will not be guided by a Christian concept of the person but by a secular humanist concept that may express itself not in concern for neglected persons but in catering to the wants of the privileged (Hardin 1993).

Therefore, eventually some national health care program will probably be enacted in the United States as the only practical way available to extend care to the neglected of society (www.pnhp.org/). The Democratic congressmen Dennis Kucinich (2005) of Ohio and John

Conyers of Michigan have introduced in the Lower House what they call "Enhanced Medicare for All" (H.R. 676), describing it as: "a universal single-payer system of national health insurance, carefully phased in over 10 years. It addresses everyone's needs, including the 45 million Americans without coverage and those paying exorbitant rates for health insurance. This approach to health care emphasizes patient choice, and puts doctors and patients in control of the system, not insurance companies. And it does not cost any extra money. Coverage will be more complete than private insurance plans, encourage prevention and include prescription drugs, dental care, mental health." There are also numerous proposals for single-payer health care systems at the state level, for example, as enacted in 2006 in Massachusetts. Advocates of such systems point out that the United States spends 40 percent more per capita than any of the other twenty-nine industrialized countries that have universal health care systems (Battista and McCabe 1999; Geyman 2005; see also http://americanhealthcare reform.org), yet is outranked by many in the actual health of its citizens, as it is ranked seventeenth among them (Friedman 2001).

Although such proposals share many of the health care goals that Christians support, we should not have any illusions about their chances of success. The German system, long celebrated as one of the most sophisticated and effective of such plans in Europe, now seems to be in trouble (German Culture 2005; Gajer 2005). Therefore we must be willing to experiment to fit U.S. conditions and keep working to incorporate into these plans as many functionalist features as possible. Above all, a concern for distributive justice should permeate any new design for health care. For example:

1. Comprehensive health care should aim primarily at the promotion of positive health, not merely at the cure of acute disease or the prolongation of life through sophisticated techniques. Therefore, it should work for (a) removal of the environmental and social causes of ill health, including the commercial encouragement of unhealthy patterns of living, and (b) provision of preventive health education that will give persons control over their own health.

2. Priority should be given to the problems of the most powerless, poorly informed, and least able to pay. These persons should not be cared for paternalistically, but should be admitted to participate in the power of decision about their own health needs.

3. Decision-making power should not be confined to a government bureaucracy, or to autonomous professionals, but should be shared by all concerned in mutual interdependence.

4. Planning should proceed in such a way as to avoid tendencies to increase dependence on higher levels and to promote a gradually increasing decentralization in both control and funding. This decentralization, however, should not be used as an excuse for the government to neglect the monitoring of health care and the supplementation and correction of defects at lower levels of organization.

5. Planning must be a continuous process of decision making that adapts to experience and new needs rather than a fixed plan based on projections that may be mistaken.

Christians may find support for various items of a functionalist program from different and opposed ideological camps. For example, ecology-minded people are convinced that environmental and social factors are the major cause of poor health conditions, but others defend the medical profession against the charge that it is responsible for these conditions. Again, the rights of health consumers are defended not only by civil rights and consumer advocates but also by individuals who believe that the free market is the best method of controlling health costs. Consequently, Christians should attempt to transcend ideological biases and use a strategy of coalition to promote particular goals.

Above all, Christians should work together through various church agencies to influence the health education of consumers and the medical education of the professionals. Catholic schools, medical schools, and teaching hospitals especially should teach a person-centered approach to health and to the objectives of the medical profession. Catholic institutions must protest against the many current forces that tend to absorb them into the centralized, bureaucratic structure of society dominated by secular humanism. At the same time, Catholics should approach secular humanists with a genuinely ecumenical spirit, which seeks through dialogue to find grounds of agreement and cooperation.

7.7 HEALTH CARE ETHICS AND PUBLIC POLICY

As the major funding source for health care in the United States, the federal government establishes ethics commissions and boards that promulgate ethical guidelines to regulate medical research and therapy. Thus, in 1974, in response to revelations about the unethical treatment of four hundred African American men in the now infamous Tuskegee syphilis studies, the U.S. Congress passed the Human Research Act. This act created the National Commission for the Protection of Human Subjects of Biomedical and Behavioral Research, which operated under the auspices of the then Department of Health, Education and Welfare (DHEW). The act also mandated that institutional review boards (IRBs) approve all federally funded proposed research involving human subjects. In 1978, the commission issued the *Belmont Report: Ethical Principles and Guidelines for the Protection of Human Subjects of Biomedical and Behavioral Research*. This report called for observance of three basic ethical principles in the conduct of any and all research involving human subjects: respect for persons, beneficence, and justice. In 1978, upon recommendation of the National Commission, the secretary of DHEW established the Ethics Advisory Board (EAB). The EAB was a multidisciplinary group convened to grapple with controversial ethical, legal, and social issues associated with biomedical research protocols, particularly those dealing with research on fetuses and pregnant women and with the expanding technology associated with in vitro fertilization. In 1979 the board published *Research Involving Human In Vitro Fertilization and Embryo Transfer: Report and Conclusions*. The report and subsequent dissolution of the EAB began a fifteen-year moratorium on embryo research.

Even as the EAB was carrying on its work, Congress was creating the successor to the National Commission, the President's Commission for the Study of Ethical Problems in Medicine and Biomedical and Behavioral Research. This commission, which worked independently from 1980 to 1983, was intended to provide a forum for debate on emerging ethical concerns. The issues the commission studied and wrote about included informed consent, the definition of death, genetic screening and counseling, differences in the availability of health care, life-sustaining treatments, confidentiality and privacy, genetic engineering, compensation for injured subjects, and whistle-blowing research.

In 1985, Congress instituted the Congressional Biomedical Ethics Advisory Board composed of representatives and senators, who were to be assisted in their work by a fourteen-member advisory committee of scientists, ethicists, and lawyers. The board was to have remained in existence until further legislative action was taken. Selection of the advisory board was delayed because, like every other dimension of American life, the process had become highly politicized. Though funding was allocated for this board and senators were selected to serve on it, a panel of experts was never selected because of intense lobbying of special interest groups and reluctance of Congress to displease constituents, and no studies were undertaken.

In 1996, President Clinton issued an executive order establishing the National Bioethics Advisory Commission (NBAC). While the commission's initial focus was to be on the protection of human subjects and the ethical issues raised by use of an individual's genetic information, that agenda was sidetracked by news of research into somatic cell nuclear transfer, or "cloning" (AMA 1996). During its tenure, 1996 to 2001, this commission produced documents on such ethical issues as those raised by possible cloning of human beings, research on persons with mental illness, and human stem cell research.

In November 2001, President George W. Bush created the President's Council on Bioethics. In its role of advising the president on ethical issues emerging from developments in biomedical science and technology, the council has turned its attention to a wide range of issues including embryonic stem cell research, genetics, and end-of-life care (PCB 2002, 2003, 2004a, 2004b, 2005).

The vast work of these various commissions can be accessed easily via the Internet (www.bioethcs.gov). While we make no attempt here to evaluate the various documents they have generated, we do offer the following general observations:

1. The very fact that Congress and government officials recognize the need for ethical guidance in the field of biomedical research and technology is a step forward. For the most part, the norms set forth by the commissions are useful and protect the rights of all persons as well as those of researchers and scientists.

2. The proposals of these commissions are made with our highly pluralistic society in mind. As a result the norms and principles they enunciate are those on which most scientists, politicians, and religious thinkers can agree. Moreover, the agenda of these commissions focuses primarily, although not exclusively, on ethical issues related to medical research and evolving technologies. Thus many of the broader and perhaps more important ethical issues, such as when human life begins, the purpose of care, and the need to ration health care explicitly, are not addressed by the work of these groups.

3. Because the work of these commissions attempts to appeal to a secular, highly pluralistic culture, there is no attempt to reflect an appreciation of the true nature of the human person, the covenantal character of the patient-physician relationship, the contours of a just society, or religious teaching. Rather, the work of these groups attempts to appeal to what is acceptable to the majority of the American public. As a result, the conclusions are pragmatic and usually balance rights rather than defend them. Proposing ethical guidelines in this manner is dangerous because it may justify whatever is popular at the expense of what is ethical.

4. Compliance with the norms and principles proposed by these groups is sought almost solely by the threat of withholding federal funding for proposed research. Thus, the "ethical" guidelines do not appeal to the altruism or virtue of those seeking funding.

Appeal is primarily to self-interest, whether individual or institutional. This is true particularly with regard to the work of IRBs that at present are proving to be fraught with many problems as they attempt to ensure that human subjects are protected in proposed research (Emanuel et al. 2004).

At the private level, there is also an extensive effort to influence public policy. At present, more than fifty private centers are sponsored by universities or corporations that seek to educate people in one way or another concerning ethical issues. Although most of these centers serve a local or regional constituency, some seek to serve a national audience. For example:

1. The National Catholic Bioethics Center (NCBC), established in 1972 as the Pope John XXIII Medical-Moral Research and Education Center, conducts research, consultation, publishing, and education to promote human dignity in health care and the life sciences and derives its message directly from the teachings of the Catholic Church.
2. The Hastings Center is an independent, nonpartisan, and nonprofit bioethics research institute founded in 1969 to explore fundamental and emerging questions in health care, biotechnology, and the environment. The *Hastings Center Report* and *IRB: Ethics and Human Research* bring the best scholarship and commentary in bioethics to *members* and other readers worldwide (http://thehastingscenter.org/about.asp).
3. The Kennedy Institute of Ethics at Georgetown University, Washington, D.C., publishes the *Encyclopedia of Bioethics,* sponsors the National Reference Center for Bioethics Literature, and produces *The Bioethics Line,* a computer-assisted method of searching for literature on questions of ethics and public policy. The Kennedy Institute also publishes the quarterly *Kennedy Institute of Ethics Journal.* Since its inception in 1971, scholars at the institute have addressed issues such as the protection of research subjects, feminist bioethics, care at the end of life, health care justice, intellectual disability, cloning, gene therapy, and eugenics. Recently, institute faculty have been pushing the boundaries of bioethics to include issues such as racial and gender quality, international justice and peace, and other policies affecting the world's most vulnerable populations.
4. The Neiswanger Institute for Bioethics and Public Policy at the Stritch School of Medicine, Loyola University, Chicago, sponsors an online M.A. program in bioethics for health care professionals who are members of ethics committees and other interested persons.
5. The Center for Health Care Ethics at Saint Louis University specializes in health care ethics as related to clinical situations and current social issues. Working in the Catholic tradition, it seeks to interpret this tradition for the pluralistic society. The center publishes *Health Care Ethics, USA,* in conjunction with the Catholic Health Association.

7.8 RESPONSIBILITIES OF CATHOLIC HEALTH CARE FACILITIES

The Catholic Church provides health care as an integral member of the health care system in the United States. In order to fulfill this mission as faithfully as possible, these facilities establish ethics committees and strive to maintain and foster Catholic identity.

The Need for Ethics Committees

Ethics committees in hospitals received their greatest impetus from the Supreme Court of New Jersey with the decision of the Karen Ann Quinlan case. The court, assuming erroneously that most hospitals had ethics committees, declared that such committees, rather than courts, should be involved in decisions concerning the withdrawal of life support. The President's Commission on Ethics in Health Care and Research (PCEMR), writing shortly after the Quinlan decision, recommended the establishment of ethics committees in hospitals of any size. Thus, by 1980, the trend to appoint ethics committees, especially in large hospitals, was well established.

In the 1980s two other influential organizations supported the founding of ethics committees: the American Hospital Association (AHA) and the Joint Commission for Accreditation of Health Care Organizations (JCAHO, 1993). The JCAHO required that if the health care facility did not have a committee, "The organization should have in place a mechanism for the consideration of ethical issues and to provide education to caregivers and patients on ethical issues in health care." Over the past twenty years, this new type of committee has become a fixture in health care facilities of any size. Even large long-term care facilities have ethics committees.

The purpose of an ethics committee is educational, not jurisdictional (Dougherty 1995). It accomplishes its purpose in three ways:

1. Through education programs for the committee itself and for the various members of the health care facility. For example, a few years ago the federal government set forth certain regulations in regard to advance directives (McClosky 1991). It was the responsibility of ethics committees to organize lectures and discussions to explain these regulations and to strategize for their application.
2. Through framing ethical policies concerning various aspects of the facilities' activities. Usually these policies are promulgated by higher authorities, for example, the board of trustees or the medical staff. For the most part, these policies are concerned with issues in clinical medicine, such as informed consent or removal of life support. Conversely, often issues concerning social justice will require the establishing of policies, for example, how to settle grievances within the work force.
3. Through consultations, which are usually requested by health care professionals and sometimes by families. The committee will usually respond to these requests through subcommittees in order not to overwhelm the people who have requested the consultation. These consultations are not decision-making endeavors on the part of the committee. Rather, the committee members help the decision makers, whether patients, family, or health care professionals, to discern the ethical issues, the options for action, and the course of action that seems to be better in the present situation, all circumstances being considered (Minogue 1996).

Ethics Committees as Educational

The primary purpose of an ethics committee is educational. Education may be fulfilled in many different ways, but a significant function of the committee is to educate its own members. Usually many of the people called to serve on an ethics committee have little formal formation in the discipline of ethics. Developing a common method of considering ethical issues, whether in regard to lectures, policies, or consultations, is most important. A common method cannot be developed unless there is some effort on the part of the committee to understand the purpose of ethics and the various methods used in considering issues or proposing solutions.

Ethics committees in Catholic health care facilities do not start at the beginning in their deliberations. Rather, each ethics committee has a set of general norms, the *Ethical and Religious Directives for Catholic Health Services* (ERD 2001). Study of the ERDs is a high priority for members of ethics committees in Catholic health care facilities. In fact, all people associated with Catholic health care facilities should be familiar with the ERDs, because they lay out a breadth of ethical responsibility that is wider than issues usually associated with medical ethics. For example, the new ERDs consider the ethical norms for social justice and cooperation among health care facilities, as well as the norms for using or removing life support.

Moreover, a method of decision making that is directed toward enhancing the dignity of the human person is also traditional in Catholic teaching. This characteristic Christian method of decision making rejects proportionalism and pragmatism and grounds moral decision making on an analysis of the moral object of a human act (John Paul II 1993, esp. 70–82). Thus certain kinds of actions such as adultery, lying, and theft must be judged to be morally wrong, no matter what the circumstances or the purposes for which they are performed. Hence there are some universal, concrete, negative norms that any ethics committee ought to insist can never be ethically violated. The traditional Hippocratic oath was based on such absolute norms, and its recent abandonment by many medical schools is a sign of the corruption of sound professional attitudes by pragmatism and moral relativism.

Yet even though there are norms and methods consistent with the Catholic tradition, there will often be discussion and difference in how to apply them. For example, it is a well-accepted norm of Catholic ethics that workers should receive a just wage (ERD 2001, D. 7). But how does one determine a just wage? Another norm concerns the use of extraordinary and ordinary means in sustaining life. But when does intubation become an extraordinary means? The intelligent, sensitive, and honest application of the ERDs to such problems is not easy and requires serious and respectful discussion and debate.

Proposing that ethics committees in Catholic health care facilities have norms and a method to guide them may seem doctrinaire in a pluralistic society (Siegel and Orr 1995). However, "the purpose of the committee is to serve the institution and patients within the framework of the Catholic tradition" (Brodeur 1984). Logically, then, ethics committees in Catholic health care facilities are to work within the ERDs and help people make ethical decisions in accord with its norms. This conclusion is implied in the ERDs (2001) in the following statements:

> Within a pluralistic society, Catholic health care services will encounter requests for medical procedures contrary to the moral teachings of the Church. Catholic health care does not offend the rights of individual conscience by refusing to provide or permit medical procedures that are judged morally wrong by the teaching authority of the Church. (part I, introduction)
>   . . . Catholic health care services must adopt these Directives as policy, require adherence to them within the institution as a condition for medical privileges and employment, and provide appropriate instruction regarding the Directives for administration, medical and nursing staff, and other personnel. (no. 5)

Hence, in the Catholic tradition, there is an assumption that moral reasoning can reach definite conclusions regarding good and bad actions aside from emotional influences. Moreover, in this tradition some actions, such as killing the innocent, are always wrong. The morality of these actions does not change due to circumstances or changing attitudes in society. Because of the relativism and consequentialism in our society, discussions in health care ethics are becoming abstract exercises in linguistic analysis rather than discussions about patient benefit in light of norms for preserving and promoting human dignity. Maintaining the identity of Catholic health care services will require that the ethics committee accept and apply the traditions of its Catholic heritage.

There should be a wide perspective represented in the committee. Members of the various health care professions should be represented, as well as persons for administration and other support services. The ethics committee is not concerned with risk management or with avoiding malpractice litigation. For this reason, if lawyers are members of the committee, their presence will be helpful only if they concentrate on patient benefit, not on keeping physicians or the institution out of court. Ordinarily, the ethics committee should not be considered a function of the medical staff, because the medical staff does not have exclusive responsibility for the ethical dimension of the health care facility. Rather, the ethics committee should be responsible to the board of trustees in order to show its concern for all ethical aspects of the corporation's activities. The ethics committee should have a budget that enables it to perform its functions successfully. Too often, its chair is supposed to fund the various needs out of some other budget. But if an ethics committee is to perform its tasks adequately, it needs secretarial help, stipends for speakers, and adequate funding for books and videos to help educate the committee members.

Striving for Catholic Identity

Catholic health care made its debut in the United States well over 150 years ago when members of religious congregations, primarily of women, sought to respond in the manner of Jesus to persons who experienced ill health. The stories of heroic women caring for the victims of cholera and yellow fever, for wounded men and boys on both sides in the Civil War, and for persons in need as the American frontier expanded have been chronicled well (CHA 1994; Kauffman 1976, 1978). In addition, this early response was prompted by the fact that immigrant Catholics were in the minority in many areas of the country, and there was concern that they receive care consistent with their beliefs in a nondiscriminatory environment (Steinfels 2003).

It is difficult to believe that those pioneering efforts are directly related to twenty-first-century Catholic health care in the United States. Today, there are sixty Catholic health systems and more than six hundred Catholic hospitals constituting about 12.5 percent of all nonfederal community hospitals. Thousands of long-term care facilities, clinics, community outreach programs, home health agencies, psychiatric agencies, and other specialty services along the care continuum make up Catholic health care today (Ascension Health 2006). These various expressions of Catholic health care are the direct descendants of those early efforts to respond to the health needs of persons in a manner consistent with the healing mission of Jesus.

Although Catholic health care appears to be a vital force within the broader health care arena, many people question the ability to sustain health care *as* Catholic for a variety of reasons. First, secular humanism as a philosophy of life challenges the basic right to operate institutions as faith-based organizations within our highly pluralistic society. Second, the ethos of the market that drives the broader health care industry is very difficult to resist (Steinfels 2003). Today, the fundamental commitment to care for persons who are poor and vulnerable competes with the drive to attain higher and higher profit margins in an increasingly competitive health care marketplace (Barr 2005). Third, evolving medical technologies, particularly in the areas of genetics and stem cell research, pose significant challenges for Catholic health care now and well into the future. With regard to the former, the question for Catholic health care will be how to use the fruits of the genetic revolution while avoiding the morass of ethical issues inevitably bound up with it, such as questions about genetic counseling, how to maintain confidentiality, and how to provide access, to name only a few. With regard to the latter, certainly the Church's stand on abortion precludes any participation in embryonic stem cell research. Seemingly it would also preclude any use of the hoped-for outcomes of that research for regenerative medicine. This could put some Catholic health care organizations at a distinct competitive disadvantage in the future, unless we do the research necessary to solve these problems in ethical ways. Fourth, the drive to sustain Catholic health care in many communities across the country over the past decade has led to many mergers with or acquisitions of other faith-based or nonsectarian organizations. Between 1990 and 2001, there were 171 such transactions ("Integrating Cultures"). When this transition occurs, the nonsectarian hospital is generally expected to act as if it were Catholic and to observe the ERD. Two outcomes of this approach are troubling. First, requiring observance of the ERDs by the merged or acquired facility means that certain reproductive services to which the community was accustomed will no longer be available. This has led to a strong backlash against Catholic health care in many communities and organized efforts across the country, such as Merger Watch, to discredit Catholic health care and undermine its ability to serve. Second, the assumption that a nonsectarian hospital can be converted into a Catholic organization simply by virtue of a contractual agreement and observance of the ERDs belies a very feeble understanding of what it means to be "Catholic."

Change in Leadership

Over the past two decades, the leadership in Catholic health care institutions has changed markedly. Positions once filled by members of the religious congregations sponsoring these institutions now are held by laymen and women, many of whom are not Catholic. Whether Catholic or not, many leaders in Catholic institutions today have little understanding of the theological foundations grounding the ministry or of the contours of Catholic culture that should provide the context within which care is provided. This makes the challenge of living up to and delivering on the claim to be "Catholic" quite daunting. It is important to note here a sign of hope with regard to this reality. Some of the larger Catholic health care systems today are beginning to take quite seriously the need to *form* lay leaders both spiritually and theologically so that they can ensure the integrity and existence of Catholic health ministry in the future (Ascension Health 2006).

In recent years the Catholic Health Association (CHA) of the United States, in collaboration with its members, produced a statement of shared identity intended to express the fundamental commitments of Catholic health *as a ministry* of the Church. Accordingly,

Catholic health care is to "promote and defend human dignity, attend to the whole person, promote the common good, act on behalf of justice, care for poor and vulnerable persons, steward resources and act in communion with the church" (CHA 2005). While the commitment statements are succinct, their implications are sweeping with regard to every aspect of a Catholic health care organization's life.

In addition to these expressed commitments, Catholic health care institutions share the following characteristics:

1. *Catholic sponsorship.* Until quite recently Catholic health care organizations were considered "Catholic" solely by virtue of their connection with the religious congregations or dioceses that founded, nourished, and sustained them. Because religious institutes and dioceses had canonical standing as public juridic persons in the Church, that is, they could carry out their activities in the name and on behalf of the Church, so did the institutionalized ministries associated with them. Over the past decade, as many Catholic hospitals have become organized into large systems, there has been increasing involvement of laywomen and men in the role of sponsor. This involvement of the laity requires formal approval from the Vatican allowing them to act publicly in the name of the Church. This trend toward lay sponsorship is certain to continue into the future (CHA 2004).

2. *Attention to spiritual care.* Catholic institutions offer spiritual care to patients, health care professionals, and others by ensuring the presence of competent and qualified interdenominational pastoral care professionals. In addition, ordained Catholic clergy are called upon to preside at the celebration of the Eucharist and to make the other sacraments available as needed.

3. *Attention to the development of a Catholic culture.* Catholic institutions are usually marked by various Catholic symbols including crucifixes, statues, and works of religious art. In addition, time for prayer often is taken before meetings, at the beginning and end of the day and at other appropriate times. Ritual is increasingly a part of the life of Catholic health care organizations, marking times of grief, loss, transition, and celebration.

These characteristics are more than superficial. They express the character of the health care organization as a ministry of the Catholic Church.

There is something deeper, however. Catholics essentially conceive of the healing ministry as an extension of the ministry of Christ (USCC 1981; John Paul II 1995). Jesus was prophet or teacher, king or shepherd, priest or sanctifier. The Second Vatican Council has taught that this threefold ministry should be reflected in all the works of the Church and in every member. Healing is part of the shepherding function of the Christian community, because building this community entails concern for each weak member who needs restoration to vital life and participation.

Jesus healed people *radically* by penetrating to the spiritual core of the human personality and liberating the person from original or social sin and also from individual, personal sin, with the more superficial but real effect of healing them also psychologically and physically. A Catholic health care facility, therefore, is also concerned with the radical healing of those for whom it cares. The experience of sickness and healing in such a hospital should also be an experience of personal spiritual growth through suffering and redemption. One of the main methods of ensuring that the Catholic organization, whether a facility or corporate entity, seeks to foster and protect its Catholic identity is the ethics committee.

7.9 CONCLUSION

The social organization of health care determines the manner in which health care is provided as well as the overall health of people. While we have sought to consider the principles in the social provision of health care and the associated ethical responsibilities, there is no doubt that the methods of providing health care are changing and that ethical responsibilities will change as well. A firm foundation for ethical analysis in regard to new developments may be derived from the Church's emphasis on the dignity of the human person, "the manifestation of God in the world, a sign of his presence, a trace of his glory," (John Paul II 1995, no. 34). Social organizations and agencies will be no more ethical than the individual people responsible for their existence and services. Hence the social aspects of health care depend on individuals dedicated to preserving the dignity of the people they serve. This truly is the bedrock principle for formulating social policy and organizations involved in health care.

Chapter Eight

PASTORAL CARE

OVERVIEW

AS WE HAVE ARGUED THROUGHOUT THIS book, bioethics, like health care itself, must always keep in mind not only physical health and medical care of the sick but also the care of the whole human person. Hence in this final chapter we will consider the problems that arise for the spiritual health of both those who are cared for in hospitals and the professionals who care for them. Therefore, we consider the history of pastoral care and its goals today, the pastoral care of the professional health care staff, the ethical counseling of both the staff and those who are ill, their spiritual counseling, and the celebration of the Christian sacraments as the healing work of Jesus Christ ministered through his pastoral ministers. Addressing these issues sums up our whole theological approach to the ethics of health care.

8.1 THE GOALS OF PASTORAL MINISTRY

If Christian ministry is to be Christlike, care for the sick undoubtedly is an essential part of it. At least a third of the Gospel according to St. Mark, aside from the passion narrative devoted to Jesus's own suffering and death, is devoted to accounts of how Jesus healed the physically and mentally sick. His care for the sick seems to have been the clearest evidence to others of his mission from the Father and of the life-giving truth of his preaching. Studies devoted to the history of pastoral care (Holifield 1983; Wilson et al. 1996; Lynch 2005) conclude that, traditionally, religious ministry has four functions: (1) to heal, (2) to sustain, (3) to guide, and (4) to reconcile. Whereas by healing and sustaining they have in mind something broader than physical and psychological healing and encouragement in times of sickness, it is obvious that ministers cannot heal and sustain if they are not intimately concerned with problems of physical and psychological health. Furthermore, we show in later sections that guidance and reconciliation are in some respects especially effective when they occur in times of health crisis. The *Ethical and Religious Directives for Catholic Health Care Services* (USCCB 2001) state, "Directed to spiritual needs that are often appreciated more deeply during times of illness, pastoral care is an integral part of Catholic health care. Pastoral care encompasses the full range of spiritual services, including a listening presence; help dealing with powerlessness, pain, and alienation; and assistance in recognizing and responding to God's will with greater joy and peace" (part II, introduction, p. 12).

The hospital in Western culture originated in the pastoral care of the sick, and only with the rise of humanism in the eighteenth century did it begin to subordinate that concern to purely medical care. In the nineteenth century, however, the nursing profession in its modern form was the creation of Florence Nightingale, her work inspired by the Christian ideals of the Anglican Church and guided by the tradition of the Catholic nursing sisters (Dossey et al. 2005).

Today, however, in many hospitals, pastoral care is left to occasional visiting ministers who are treated much as any other visitor. In others, a chaplain is provided, but he is regarded by the medical staff simply as a convenience to those confined to the hospital, just as are the hospital barber or proprietor of the gift shop. It is becoming much more common, however, even for public hospitals to include a department of pastoral care as a recognized part of their therapeutic work. The members of such a department are still often regarded as somewhat less than professional colleagues of the medical staff, who think of them according to outmoded stereotypes.

The first reason for this situation is the secularization of the medical profession, which believes itself neutral to religious concerns. This is the case even in many, perhaps most, Catholic and other church-affiliated hospitals, where a large part of the medical staff may not be members of the sponsoring church (Guinan 1999; Lee 2002; Capizzi 2003). Even when a Catholic hospital has a largely Catholic medical staff, these health care professionals may still conceive their own tasks as rigidly separated from the concerns of pastoral care. We, however, have insisted throughout this book that modern secularization of institutions can be reconciled, if the proper effort is made, with due respect for all reasonable worldviews and values systems, including both secular humanism and true Christianity (Ashley 2000b; Engelhardt 2001).

Thus the question arises as to whether a purely secular hospital serving principally persons more influenced by secular humanism than the traditional religions (who make up probably at least 40 percent of the American public) should have a pastoral care department and, if so, what its character should be. We believe that such a health care facility would still need a pastoral care department, although it probably should have a different name more in keeping with the symbolic system of humanism. The purpose of such a department would be to help persons deal with these existential (spiritual) problems that arise so acutely in times of illness or dying. The continual spate of books and articles on death and dying since the pioneering work of Elisabeth Kubler-Ross (1969), many written from a purely humanist point of view, are evidence of this concern (McCarthy et al. 2000). Also, this need cannot be met adequately by psychotherapists or social workers who are not usually able to treat strictly spiritual problems.

In a Catholic hospital, pastoral care should be thoroughly Catholic, but as the Second Vatican Council has taught, being truly Catholic requires accepting pluralism and ecumenism. Thus Catholic hospitals should provide counseling for the large number of their clientele who say they "have no religion," are "not interested in religion," and so forth (ERD 2001, D. 22). Such counseling should respect the system of values by which their clients live and should avoid denominational pressures. At the same time, it should not neglect the need of such nonreligious persons to deal with the problems of suffering, death, alienation, and loneliness on their own terms (Natural Death Center 2003).

A second reason for the ambiguous situation of pastoral care in many hospitals is that in fact the chaplain or others occupied in pastoral care lack specialized professional training to work with the sick. All ministerial education requires general skill in pastoral health care, and for this reason assignments to a chaplaincy or pastoral care department in a modern hospital require specialization. Catholic hospitals have moved away from the time when the local bishop supplied the hospitals of his diocese with a chaplain priest, often one unable to accept a regular pastoral assignment because of age or illness, but who could reside at the hospital and administer the sacraments. Catholic hospitals are now hiring only those chaplains certified for special training and competency in health care.

In Catholic hospitals, the pastoral care staff usually includes at least one priest or deacon, several religious or laypeople, and in most large facilities, pastoral representatives of churches other than Catholic. All members of the pastoral staff are designated as chaplains, even though at one time this term was reserved for clergy (NACC 1995). The ERDs require that priests and deacons be appointed to the pastoral care staff of Catholic health care facilities by the local bishop, in collaboration with the administration of the institution (NCCB 2001, D. 21). Religious and laity are appointed by the administration of the facility, as is the director of the pastoral care team. If the director is not a Catholic, however, his or her appointment must be approved by the local bishop (D. 22). Although the appointment of pastoral care personnel is recommended in Directive 22, the process of appointment is to be "left to diocesan policy." Because few dioceses have policies in this regard, the freedom of the administration to appoint people to this position seems reasonable. Finally, it seems that appointment to the pastoral care staff, either by the local bishop or by administration, carries with it the special designation needed to constitute one as a minister of the Church (USCC 2001; Sheehan 2005). For this reason we use the words "chaplain" and "minister" interchangeably (www.acpe.edu).

Preparation of Pastoral Care Professionals

The development of *clinical pastoral education* (CPE) was the result of the pioneering work of Anton Boisen (1876–1965), a Protestant minister who had himself suffered psychotic episodes but learned from them the need for a more psychotherapeutic approach to the care of the sick (Hall 1992; see www.acpe.edu). A national association, the Association for Clinical Pastoral Education (ACPE), now accredits programs for preparing priests and lay ministers in this approach through supervised experiences in health care facilities, which have proved very successful although sometimes criticized for theological deficiencies. Catholic ministers also need a good understanding of what John Paul II (1997; Ashley 1996b) called "the theology of the body."

This new psychotherapeutic emphasis on pastoral counseling agrees in some respects with the traditional Protestant emphasis on pastoral counseling, but it also produces a certain tension in ministerial identity for those who find it hard to reconcile the moralistic and evangelistic emphasis of their tradition with modern psychotherapy's stress on guilt-less self-expression. Catholics, because of their emphasis on sacramental ministry in which counseling was often largely restricted to hearing confessions, were slower to accept the new psychotherapeutic approach. After the Second Vatican Council, however, CPE began to be a regular part of priestly formation in many seminaries, and the National Association of Catholic Chaplains began to develop its own programs and certification in specialized pastoral ministry. Here again the tension between traditional types of ministry and psychotherapeutic emphasis has not yet been completely resolved (Powell 2000).

Although CPE or its equivalent has served to make ministers of pastoral health care more professional and has thus somewhat improved their status with medical staffs, it has also raised the question as to whether pastoral care is simply another form of psychotherapy and social work. Until pastoral care people themselves have a clearer theology of pastoral care and a surer sense of their specific identity, they will have difficulty being accepted as professionals by hospital administrators and medical staffs. The ERD states, "Catholic health care organization should provide pastoral care to minister to the religious and spiritual needs of all those it serves. Pastoral care personnel—clergy, religious, and lay alike—should have appropriate professional preparation, including an understanding of these *Directives,* D.10" (Council of Collaboration 2004).

Pastoral Care in Relation to Other Health Care Services

In seeking their proper role in health care, clergy often claim that they deal with the whole person or the "patient" as a person, whereas other health care professionals are more concerned with special parts of the person (Estadt, Blanchette, and Compton 1991; Clinebell 1995). In contrast, some physicians believe that the medical doctor, who is the only complete health care professional, must therefore head the health care team and make the final decision in all matters. Thus the physician deals with health care as a whole, while other members of the team, including the minister, deal only with special or incidental aspects of the client's health problem. Thus sometimes the physician considers the ministry of the clergy to the sick merely as partial, auxiliary, or incidental and resents as presumptuous and intrusive any claim on the clergy's part to deal with the whole person.

This controversy about whole and part can be clarified by realizing that different wholes are in question. In viewing the client under the aspect of *physical* health, the physician is the chief of any health care team and de jure has the ultimate decision in presenting to the sick person an evaluation of a possible course of treatment, although de facto a nurse, dietician, physical therapist, or pharmacist may actually know more about the sick person. The ultimate decision, however, remains with clients, or those responsible for them if they are incompetent.

When making decisions about how to use the services of the health care team, persons must take into consideration other aspects of personality than physical health; they may also need the help and counsel of the psychotherapist, the ethical counselor, or the spiritual guide (Kirkwood 1995; Topper 2003). Sensitive physicians are quick to realize this and are happy not to stretch their responsibility beyond their professional competence for physical or, perhaps, mental health.

Thus, on behalf of the whole person, the first task of the health care ministry is to help clients understand the several dimensions of any health decision. In a hospital it is reasonable that the pastoral care department play a significant role in receiving and discharging. Those entering a hospital for care need to look forward to their experience in the hospital as one over which they have genuine control, and they should leave it feeling they are prepared to go on with normal life. Ministers can help them achieve this sense of self-control at a time when they often feel utterly helpless.

The foregoing tasks of the health care ministry, however, important as they are, remain secondary to its specific and central task of helping those they care for grow through their experience of sickness and convalescence or of death. But before discussing this principal work of the health care ministry, we must discuss the responsibility of the pastoral care people for the other members of the health care team.

8.2 PASTORAL CARE OF THE HEALTH CARE STAFF

The sick are not the only persons in need of pastoral care: so also are the members of the administrative and medical staffs and all the auxiliary personnel. Today it is well recognized in hospitals that the mental health of the staff is an important factor in the therapy of the ill. They are, as Henri Nouwen titled his well-known book, "wounded healers" (1979; Ross 2005). In fact, in any health care facility the effectiveness of health care depends in large part on the type of interpersonal relations that exist among its staff. Ultimately, this is a spiritual problem, because physicians, nurses, and others engaged in the very difficult vocation of caring for the suffering and confronting the crises of life and death are engaged in their own spiritual struggle (Levey 2001; Booth et al. 2002; Stanton and Cann 2003).

Staff members need help to maintain their sense of dedication, their courage, and their human compassion against all temptations of routine, cynicism, callousness, and ambition. If the Catholic Church from a long and often bitter historical experience has accepted the motto *ecclesia semper reformanda* ("the Church needs constant renewal"), this is equally true of hospitals and the health care profession. Only on the basis of this constant effort to renew Christian humanism within the staff is there any real hope of sound ethical judgment in the care of those who are ill.

In order to incorporate fully the pastoral care team into the life of the hospital, we suggest that the chaplain or director of the pastoral care department or some representative of that department who is especially competent should be included on the ethics committee of the hospital. This will provide a channel for raising ethical issues of an organizational nature as well as those that affect personnel of the facility. For example, the ethics committee handbook of one medical center (University of Kansas Medical Center 2002) reads, "The committee membership will be multidisciplinary. A majority of the membership will be non-physicians. Additional membership will include as available at least the following disciplines: nursing, social work, pastoral care, clinical ethics, law, respiratory care, and dietetics and nutrition" (3).

Moreover, the staff should be thoroughly informed of the religious and counseling services that the pastoral care department is ready to provide to them. It is important here, for example, that a Catholic hospital let the personnel know that they are welcome at the Eucharist and for personal confession or counseling. It is also important (and often neglected) to let non-Catholics know that the department has considered their needs, inquired about them, and made some provision for them in a way that is convenient and free of embarrassment.

The director of pastoral care should have a recognized procedure by which discussion can be facilitated with the administration, with the medical staff, with whatever group represents the nurses, and with the union or other representative body of the hospital employees concerning issues of interpersonal relationships that the members of the pastoral care department may have observed are affecting the welfare of the sick or of the institution. Naturally, administrators may be reluctant to give the director this formal access to groups in the hospital with which the administration may be at odds. Unless such recognized access exists, however, the director or chaplain will not be able to play that role of arbitrator and peacemaker, the existence of which must be a primary and spiritual ethical concern of any truly human institution. Ethics is always concerned about the tension between justice and social harmony. It is absurd to speak of an institution's concern for medical ethics if it does not recognize the need for this type of peacemaking as a truly ministerial function.

Coministry

If the pastoral care department is to fulfill this role, its members must have a profound respect for those who dedicate their lives to the healing profession and should acknowledge that spiritual ministry to the sick is not a monopoly of the pastoral care department. For Catholics, the Second Vatican Council (1965) reemphasized the ancient concept of "the universal priesthood of the believers," according to which Christ's ministry is not confined to ordained clergy. In its threefold function of teaching, shepherding, and worshiping, this ministry is shared in a variety of ways by every member of the Christian community so that all Christians are ministers along with Christ, who himself is the Servant of the Father (NACC 1996; Sheehan 2005). Consequently, all Christians also share in pastoral ministry to the sick. Jesus made this one of the responsibilities for love of neighbor on which all persons are to be judged (Mt 25:31–46).

In a very special way, therefore, the physicians, nurses, administrators, and all the members of a hospital staff are carrying out not merely a secular service but a genuine Christian ministry of healing, deriving its authority from Christ's own healing work and witnessing to his continuing presence in the world (Flanelly, Weaver, and Handzo 2003). Thus the priest-chaplain and the whole pastoral care department not only should refrain from monopolizing the religious aspect of health care but should also carry on an educational effort to help the hospital staff appreciate the spiritual and ethical values of their own professional work. Finally, it is important that the pastoral care department itself provide a model of true humanity and good interpersonal relations. The American Medical Association's *Principles of Medical Ethics* (2001) states, "IV. A physician shall respect the rights of the sick, colleagues, and other health professionals, and shall safeguard patient confidences and privacy within the constraints of the law" (XIV). Not infrequently, the chaplain is the most difficult person on the staff, not because he plays the role of prophet, but because he is a warped personality constantly defending his own clerical status. Needless to say, in such cases the administration should not let respect for the clergy stand in the way of seeking a reeducation or a replacement of the chaplain.

8.3 PASTORAL CARE AND ETHICAL COUNSELING

The primary task of pastoral care is *spiritual* guidance and celebration, yet the purpose of this book has been to deal with *ethical* questions confronted not only by the sick but also by health care professionals in dealing with the sick. Therefore, before discussing spiritual counseling, we deal with ethical counseling. But how can a minister be an ethical counselor to persons who, in a pluralistic culture, are committed to such different value systems (John Paul II 1981, no. 10; Farris 2002)?

Different value systems cannot be simply reduced to some common denominator, but rather are *analogous* to each other, that is, fundamentally different yet having much in common. This is especially true of the value systems of cultures and social situations that may be very foreign to the counselor's experience (Wicks and Estadt 1993; Wilson et al. 1996; Lartey 2003; Furniss 2004). Consequently we believe that in pastoral care it is possible to proceed ecumenically to find a common ground for ethical decisions between different value systems of the counselor and the person counseled. Such an ecumenical method depends on (1) the counselor's clarity about her or his own values and fidelity to them, (2) respect for the values of others and their fidelity to these, and (3) a common effort to find a basis for mutual dialogue and action (Steinhoff-Smith 1999). Today most people remain in the hospital only a short time, so they are not in any condition to rethink their whole outlook on life (Stone 2001; Bidwell 2004). Hence an ethical counselor should in general not disturb the client's basic commitment unless it becomes apparent that such issues at the spiritual level have to be faced because the sufferer is already struggling with them. Consequently the counselor usually can only deal with a Jew within the Jewish ethical tradition, a Baptist within the Baptist tradition, a humanist within a humanistic set of values. Pressure to proselytize persons during illness to one's own faith is an unfair exploitation because it fails to respect the freedom required for a true conversion.

What then should be the goal of such short-term ethical counseling? How in the hospital situation can persons be helped within the context of their value system to achieve a free and informed conscience and to arrive at prudent ethical decisions? While human decisions to be ethical first must be free, the sick suffer from various limitations of their psychological freedom. When their illness is mental, this freedom is severely restricted or even eliminated by neurosis or psychosis. When it is physical, however, the sick still suffer some degree of constraint because of weakness, mental confusion, depression, and so forth, consequent of their physical condition and also because they are confined to a narrow and unfamiliar social situation. Thus the sick person is often not able to think clearly and realistically.

Ethical counseling of the sick, therefore, must first aim at creating an atmosphere in which the client's freedom is maximized. Until some area of genuine freedom opens up for the client, ethical discussion is useless. When such an opening is achieved, the counselor must strive to keep ethical discussion confined to just that area of freedom and not waste time with what seem to be ethical arguments but are in fact only the expression of emotional conflict. The means to achieving this increased freedom are essentially the techniques of psychotherapy, which the minister needs to understand and use in a modest way, referring more difficult problems to members of the health care team who are professionally skilled in such therapy (Ciarrocchi 1993; Vaughan 1994). Religious ministers have something special to contribute to this freeing process, however, because they can help to lift the burden of existential fear or hopelessness that may be one of the chief obstacles to freedom (Capps 1995; Howe 2003). Persons who are confident of God's loving and forgiving care have a peace of mind even in the face of suffering and death that makes it possible for them to face difficult decisions with serenity and sanity.

In the ethical counseling of medical professionals who ask a minister for advice, especially on bioethical matters, the same principles should be followed as for sick clients, although the freedom of such professionals is not limited by illness. They too, however, suffer from certain biases and conflicts of attitude, and many have value systems very different from those of others, including the minister. Consequently the minister should express his or her own honest opinions and be willing to engage in respectful dialogue with the staff persons, seeking a common ethical ground.

Subjective and Objective Morality

Once the counselor is assured that the client is sufficiently free to deal with an ethical decision, the counselor's next objective should be to help the sick person arrive at a decision that is prudent and thus at least *subjectively* good, that is, according to the client's honest conscience, even when the counselor is not convinced that this decision is *objectively* good (see chapter 2, section 2.4). There are three reasons why such a gap between subjective morality and objective morality may occur or may seem to the counselor to exist: (1) seriously ill counselees may have a different value system than the counselor, (2) the counselor's judgment may appear inconsistent with the patient's own value system, and (3) the counselee's decision may be inconsistent with the facts of the situation as the counselor perceives these facts.

In the first case, as already stated, the counselor generally should not attempt to convert the counselee to the counselor's own value system, but should help the patient to make decisions consistent with the counselee's own values. If, of course, there is more time and the counselee's condition permits the counselor, if the counselor thinks the counselee's value system is faulty, he or she may find opportunity to encourage the counselee to seek the objective truth about values. In the second case, the counselor should do what is possible to help the counselee to make a self-consistent decision, because only then will the decision be conscientious and subjectively right. In the third case, the counselor should try to help the counselee perceive the facts of the situation correctly. Nevertheless, in this last case, the counselor should remember that one's perception and interpretation of facts is influenced by one's value system and personal experience, so that it may not be possible for counselee and counselor to come to an agreement on the facts.

The reason that the counselor first should be concerned to help a client come to a subjectively honest decision is twofold: because a person always retains primary responsibility for health decisions and because the proximate norm of all moral decisions is the conscience of the agent. Ethically it is more important that persons do what they sincerely believe to be right at a given stage of their moral development than that they do what is objectively right. Because we live in a sinful world, and each of us suffers from the darkness of mind and hardness of heart resulting from our own sins, the word of God is received by us in obscurity. Only little by little do we move forward into the light, as is so eloquently witnessed in the Old Testament by the history of the "chosen people." What is most essential is that we keep moving forward, even if our steps are frequently missteps. For those who make mistakes in good faith, experience is self-corrective.

The New Testament shows how Jesus (unlike the Pharisees) is more concerned with the faith and goodwill of sinners than he is with their conformity with a law of which they are often ignorant and with which they do not know how to comply. St. Paul (1 Cor 8) also urges respect for the conscience of others, even when they are mistaken and immature in their moral understanding. This was also the teaching of John Paul II (1981, no. 9) on the "gradualness" of moral conversion, that must be carefully distinguished, however, from the "gradualism" of proportionalism.

The task of the counselor, however, does not stop with helping a client arrive at a subjectively prudent and conscientious decision. The fact that a decision is honest does not prevent it from being harmful to others or even to the one who makes the decision when it is actually an *objectively* wrong decision. Honest mistakes do not injure moral integrity, destroy spiritual relations to God and neighbor, or prevent some spiritual growth, but they do have consequences from which we and others suffer. Moreover, Christian morality is creative; it is a response to God's call to move forward toward him and to share in his redemptive work. This divine call is often present in the crisis of sickness and dying. Consequently, the counselor cannot be content simply to ratify, as it were, decisions made by a client within the narrow limits of the client's routine morality.

On the one hand, if the counselor sees that the counselee's decision may in fact be clearly injurious to the counselee or to others (e.g., if he or she is thinking of suicide or abortion), the counselor has to do what is possible to prevent this harm, even when the counselor is convinced of the subjective honesty of the decision (John Paul II 1981, no. 8). On the other hand, the counselor may judge that it is necessary in particular cases to confront the sick person with the challenge inherent in the decision that has to be made. Thus the counselor must raise disturbing questions that ultimately go beyond the ethical level to the spiritual level of the person's value system. Obviously counselors must be very cautious about disturbing sick people in this manner, yet they should have the courage to do so when their behavior signals that such probing and confrontation are necessary. The wonderful scene of Jesus and the Samaritan woman (Jn 4:4–30) shows how the spirit of God can be at work in the human conscience, revealing itself by the uneasiness, the denial, the defiance, and the disguised cries for help that a spiritually sensitive and experienced counselor can recognize. In these cases the apparent subjective honesty of the client masks a hidden conflict of conscience that cannot be resolved without probing that goes beyond the subjective to a new and deeper perception of reality. This incident also reminds us that women and men, because they have somewhat different life experiences, also require nuanced approaches in making ethical decisions (Stevenson-Moessner 1996; Neuger 2001; Gorsuch 2001). It is no simple matter for a counselor to balance these two counseling aims of subjective and objective conscience (Lebacqz and Driskill 2000).

Formerly, it would seem that the clergy were too quick to impose objective moral standards on people, with little sensitivity to the moral development or experience of different individuals. Today, with the growth in psychological understanding of individual differences and of the developmental aspects of morality, it would seem that the opposite temptation prevails. The axiom "people must make their own conscientious decisions" has often been pushed so far that some ministers have lost interest in objective morality. For example, because of the present campaign to legalize "assisted suicide," some counselors and some physicians think that if people want to kill themselves and are sincere in their decision, they should be assisted in carrying it out. Rather, the minister should do what is possible to prevent objective harm and to challenge the judgment of the sufferer or the professional when signs indicate that such challenge may be an opportunity for successful moral growth or improvement of the hospital's bioethical policies.

In carrying out this educative task, ministers should first emphasize, as we have attempted to do in this book, the primary values and principles of Christian living as they apply to the healing process. These principles should not be presented as rules but as goals to be creatively achieved in a loving and generous response to the grace of God, after the pattern of the Good Samaritan (Lk 10:25–37), who saw in the injured man in the ditch the call of God. The professional or the patient who have these goals at heart and use the knowledge and imagination available to reach them will act in a truly humane and Christian way, enlightened by the Holy Spirit. The analogy between the physician and the moral guide should be stressed: as the physician diagnoses not to blame the sick persons but to prevent or heal physical ills, so the ethical counselor diagnoses moral evils not to blame the counselee but to help them avoid harm to themselves and others and to lead a more genuinely happy life.

Christians open to the Spirit in this way are not negligent of or ungrateful for the guidance given by the pastors of the Church, whether that guidance has the certitude of the Gospel or simply the authority of pastors doing what they can to apply the Gospel in a given time or place according to the lights they possess. Alternatively, mature Christians know that God requires of them personal decisions based not only on pastoral guidance but also on their own gifts and experience.

The final task of ethical counselors, therefore, is to help those they counsel mature in conscience and live in peace with the responsibility for their own decisions, content with the assurance that God calls us to share in his task of healing a wounded world (Ciarrocchi 1995). Indeed, all those engaged in health care can be confident that the words addressed by Jesus to the apostles apply also in a very real way to them, "Proclaim the kingdom of God and heal the sick!" (Lk 9:2) and also expressed elsewhere, "Amen, I say to you, whatever you did for one of these least brethren of mine, you did for me" (Mt 25:40).

8.4 SPIRITUAL COUNSELING IN HEALTH CARE

So far in this chapter we have discussed some of the functions that the religious minister can perform as an integrator of health care in the interests of the total health of the human person, but we have not yet discussed the specifically spiritual role of the minister (Walters 1995; Ashley 2000b; Williams 2002; VandeCreek and Burton 2005). The reason that some have confused pastoral care with psychotherapy or are unable to appreciate CPE is because they are uncertain about what "spiritual ministry" really means or how it can contribute significantly to the ill person's healing. Today the term *spirituality* is used in very confusing ways so that some even speak of a "materialist spirituality" (Center for Naturalism 2005). To discuss this problem, we first begin with the question of how spiritual counseling differs from psychological counseling as these occur during a person's stay in a hospital or long-term care facility.

Persons who are ill are faced with potentially serious problems:

1. They may fear suffering and death.
2. They may face the uncertainties of diagnosis and prognosis and fear about the pain of embarrassment of various testing or treatment procedures unfamiliar to them or all too painfully familiar.
3. They may face the tedium of a long stay in the health care facility under circumstances they find either boring or excruciating.
4. They suffer separation from their regular work, friends, and family and are not comfortable in the new situation.
5. They may be worried and perhaps feel guilty about the various responsibilities at home that they cannot handle.
6. They suffer from a sense of deprivation of privacy and of freedom, almost as if they were imprisoned.
7. They may feel puzzled about why this is happening to them and may interpret their sickness as punishment for moral guilt or experience the "silence of God." They may also anticipate further guilt through a lack of courage or hope.
8. They may feel alone and deserted in meeting all the forgoing, and their sense of dignity, worth, and membership in the human community may be diminished by real moral guilt for which God's forgiveness is truly needed.

Spiritual ministers in their own proper role are called on to help the sick persons in these struggles and may also be called on to help members of the health care team who are faced with similar problems both in their personal lives and in their professional involvement with clients. The first task of the spiritual guide is to establish *trust*, but this trust differs from that on which most professional relations are based, because it has a type of ultimacy (Hall 1995; Dayringer 1998; Allen 2002; Quinlan 2002; Howe 2003). People often seek out a minister to confide in when they can no longer trust their lawyer, their physician, or even their psychiatrist. The different experiences of women and men must also be taken into account and is often overlooked (Stevenson-Moessner 1996; Neuger 2001; Gorsuch 2001; Malony 2001). Ministers must build up trust on the foundation not of words but of behavior. A minister must keep promises, maintain contact, and be available to help in whatever difficulty is bothering their clients or to look for someone who can help. A minister must also be nonjudgmental, empathetic, and very careful about confidentiality. Finally, a chaplain's care is expected to extend beyond those cared for to their families.

Nevertheless, as in other counseling, this trust has its limits, and ministers must make clear to those they serve that a spiritual counselor has limited powers. Otherwise the trust between chaplain and client will soon appear to be violated. Thus chaplains should explain that they cannot work miracles at will, change hospital policies or structures, or get the client discharged and that their role is primarily that of a listener, counselor, and celebrant of the sacraments. All this should become clear in the implicit or explicit counseling contract. It is up to counselors to set these limits tactfully and to remember that they are dealing with persons who in their weakened condition have undergone considerable psychological regression, which makes them as dependent and demanding as a child in relation to its parents. The minister should give the seriously sick permission for this dependency, but only a limited permission. If such limits are not set, the minister will soon find that the counselee interprets much that the minister does as a betrayal of trust.

Caring in the Name of the Christian Community

This trust between a spiritual guide and the spiritual pilgrim takes its special character first from the charisma of the minister as a designated representative of the Christian community. The spiritual guide is an "apostle," that is, one sent by the church in the name of God on whom the spirit of God has been invoked by the prayers of the Christian community. Even when spiritual guides are not ordained, their ministry must somehow be authorized by the Christian community if it is to be given that special trust that should characterize it. Physicians and psychotherapists in their white coats are often invested with an analogous charisma, but this is only an analogy to the charisma of the spiritual guide.

Therefore spiritual counselors need to reflect constantly on two realities: first, that God is acting through them to accomplish what is quite beyond their own abilities and, second, that unless they acknowledge their own human limits, they will be placing obstacles in the way of God's work. Ministers who have this correct perception of their own role will not attempt to put themselves under impossible strains or feel guilty at an inability to solve all the problems of all for whom they care. Alternatively, they will feel and communicate to the suffering unlimited hope in the loving power of God and a sense of each one's dignity in God's eyes and their own (Capps 1995). They should make a special effort to make sure, if possible, that when after diagnosis or treatment persons leave a facility they will retain a connection to the Christian community or know how to form such a connection if it has not existed before (Linn, Linn, and Linn 1993).

Some ministers are so secularized that they feel more comfortable in a psychotherapeutic role than in a spiritual one and thus fail their clients by refusal to speak in God's name. They avoid talking with the sick about spiritual issues, praying with them, or inquiring about their need for the sacraments, as if these were forbidden or offensive topics. The sick may very well read this as a lack of faith on the minister's part and thus as a threat to the patient's own faith, which is already sorely tried by doubts and anxieties raised by his or her condition. Ministers who find themselves in a quandary about their own pastoral identity should attempt to resolve this ambiguity through spiritual guidance and perhaps psychotherapy if they are going to fulfill their responsibility of helping the sick through *their* quandaries (Capps 1990; Mosgofian and Ohlschlager 1995).

Discernment

The minister, just like a psychotherapist, is a listener and a reflector through whom the realities of the client's situation become clearer to the client and more manageable. Furthermore, as with the psychotherapist, the minister listens not just to what the client seems to be saying superficially, but to what he or she, perhaps unconsciously, is trying to say nonverbally and symbolically (Clements 1983). The psychotherapist, however, is listening for the message that rises from the client's subconscious emotional drives, whereas the minister as a spiritual therapist is listening for a message that comes from a still deeper level, from that place the scriptures call the "heart," that is, from the spiritual interior of the person's being where the person is committed to some sort of ultimate values and to some fundamental insight into reality (Hall 1992; Ciarrochi 1993; Lester 2003). In most persons this commitment and vision is dim and confused indeed; yet it is the source of all personal life, where people really live and where they really die. "Out of the depths I call to you O Lord, O Lord hear my voice" (Ps 130). It is this voice de profundis to which the minister must listen. Moreover, a spiritual guide is not looking, as is the psychotherapist, for the psychic energies and motivations that flow from human instinctual needs, but for the work of the Holy Spirit in the sufferer; the signs of faith, hope, and love; and the spiritual forces of sin and alienation that oppose these (Walters 1995). This is the spiritual level of human functioning.

The patient may raise these questions directly by saying, "Why has this happened to me, Father? Have I sinned? Am I going to be punished? What will happen to me if I die?" or "I don't seem to be able to pray now that I am sick," and so forth. Today, in a secularized society, however, such questions are seldom asked *directly* (Conn 1998). Even if they are, the chaplain may very well suspect that they do not really come from the spiritual level of personality but are merely the pious language that some people (especially those who are from a fundamentalist religious background) use in speaking of purely physical or psychological problems. Also the sick person may think that this is the way you are supposed to converse with a minister, who is supposed only to talk in a type of religious language (Harding 2000). Therefore the counselor has to listen to religious questions inherent in pseudo-religious language (Cleary 1999). In both cases, ethical counselors must go deeper to find the really spiritual level in the person and, if in fact it is spiritual, deal with it in spiritual terms, or if the counselor is not prepared to do this, refer the person to a proper spiritual counselor.

This requires patience, and it is usually a mistake to begin asking spiritual questions of a client with whom the needed level of trust has not yet been established (Moran 1997). Alternatively, experienced spiritual counselors learn how to cut through levels of small talk and psychological talk to the issues with which they have to deal. Simple directness is ordinarily not resented by clients. *Directness* is not bluntness or insensitivity. It is rather a form of respect for a client, a refusal simply to play games.

This respect for the person demands that the minister not take advantage of the sick person's weak condition. It is unethical to try to force sick persons to repent, accuse them of supposed sin, make demands for prayer or faith, and so forth. It may seem incredible that some ministers carry on such a preaching attack on helpless people, but many victims will report unpleasant experiences of being confronted by zealous ministers in a hospital and being embarrassed or pressured. Reports of such experiences have done much to prejudice physicians and nurses against the ministerial profession.

The minister who exerts this pressure fails to trust in God's providence, by which God is using an experience of illness as an occasion of possible spiritual growth. The spirit of God is already at work in the sufferer in ways that are not labeled religious. The minister must recognize this growth process and cultivate it, helping persons to understand what is going on in their own terms.

A specific responsibility for ministers is not only to deal with the sick person's spiritual problems as an individual but also to help him or her become vividly aware of the real presence of God and of the church as the people of God in the individual's life in this very event of sickness where the sufferer may feel abandoned and isolated. Ministers are themselves a visible sign or sacrament of this presence, incarnating God, as it were, in a tangible, human, imperfect, but real form.

Also, it is not enough that ministers provide this witness of God's presence only to members of their own church. Too many ministers assume that they have responsibility only to their own parishioners or to those of their own denomination and that others will resent their presence. Usually, however, this is not the case. Most laity are less ecclesiastically defined than we think. For them any minister, even a rabbi, is still a "man of God" and as such ought to have some interest in them as "children of God." Even the humanist is seldom content with the silence of humanism in the face of the ultimate questions and is resentful if the religious minister writes him off as a nonbeliever.

Objectives of Spiritual Care

As a spiritual adviser, the minister's primary task is really a very simple one, but not easy one. This task is to say, as much or more by presence, attitude, and nonverbal symbols as by the exhortatory word, that God is present to sick persons in their fear or suffering. The spiritual guide must manifest that God is a loving, caring father, a cosuffering Lord Jesus, a healing spirit present as the one God actively loving the sufferer, but this is a presence in *mystery*. That is, it exceeds human rational empirical comprehension because it leads to an open future. This implies a spiritual awe before the *mysterium tremendum* (Van Kaam 1995). The sick person, as did Job, feels guilty and yet is not clear how he or she is guilty. There is a sense of *judgment*, the perception of one's responsibility for the consequences of one's misuse of God's loving gift of free will and of the grace to use it well that one has rejected. The minister should not deny this. Indeed, a minister symbolizes this judgment. The minister also overcomes judgment, however, by being a sign of mercy and reconciliation (John Paul II 1999, no. 7).

Sickness may be the time of genuine conversion in which persons truly find God for the first time in their lives or after a long time of forgetfulness and separation. For the survivor of a deceased person it also may be the occasion of conversion, but often instead leads to despair (Oates 1997). The minister must affirm the reality of suffering or death as an invitation of divine mercy, but that is not the whole of the minister's responsibility. Conversion is the beginning of a new life, but that life has to be lived authentically or it will be lost again. Consequently, one of the chief aims of spiritual counseling is to assist converts to begin to grow daily in the Christian life and to plan practically to continue that growth once they have returned to the routine situations of everyday life.

It is important also that the minister, in helping sick persons realize God's presence, make vivid to them that the minister is a sign of the concern of God's people, of the Christian community or church, for a suffering brother or sister. Sickness is in Old Testament terms a type of "uncleanness," and a sick person may experience a "leprosy" of loneliness, alienation, and "excommunication" as an outcast from life and the human community. This is especially true of persons with acquired immunodeficiency syndrome (AIDS). The minister removes this excommunication and reunites the lonely one with the community that is praying for him or her. Recall how Jesus, healing a leper, sent him to a priest to be readmitted to the Jewish community (Mk 1:44). Recall, as well, how Jesus might indicate that the cured person should "sin no more," but he never asked people how they became sick or how they contracted their pathologies.

8.5 CELEBRATING THE HEALING PROCESS

The specific spiritual task of pastoral care is not exhausted simply by counseling. It must not be confined to talking about the presence of God, but it must deepen into *experiencing* that presence in prayer, worship, celebration, and communion (CCC 2000, 1135 ff.).

Today, when most chaplains and other ministers as well are training in CPE programs, they sometimes feel a tension between the model of the chaplain as a pastoral counselor, whose main task is to engage in a therapeutic psychological process with the sick person, and the model of the pastor, one who presents the sacred scripture, prays with and inspires the sufferer, and administers the sacraments. These two models of ministry at times may seem opposed to each other. In particular, one seems aimed at removing feelings of guilt and giving feelings of interpersonal warmth and confidence and getting clients "in touch with their feelings," whereas the other might impose a formalized religious response that covers up a client's real experience (Oates 1985).

Actually the two models, when they are well understood, are complementary and can reinforce each other. We have already shown how pastoral counselors by their own presence are already a *sacrament*, that is, a sign of the presence of God (Anderson 2003). The word of God first came to human beings not in the text of the Bible that recalls his coming but in the incarnation of Jesus Christ, who came to the sick and suffering, shared their suffering, and healed them by his touch (Mk 2:1–12). Ministers, because they are sent by Jesus, are living witnesses, "other Christs," and a sign of Christ's care for the patient. Therefore everything that the minister does to witness this tender concern, this ability to empathize, to listen, and not to judge—except in the sense of diagnosis of spiritual ailments to heal the spirit as a physician diagnoses physical ailments to heal the body—is a sacrament of Jesus's presence. Even humor and light banter, if their purpose is precisely to establish real communication, resemble the wit that Jesus constantly displayed in his preaching and parables. Above all, the down-to-earthiness—the freedom from stuffiness, self-righteousness, and elitism that can be the curse of the clerical state—is in imitation of Jesus, who did not hesitate to eat with sinners in simple fellowship (Mk 2: 16–17).

Thus, when ministers read the scripture with the sick, they should already have placed the scripture in a human relational context in which the word of God can be truly understood. Prayer also must grow out of this living context; that is, it should be natural for two people who have come to share a common concern to give it prayerful expression. A minister should not be praying in front of an embarrassed person who feels as if something is "being laid on him," in which he has no part. An opening for prayer will come, however, only if the sufferer senses that the minister's concern for him or her goes *deep*, deeper than the mere professional interest. The scriptures used should be chosen just because they help to make real the presence of Jesus, especially in his power to forgive, heal, and lead one into the fullness of life (Wimberley 1994; McArthur and Mack 1997; Sande 2004).

The Catholic priest is more likely than the Protestant minister or the rabbi to be concerned about the administration of the sacraments in the hospital setting. These too must be understood not as some sacred sign intruding into a real situation, but as a ritual of a process of healing that is already occurring. The primordial sacrament is the touching Jesus used when he healed the leper. "Moved with pity, he said to him, 'I do will it. Be made clean.' The leprosy left him immediately, and he was made clean" (Mk 1:41–42). It indicates the intimate presence, the care, the community, the power of life between Jesus and the sick and outcast. When a chaplain does what is so natural, namely, to hold the hand of sick persons to give them reassurance that the minister is there, that they are not alone, that is the primordial sacramental rite on which all the other sacraments are based—*human bodily contact* as a sign of *spiritual presence.*

Anointing the Sick

What ministers have done as good pastoral counselors, they now deepen and intensify by a sign that combines the verbal word of scripture with the nonverbal sacramental act. The rite of anointing of the sick brings this out clearly (Paul VI 1972) It is not merely for the dying, as formerly, but for any person seriously ill (Graumann 2002), when the person's condition is "serious," which should be judged not merely in physical terms but also in psychological terms. Thus, when anyone is sick enough that the minister suspects that the thought of possible death with its deep anxiety has entered his or her mind and produced fear and the threat of despair, then the spiritual and perhaps physical healing of the sacrament is needed and should be given. Whenever there is question of major surgery or of any disease that sick persons know sometimes leads to death and thus raises this fear in their own minds, ministers can anoint. They should not anoint when the illness is one in which recovery is assured and that consequently does not appear to contain any serious threat.

What is the meaning of this rite? First, it is not merely something done by a priest to a sufferer. Even when ministers are alone, they are there to represent not only God but also the Christian community (Rahner 1963). In fact, God is the center of the Christian community, so the minister is there to represent the Trinitarian community into which all Christians are incorporated in the second person incarnate by their baptism. The anxiety of sick persons is that by their illness they are outcasts, aliens to this community. The sick experience this in their isolation from usual daily life and by the threat of death that might take them away forever. What such sufferers need is the reassurance that their people and their God are still with them. The priest supplies the sign of this by *touching* a sufferer. This touch means "presence" and "acceptance" and as such is common to all the sacraments. It is a special type of touch in this case, however, a *healing* touch because it is the "anointing with oil," a common form of healing remedy that has the sense of soothing pain and infusing life and movement. Its significance as a spiritual healing is given by the words spoken.

This actual form of the sacrament is also preceded by brief scriptural passages that can be expanded. This is in keeping with the general principle that each sacrament should begin with a proclamation of the word of faith, because it is faith that opens the person to God's work and is the beginning of God's gifts.

Communal Nature of the Anointing of the Sick

Although the sacrament is valid with only the priest and the recipient present, this is not the ideal way to perform it. The sacraments are not performed merely in the ritual moment. Rather, they are the celebration of a culminating moment (not necessarily the last) of the saving work of God that has gone on for some time through what are apparently merely secular events. Therefore it is fitting not only that physicians and nurses be present at the anointing but also that they participate in it by reading the scriptures or saying some of the prayers and by imposing hands on or making the sign of the cross.

If the sacrament is not to mark the end of life but to help in the healing process, both physical and spiritual, it is certainly not separated from or in competition with the medical work of the hospital (Lysaught 2005). Rather, it is part of that healing process. In fact, it is a celebration of God's healing work, which God performs not only through the ritual but also through the *ministry* of the physicians, nurses, and administration. Priests are not the only ministers of health; they are part of a psychosomatic healing *team,* every member of which is called by God to a healing work and empowered by him through their natural gifts and education. The priest's special role on this team is to make explicit and eucharistic (thankful) the work of all.

Priests, in their instruction and commentary and by additions to some of the prayers, if necessary, should thank God for the healing gifts and work of the medical staff. It would be very appropriate for sick persons also at this time to express their thanks to the physicians and nurses. This expansion of the ritual can best be done when the sacrament takes place at the Eucharist in the hospital chapel, but it can also be done in the hospital room or ward when the physician can be present.

The proper rite for the dying is not the anointing of the sick but the reception of *Viaticum*, or final communion (NACC 1993). This is the expression of the sick person's communion and unity with the Church on Earth, which prays for his or her swift passage to the eternal banquet. Thus this communion should be shared with others present if possible.

When an emergency arises and someone must be anointed quickly, if the person whose life is endangered recovers consciousness, it is possible to hold a healing service of prayer so that he or she can more fully participate in the fruits of the sacrament. In the case of a person who is doubtfully alive, the sacrament of anointing should be administered, but the ritual forbids it to be given to someone who has already died. Previously priests were advised to administer the sacrament to someone who had recently died—up to two or three hours—if the death had been sudden. The ritual no longer prescribes this. A Catholic family may be very disconsolate to hear that the sacrament was not received by a member of the family who has died as the result of a fatal accident. If there is some doubt, even minimal, that life still remains, the priest may choose to anoint the patient conditionally. Perhaps a better procedure is to assure the family that the patient received the proper rites of the Church, meaning by this that the priest has prayed for the departed and blessed the body, because in such circumstances these are the proper rites according to the present discipline. In these ecumenical times, chaplains *also* should not hesitate to administer anointing to non-Catholics who might present themselves reverently at a general anointing service, because they probably are baptized and in good faith. If they are not already baptized, the sacrament still constitutes a prayer for the person's healing.

The Sacrament of Reconciliation

Sickness is sometimes the reminder that we need that the sacrament of reconciliation, or penance, is an apt means to facilitate conversion. Jesus's message was "This is the time of fulfillment. The kingdom of God is at hand. Repent and believe in the good news!" (Mk 1:15). The "good news" is that God through his ministers helps us to repent and believe and thus opens up to us the joy of belonging to his kingdom. Those who have deeply experienced this joy of forgiveness and new hope can make sickness into a blessing.

In his post-synodal apostolic exhortation "On Reconciliation and Penance," Pope John Paul II (1984, no. 31, III) has given a full explanation of this sacrament and has informed us of "contrition," or the sorrow for sin that it requires:

> *Conversion* and *contrition* are often considered under the aspect of the undeniable demands which they involve and under the aspect of the mortification which they impose for the purpose of bringing about a radical change of life. But we do well to recall and emphasize the fact that *contrition* and *conversion* are even more a drawing near to the holiness of God, a rediscovery of one's true identity which has been upset and disturbed by sin, a liberation in the very depth of self and thus a regaining of lost joy, the joy of being saved, which the majority of people are in time no longer capable of experiencing. . . . It is an act of honesty and courage. It is an act of entrusting oneself, beyond sin to the mercy that forgives.

This sacrament of reconciliation, or rite of penance, for the sick can be celebrated in the form of a penance service in the hospital chapel or even in the ward, with the invitation to all who wish to make individual confession and receive absolution. Such a service is an opportunity for the priest to deal with the question of sin and guilt and the meaning of suffering and of mercy and hope. When confession is made in a ward, it should be remembered that if it is difficult to achieve sufficient privacy, the penitent can be instructed simply to make a general acknowledgment of sins and to speak of them in detail in a future confession.

Baptism

Most of the questions concerning baptism in hospitals are concerned with the baptism of infants or the baptism of unconscious adults who are dying. In regard to baptism, the *Catechism of the Catholic Church* (CCC 2000, no. 1257) teaches:

> The Lord himself affirms that Baptism is necessary for salvation [Jn 3:5]. He also commands his disciples to proclaim the Gospel to all nations and to baptize them [Mt 28:9–20]. Baptism is necessary for salvation for those to whom the gospel has been proclaimed and who have the possibility of asking for this sacrament. The Church does not know of any means other than Baptism that assures entry into eternal beatitude; this is why she takes care not to neglect the mission she has received from the Lord to see that all who can be baptized are "reborn of water and the Spirit." *God has bound salvation to the sacrament of Baptism, but he himself is not bound by his sacraments.*

Thus the Catholic Church does not deny that the grace of Christ in ways known only to God can be given to anyone in the world without baptism, but it strives to fulfill its commission from Christ to preach the Gospel to all and to offer baptism to those who accept it and to their children. Moreover, the *prayer* of the Church for all persons is often efficacious even when it cannot be ritually expressed in the sacraments (see 1 Cor 7:9). The *Catechism of the Catholic Church* says (CCC 2000, no. 1261):

As regards children who have died without Baptism, the Church can only entrust them to the mercy of God, as she does in her funeral rites for them. Indeed, the great mercy of God who desires that all men should be saved, and Jesus' tenderness toward children which caused him to say: "Let the children come to me, do not hinder them," (Mt. 19:14) allow us to hope that there is a way of salvation for children who have died without Baptism. All the more urgent is the Church's call not to prevent little children coming to Christ through the gift of holy Baptism.

Nevertheless, it still is obligatory to administer baptism to children to manifest the concern of the Church and thus to keep alive the consciousness of the dignity of the human person from the first moments of existence (CCC 2000, no. 1250). Consequently, nurses and physicians should baptize infants who are in danger of death and even miscarried fetuses who exhibit human form and some sign of life. They should pour water on the child (on the head, if possible) so as actually to touch its skin and should say, "I baptize you in the name of the Father, the Son, and the Holy Spirit." In this way they express Christian reverence and fellowship with this little person who will forever be part of the Trinitarian community. If the infant is surely dead, baptism should not be administered, but the family of the infant may be assured that God's mercy has been implored through the prayers of the Church.

For the dying unconscious adult, it is permissible also to perform such a baptism with the condition, "If you are not baptized, I baptize you." Clearly this is not a grave obligation unless the person has asked to be baptized before lapsing into unconsciousness. This should not be done in a merely mechanical manner (trying to baptize everyone in the hospital) but only when there is some sign or probability that the person if conscious would be receptive of the sacrament. In our U.S. culture, secularized as it is, surveys have nevertheless shown that the great majority of people have at least some belief in God and reverence for Jesus and thus would be open to whatever help the Church has to offer in prayer and sacrament. As part of the physician's and nurse's care for particular persons in their charge whom they believe have given some indication that they might wish such baptism, they may confer it on dying infants or conditionally on unconscious persons provided this can be done without offense to their families. Again, this shows the Church's concern for a person who has providentially come under the care of the Catholic community.

Eucharist

The Eucharist is the supreme sacrament and sign of the Christian community, indicating that such patients remain a part of that community, even when absent from the public worship assembly, and that they are destined for eternal life with the community (CCC 2000, nos. 1211, 1374; John Paul II 2003). It is a life-giving, health-giving sacrament, as the eating of bread and drinking of wine are the basic symbols of the power to live and under these signs Jesus, the Lord of Life, is himself present to give us eternal life. Today the Eucharist is often distributed by auxiliary ministers, not by the priest. This is appropriate, because in the earliest days communion was taken from the public assembly to the homes of the sick. In a hospital it would be appropriate when possible to have the sick who are able and who wish to listen to the mass in the chapel on closed-circuit radio or television then to be brought communion immediately after the mass. In this way the union between mass and communion would be emphasized. It is essential in any case that communion in the health care facility should not be reduced to a routine in which someone pops in and out of a room to place a wafer in a sleepy sick person's mouth. We suggest at least a card containing a scripture reading and prayers that such persons can use while preparing for communion.

Lay Ministers

Today religious sisters and brothers and laypeople share in the sacramental ministry (CIC 1983 [2000], c. 910, para. 2). We have already mentioned that anyone can administer baptism who intends to do what the Church does in this most necessary of all sacraments. It is permitted, furthermore, for deacons and nonordained persons, men or women, to hold a service of healing (USCCB 1979). This can consist of scripture readings, prayers, and the laying on of hands for the sick. They can also make use of blessed oil as a sacramental. It would seem, however, that in such services it should be made clear to all that what is taking place is not a sacrament in the strict sense. This does not follow, however, that the prayer is inefficacious. Jesus said, "Where two or three are gathered together in my name, there am I in the midst of them" (Mt 18:20). Thus it is *preparatory* to the full public visit of the priest to the sick as a representative of the whole Christian community. Just as the physician's arrival completes the care given to patients by nurses, even if the physician does nothing additional except to approve and confirm what has already been done, so the priest approves, confirms, and completes the healing prayer of a local group and of auxiliary ministry. This is not a mere formality but an expression of the unity and public witness of the Church.

It should be remembered, too, that deacons, sisters, brothers, and other visitors, although they cannot give sacramental absolution, can truly help a sick person to conversion and reconciliation with God and neighbor in an efficacious way. We are not proposing revival of the "confession to a layman," which was common in the Middle Ages when a priest was not available, but rather are emphasizing that today in pastoral counseling such confession often takes place spontaneously. When it does, the ministers who are not priests should help such clients make an act of contrition and then encourage them to have a priest hear their confession when it becomes possible. The lay ministers should also assure them that here and now the mercy of God is truly present in prayer and that with this trust in God's mercy they should be at peace. The reason for confession later is to ratify and complete by the public acknowledgment of the priest as a representative of the Church a conversion that has already taken place. There is no reason for nonordained ministers to believe that, because they are not ordained, they cannot help patients achieve this reconciliation here and now.

The Sacraments and Bioethics

The forgoing discussion of sacramental ministry may sound liturgical rather than ethical, but it sums up the ethical message of this book. That is, medical ethics has to do not with certain rules about forbidden procedures, but with a healing process by which the dignity of every human person in all its dimensions is respected by the community and by which the sick person is restored to full life in community. Unethical behavior tends to exclude persons from the deepest sharing of communal life centered in the Trinity. Ethical behavior fosters this communion. This ethical vision with its perception of the true scale of values is summed up and expressed in the sacraments, especially in the Eucharist. A Catholic health facility that really understands the healing character of the sacraments will have a perfect model for an ethical treatment of the patients. The sacraments represent for us how Jesus, in love, went about treating sick people.

What makes a Catholic hospital different from all other hospitals? Its vision of the sick is a eucharistic vision, carried out in all details of the treatment of the sick and the mission of the healing team.

8.6 CONCLUSION

The hospital originated in Western culture because of a desire to give spiritual care to dying people. At that time, spiritual care was the only type of care that could be given to people with fatal pathologies. As time progressed, and medical science achieved the power to heal people with serious illnesses, there was also a tendency to weaken the efforts of the spiritual ministry. Indeed, various studies and anecdotal evidence seem to indicate that physicians have a very difficult time meeting the needs of dying persons. Dying and death became experiences outside the pale of medical competence. While pastoral care people are competent to help the dying, the solution of compassionate care for such persons does not lie in separating pastoral care from medical care. Rather, physicians must be convinced of the need to minister to the dying in conjunction with the pastoral care staff.

In contemporary times, inducing death is often looked upon as a solution to human problems. In the care of people suffering from fatal pathologies, because of pain, deprivation, or a feeling of absurdity, some recommend suicide or assisted suicide as reasonable choices. But human problems are not solved through killing innocent people. Hence the added emphasis needed upon excellent pastoral care ministers in all health care facilities. Preparing persons for their passage into eternity is the last step of the healing process with which bioethics seeks to establish true guidelines. It is, as the title of a book by the late Pope John Paul II (1994) expressed it—and as he gave witness in his last illness and death—the "crossing of the threshold of hope."

GLOSSARY

Agape: Greek word for theological virtue of charity; the love of God and neighbor as oneself. The unselfish and benevolent concern for the spiritual well-being of another.

Autonomy, principle of: Prominent in principalist theory. The right to make moral decisions that affect oneself and are free from interference by others. From the Christian viewpoint, limits to autonomy arise because of personal responsibilities and needs of other people that must be considered in ethical decision making. (cf. Beauchamp and Childress 2001, 120ff.)

Axiology: The study of the nature, types, and criteria of values and value judgments. Clearly, some values are more important than others.

Basic needs: The innate goals or goods of human persons: to seek the good; to prolong life; to propagate future generations; to form communities, to know the truth. (cf. Aquinas, *Summa Theologiae I–II,* q. 94, a. 2)

Beneficence, principle of: In principalist theory, the obligation of the medical professional to provide medical benefits for the patient. May lead to conflict between judgment of health care professional and patient in regard to what is beneficial. (cf. Beauchamp and Childress 2001, 259ff.)

Bioethics: Application of ethics or morality to medicine and health care.

Biologism (sometimes called physicalism): The error of basing ethical decisions on the physical act, apart from the moral object of the act. Alleged by some as a fault of sexual ethics in the Catholic tradition. This misconception of Catholic ethics arises from a mistaken notion of the moral object.

Capitation: The payment of a per-member per-month rate to cover defined health care services for a defined population.

Cardinal virtues: Fundamental moral virtues upon which all other moral virtues depend: justice, fortitude, temperance, and prudence. (cf. Aquinas, *Summa Theologiae* II-II)

Cartesian: Relating to the philosophy of René Descartes (1596–1650). A philosophy that separated the mind from the body as different substances and that stated there are clear and distinct innate ideas. Main principle: *I think, therefore I am.*

Casuistry: A method or theory of ethical decision making that relies upon similar and more obvious cases to reach ethical conclusions. Sometimes used pejoratively to indicate that an ethical conclusion lacks foundation in moral principles. (cf. Rich 1995)

Categorical imperative: Immanuel Kant's moral theory; provides no concrete moral guidance for moral action except that for an act to be good it must have the form of "categorical imperative," namely, that we act toward others as we would want them to act toward us.

Certitude, physical and moral: Physical certitude relates to matters of fact, especially in science. Moral certitude is the certitude needed to act in moral or ethical matters. Scientific certitude is not possible in ethical or moral decisions, because circumstances, which are variable, as well as general principles, must be taken into consideration. Moral certitude derived from what happens in most cases, *ut in pluribus.* (cf. *Summa Theologiae I–II,* q. 96, a. 1 ad. 3)

Circumstances of a moral act: Who, what, where, with what aids, how, when, why, and so forth can make a moral act better or worse. Circumstance "why" is the internal or subjective intention of the moral act; part of the total moral object; the *finis operantis* of the moral act. "Consequences, circumstances or intention can never transform an act intrinsically evil by virtue of its object into an act subjectively good." (cf. John Paul II 1993, no. 81)

Conscience: A judgment of reason whereby the human person recognizes the moral quality of a concrete act that he is going to perform, is in the process of performing, or has already completed. (CCC 2000, no. 1778)

Continence: In classical ethics, the firm will to maintain rational control over the pleasure from sexual activity. The disposition for chastity, which is a virtue controlling sexual desires. In medical terminology, voluntary control over urinary and fecal discharge.

Delayed hominization: Theory concerning moment of conception that maintains that human life does not begin when sperm and ovum fuse, but later on in the process of generation. Proved false by modern embryology. (see John Paul II 1995, no. 60)

Deontology: Ethical theory that emphasizes obedience to rule and precepts as opposed to the teleology of human actions.

Deposit of the faith: The heritage of faith contained in sacred scripture and tradition upon which the magisterium draws when it propose some truth as revealed by God. (cf. CCC 2000, glossary)

Development of doctrine: Growth in the understanding of God's revelation, which continues through the contemplation and study of believers, theological research, and the preaching of the magisterium. "Yet even if Revelation is already complete, it has not been made completely explicit, it remains for Christians to grasp its full significance over the course of the Centuries." (cf. CCC 2000, no. 66)

Ecumenism: Promotion of the restoration of unity among all Christians and among all Christian churches. (cf. *Decree on Ecumenism*, Vatican Council II 1964)

Eschatology: The theology of the end of history. Concerns final events in the history of the world and the Second Coming of Christ as revealed by God.

Ethical and Religious Directives **(ERD):** A body of moral principles and practical norms that are legislated by the bishops of the United States for health care facilities under their jurisdiction. The latest edition was issued in 2001.

Fee-for-service: Payment of provider for individual services rendered as opposed to payment with fixed salary for health care professional, or capitation.

Finis operantis: Of a moral action, Latin for "the goal or end (motive) of the agent." "Why" the action was performed. Accurately referred to as the motive of a human act but sometimes called the intention of the moral act. A circumstance of the moral object that receives special prominence in overall evaluation of the moral act but does not supplant the moral object (finis operis). (cf. Aquinas, *Summa Theological I–II*, q. 18, a. 6; cf. **Total moral object**)

Finis operis: Of a moral action, Latin for "the goal or end [purpose] of the work." "What" the human act effects in the moral order. Often referred to as the intention or purpose of a human act (cf. Aquinas, *Summa Theologiae I–II*, q. 18, a. 6), "the primary and decisive element for moral judgement." (see John Paul II 1993, no. 79; cf. **Total moral object**)

Formalism: See Kant's categorical imperative.

Fortitude: Courage; the cardinal virtue that controls the aggressive and endurance drive natural to human persons as embodied beings. Acquired through practice and grace.

Fundamental option: A person's deliberate commitment to a life goal.

Genotype and phenotype: The genotype of an organism is its genome at conception; the phenotype is the mature condition of the organism in which the information contained in the genome has been implemented.

Grace: "The free and undeserved gift that God gives us to respond to our vocation to become his adopted children. As *sanctifying grace*, God shares his divine life and friendship with us in a habitual gift. As *actual grace* God gives us the help to conform our actions to his will." (see CCC 2000, glossary, 881)

Hippocratic oath: A statement of fundamental ethical principles governing the practice of medicine. Original statement attributed to Hippocrates, the father of medicine (BCE 460–377). The core of the oath is to do what is best for the patient. The wording of the oath has been changed through the centuries. (cf. Rich 1995)

Humanism: A philosophical perspective that values and concentrates on secular concerns. Often divided into secular humanism, which features an agnostic or atheistic viewpoint of human life, and Christian humanism, which realizes the need to strive for social and economic well-being but retains belief in an afterlife and dependence upon God. (cf. American Humanist Association, 1933, 1973, 1999)

Incommensurable goods: A moral value that is both an end in itself and not subordinated to any higher good.

Joint ventures: Efforts of Catholic health care facilities to join with other health care facilities, whether Catholic or non-Catholic, in providing health care. Often results in a corporation, some of which have been approved by the Vatican as juridical persons in the Church. (cf. ERD 2001, section 6)

Juridical or juridic person: Distinct from a natural person or material goods, constituted by competent ecclesiastical authority for an apostolic purpose for continuous existence and with canonical rights and duties. Public juridic persons act in the name of the Church. The private juridic person acts in its own name. (cf. CIC 1983 [2000], cc. 113–23)

Justice: A cardinal moral virtue that consists in a constant and firm will to give their due to God and neighbor. *Commutative justice* respects the rights of other persons; *distributive justice* establishes fairness and equity in the community in regard to citizens; *legal justice* concerns the acts of citizens in regard to the community; *social justice* respects the rights that flow from human dignity. (cf. CCC 2000, 899)

Last rites: Sacraments given to dying patients; usually consists of sacraments of reconciliation, Eucharist, and anointing of the sick.

Legalism: An ethics based on the will and commands of a legislator, usually expressed in laws, rather than based on the needs of the human person.

Magisterium: The teaching authority of the Catholic Church whose task it is to interpret authentically the word of God and sacred tradition. Exercised by the Holy Father, by Ecumenical Councils acting in unity with the Holy Father, and by individual bishops when acting in unity with the Holy Father. (cf. CCC 2000, nos. 888–96) This teaching has four degrees: (1) infallible definitions concerning faith and morals that a truth pertains to the deposit of faith, (2) defined truths concerning faith and morals strictly connected to revelation, (3) nondefinitive teaching calling for religious submission of will and intellect, and (4) prudential interventions to protect the faith, sometimes involving conjectural or conditional elements that may in time require revision. (cf. CDF 1990)

Managed care: Contracting with health care providers to deliver health care services on a capitated basis. Several different methods, all designed to reduce health care costs.

Middle principles: Proximate moral principles, derived from fundamental moral principles, which are used to evaluate the morality of individual human acts; e.g., fundamental moral principle: love your neighbor; middle principle: do not spread scandal concerning your acquaintances. Middle principles are utilized frequently in contemporary American bioethics, often without clear reference to fundamental principles.

Ministry: The service or work of sanctification performed by the preaching of the word, the celebration of the sacraments, and striving for social justice. There are several ministries mentioned in the New Testament; Christ himself is the source of ministry in the Church. (cf. CCC 2000, 893–903)

Moral object (see also **Total moral object** and **Finis operis**): What a human act accomplishes in the moral order. Considers the physical effects of the act, but also the effects in relation to God, oneself, and other people. "The human act depends upon its object, whether that object is capable or not of being ordered to God. . . . An act is therefore good if its object is in conformity with the good of the person with respect to the goods morally relevant for him." (see John Paul II 1993, no. 78)

Mosaic law (Torah, literally, instruction): The first five books of the Hebrew scriptures often attributed to the prophet Moses. Also used more comprehensively for the entire Jewish Bible (the Old Testament), and even more broadly for other sacred literature and oral tradition (Talmud and Mishnah).

Natural law: The requirements of true human happiness achieved through an ordered satisfaction of the *innate (basic) needs* of the human person as known from human reason. Its precepts are primary, known to all; secondary, commonly known to all but often obscured by culture or education; and tertiary, known only to the educated. (cf. *Summa Theologiae I–II*, q. 94)

Natural family planning: Modern methods of controlling reproduction by abstaining from intercourse during a woman's fertile periods of menstrual cycle. Ethically justified by other moral responsibilities of the couple.

Nominalism: A philosophical theory that holds there are no universal essences in reality and that the mind cannot form universal concepts. Influential in counteracting Scholasticism.

Nonmalfeasance, principle of: From the Hippocratic oath, "first of all, do no harm." Also utilized in *principlism* method of doing bioethics. (cf. Beauchamp and Childress 2001)

Objective morality, subjective morality: Objective morality evaluates the morality of an external act; subjective morality evaluates a moral act from the perspective of the knowledge and motivation of the person acting. Most often they coincide, but possible for opposition between the two. (cf. John Paul II 1995, nos. 18, 82; 1993, n. 79ff)

Organism: A living being with multiple interdependent parts that function in accord with the good of the whole.

Original sin: The sin by which the first human beings disobeyed the commandments of God, choosing to follow their own will rather than God's will. (cf. CCC 2000, glossary, 891)

Pastoral care: The ministry offered primarily to foster spiritual well-being. "Pastoral care is an integral part of Catholic health care and encompasses a listening presence, help in dealing with powerlessness and pain and assistance in responding to God's will with greater joy and peace." (see ERD 2001, 12)

Placebo: A medication or innocuous substance used in controlled experiments testing the efficacy of another substance. Use of placebo may result in *placebo effect*: the improvement of a patient that cannot be considered due to the substance or treatment used.

Pluriformalism: A revision of classical ethics in which a supreme good of contemplation is replaced by several incommensurable goods. (cf. Grisez et al., 1987, 115–33)

Point of service: A managed care plan that allows subscribers to choose providers or specialists within the plan's network as referred by their primary care physician or to self-refer to a provider outside the network. Out-of-network services are reimbursed at a reduced rate.

Postmodernism: A theory or attitude that emphasizes the ambiguity of all human communication and argues that all claims of truth involve circular reasoning.

Principlism: An ethical method, common today in secular bioethics, and of Kantian origin, that is based on three or four middle principles of autonomy, nonmalfeasance, beneficence, and justice for all concerned.(cf. Beauchamp and Childress 1995,100–109)

Proportionalism: An ethical theory based on a principle of proportion that holds every concrete moral norm has exceptions because the circumstances or intention of the acting agent can outweigh the value of the moral object. Rejected by Pope John Paul II in the encyclical *Veritatis splendor* (1993, no. 79ff).

Prudence: The highest moral virtue; skill in judging the means to achieving the goal of individual human acts and to the ultimate end of human life; considers alternative means, concrete circumstances, and future consequences.

Prudential personalism: A teleological ethics, developed by Thomas Aquinas, in which moral judgments in concrete circumstances are governed by a hierarchy of natural needs of the human person that contribute to the final goal of happiness. (cf. **Natural law** and **Total moral object**)

Rigorism: The tendency to judge moral matters in a rigid manner, abstracting from the circumstances of the person acting. Opposed to probabilism, which allows one to follow a reasonable moral opinion, even though it is not as thoroughly proven as a rigorous opinion.

Romanticism: The judgment of moral and esthetic values on a nonrational, subjective, and emotional basis in contrast to objective facts.

Sacrament: An efficacious sign of grace, instituted by Christ and entrusted to the Church, by which divine life is dispensed to us through the work of the Holy Spirit. (cf. CCC 2000, glossary, 898)

Secular bioethics: Theory of bioethics that is founded upon materialistic or agnostic philosophy and does not base moral considerations upon responsibility to God.

Sensus fidelium (sense of faith): Not popular opinion but the witness of faithful Catholics to the truth of sacred scripture and sacred tradition. "The people unfailingly adhere to the faith, penetrate it more deeply with right judgment, and apply it more fully in daily life." (see Vatican Council II 1964, no. 12)

Sin: An offense against God as well as a fault against reason, truth, and right conscience. A failure in genuine love of God or neighbor caused by a perverse attachment to another good. A thought, word, or deed contrary to the law of God. In judging the gravity of a sin, it is customary to distinguish between serious and light sin (mortal and venial.) Mortal sin results in a loss of charity and the state of grace; venial sin weakens charity and manifests a disordered affection for created goods. (cf. CCC 2000, nos. 1849–53)

Situation ethics: A moral theory that denies the relevance of universal or general principles or conclusions because each moral judgment is different and circumstances are never repeated. Prominent proponents: Joseph Fletcher, Jean Paul Sartre.

Solidarity, principle of: Based on the equal dignity of human persons. Requires the effort to reduce social and economic inequalities. A direct demand of human and Christian charity. (cf. CCC 2000, nos. 1939–42)

Spirituality: An effort to live in friendship with God, in faith, hope, and love. Many and varied spiritualities, emphasizing various activities or principles, have been developed throughout the history of the church.

Sponsor: An entity that is a public juridic person and carries on an apostolate in the name of the Church, e.g., religious congregations or corporations formed of health care institutions.

Subsidiarity, principle of: A moral principle that fosters personal freedom and initiative within a larger social complex. "A community of a higher order should not interfere in the internal life of a community of a lower order depriving the latter of its functions but rather should support it by helping to coordinate its activities with the common good." (Pius XI 1930)

Teleological ethics: Ethical theories that judge morality by whether or not it chooses effective or counterproductive means to the goals of true human happiness.

Total moral object: The complex of elements that compose the human act considered as a unit; i.e., the moral object or *finis operis,* "What" is accomplished in the moral order; the motive, or *finis operantis,* "Why" the human act is performed; and the other circumstances that surround the moral object, e.g., who, when, what assistance, etc.

Voluntarism (deontology): Ethical theories that judge morality only on the basis of the will of the legislator without inquiring as to the teleological purpose of the law.

REFERENCES

Abrams, Richard. 1988. *Electroconvulsive therapy*. Oxford: Oxford University Press.

Aday, Luann. 1993. *At risk in America: The health and health care needs of vulnerable populations in the United States*. San Francisco: Jossey-Bass.

Adelman, Ken. 2000. Changing who we are: Gene therapy could free us from certain diseases even make us taller, stronger, smarter. But are scientists playing with fire? *Washingtonian* 35 (August): 25–28.

Adler, Mortimer. 1993. *Four dimensions of philosophy*. New York: Macmillan Press.

Aertnys, Joseph, and Charles Damen. 1947. *Theologiae moralis*. Vol. 1, no. 398. Rome: Marietti.

Agras, W. Stewart, and Robert Berkowitz. 1988. Behavior therapy. In *Textbook of psychiatry*, ed. John Talbott, Robert Hales, and Stuart Yudofsky, 891–905. Washington, DC: American Psychiatric Press.

AHA (American Hospital Association). 1986. *Cost and compassion*. Chicago: American Hospital Association Press.

Ahmann, John. 2001. Therapeutic cloning and stem cell therapy. *National Catholic Bioethics Quarterly* 1 (Summer): 149.

Alberta Consultative Health Association Network. 2003. Informed consent. www.achrn.org/informed_consent.htm

Al Khayat, M. H. 1995. *Health and Islamic behavior*. In *Health policy, ethics and human values: Islamic perspective*, ed. A. R. El Gindy, 447–50. Kuwait: Islamic Organization of Medical Sciences.

Allen, J. Timothy. 2002. *A theology of God-talk: The language of the heart*. New York: Haworth Press.

AMA (American Medical Association). 1996. New bioethics panel to study genetics research subjects. *AMA News* (June 1996): 10.

———. 2000. Attitudes and desires related to euthanasia and physician assisted suicide among terminally ill patients and their caregivers. *JAMA* 284 (19): 36.

———. 2001. *Principles of medical ethics*. www.ama-assn.org/ama/pub/category/2512.html

AMA Council on Ethical and Judicial Affairs. 1994. HIV infected patients and physicians (9:131); Withholding and withdrawing life sustaining medical treatment (2:20). *Code of medical ethics.* Chicago: American Medical Association.

American Association on Mental Retardation. 2004. www.catholic.net/RCC/Issues/Contraception/contraception.html

American Humanist Association. 1933. *Humanist manifesto I.* New York: American Humanist Association. www.americanhumanist.org/about/manifesto1.php

———. 1973. *Humanist manifesto II.* New York: American Humanist Association. www.americanhumanist.org/about/manifesto2.php

———. 1999. *Humanism and its aspirations.* New York: American Humanist Association. www.americanhumanist.org/3/HumandItsAspirations.php

American Society for Reproductive Medicine. 1999. Sex selection and preimplantation genetic diagnosis. *Fertility and Sterility* 72:595–98.

Anderson, Ray Sherman. 2003. *Spiritual caregiving as secular sacrament: A practical theology for professional caregivers.* London: J. Kingsley.

Annandale, Ellen, and Kate Hunt. 2000. *Gender inequalities in health.* Buckingham: Open University Press.

Annas, George. 1989. *The rights of patients: The basic ACLU guide to patient rights.* 2nd ed. Carbondale: Southern Illinois University Press.

———. 1998. The patients' bill of rights. *New England Journal of Medicine* 338 (10): 695–702.

———. 2002. Medical privacy and medical research: Judging the new federal regulations. *New England Journal of Medicine* 346 (3): 216–20.

APA (American Psychiatric Association). 1973. *Diagnostic and statistical manual of mental disorders (DSM).* Washington, DC: APA.

———. 1981. *Principles of medical ethics with annotations especially applicable to psychiatry.* Washington, DC: APA.

———. 1985. *Task force, seclusion and restraint: The psychiatric uses.* Washington, DC: APA.

———. 1986a. Sexual involvement between psychiatrists, their students, supervisors, colleagues, and employees. *Ethics Newsletter* 2:2.

———. 1986b. Unethical behavior, incompetency, and impairment in the ethical decision process. *Ethics Newsletter* 2:1.

———. 1994. *Diagnostic and statistical manual of mental disorders.* 4th ed. (*DSM-IV*). Washington, DC: APA.

———. 2000. Diagnostic criteria for Attention Deficit/Hyperactivity Disorder. In *Diagnostic and Statistical Manual of Mental Disorders,* 4th ed., 92–93. Washington, DC: APA.

———. 2002. Fact sheet on homosexuality. www.thebody.com/apa/apafacts.html

Aquinas, St. Thomas. 1920. Summa Theologiae I–II. *The summa theologica of St. Thomas Aquinas.* www.newadvent.org/summa.

———. 1976. *Summa Theologiae.* Ed. Thomas Gilby. New York: McGraw-Hill.

———. 2002. *Summa Theologiae* Ia, 75–89. *The treatise of human nature.* Trans. Robert Pasnau. Cambridge, MA: Hackett.

Arévale, M., V. Jennings, and I. Sinai. 2002. Efficacy of a new method of family planning: The standard days method. *Contraception* 65: 333–38.

Arias, Brent. 2004. *Birth control.* http://panoply.home.att.net/abc.htm

Arkes, Brent. 1990. On delayed hominization: Some thoughts on the blending of new science and ancient fallacies. In *The interaction of Catholic bioethics and secular society,* ed. R. E. Smith, 27–38. Braintree, MA: Pope John Center.

Armstrong, Dave. 2005. The Stephanos project: Does orthodoxy allow contraception or not? http://ic.net/~erasmus/RAZ162.HTM

Arnstein, Robert. 1986. Divided loyalties in adolescent psychiatry: Late adolescence. *Social Science and Medicine* 23 (8): 797–802.

Arraj, James. 1989. Is there a solution to the Catholic debate on contraception? www.innerexplorations.com/catchtheomor/is.htm

Arraj, James, and Tyra Arraj. 1984. *St. John of the Cross and Dr. C. G. Jung*. Chiloquin, OR: Tools for Inner Growth.

Ascension Health. 2006. *Environmental and horizon scan: A summary of key market forces, emerging trends and long range projections in healthcare*. St. Louis, MO: Ascension Health.

Ashley, Benedict M. 1972. A psychological model with a spiritual dimension. *Pastoral Psychology* (May): 31–40.

———. 1985a. Theology and the mind–body problem. In *Mind and brain*. St. Louis: Institute for the Theological Encounter with Science and Technology.

———. 1985b. *Theologies of the body*. Braintree, MA: Pope John Center.

———. 1990. Contemporary understandings of personhood. In *The twenty-fifth anniversary of Vatican II: A look back and a look forward, proceedings of the ninth bishops' workshop, Dallas, Texas*, ed. Russell E. Smith, 35–48. Braintree, MA: Pope John Center.

———. 1992. Dominion or stewardship. In *Birth, suffering and death: Catholic perspectives at the edge of life*, ed. Kevin M. Wildes, Franceso Abel, and John C. Harvey, 85–106. Dordrecht: Kluwer Academic.

———. 1995. *Spiritual direction in the Dominican tradition*. New York: Paulist Press.

———. 1996a. *Living the truth in love: A Biblical introduction to moral theology*. Staten Island, NY: Alba House.

———. 1996b. *Theologies of the body: Humanist and Christian*. 2nd ed. Boston: National Catholic Bioethics Center.

———. 1998. What is a human person? *NaPro Ethics* 3 (July): 4–5.

———. 2000a. Asceticism: Christian perspectives. Self-mutilation. *The Encyclopedia of Monasticism*. New York: Fitzroy Dearborn.

———. 2000b. *Choosing a worldview and value system: An ecumenical apologetics*. Staten Island, NY: Alba House.

———. 2000c. Spirituality and counseling, ed. Robert J. Wicks, 656–70. *Handbook of spirituality for ministers*. Vol. 2 of *Perspectives for the 21st Century*. New York: Paulist.

———. 2000d. *Theologies of the body: Humanist and Christian*. 3rd ed. Boston: National Catholic Bioethics Center. (Originally published 1985.)

Ashley, Benedict M., and Albert Moraczewski. 2001. Cloning, Aquinas, and the embryonic person. *The National Catholic Bioethics Quarterly* 1 (2): 189–202.

Ashley, Benedict, and Kevin O'Rourke. 1997. *Health care ethics*. 4th ed. Washington, DC: Georgetown University Press.

Atkinson, Gary M., and Albert S. Moraczewski. 1980. *Genetic counseling: The church and the law*. St. Louis: Pope John XXIII Medical-Moral Research and Education Center.

Austriaco, Nicanor P. G. 2002. On static eggs and dynamic embryos: A systems perspective. *National Catholic Bioethics Quarterly* 2 (4): 659–83.

———. 2004. Immediate hominization, from the systems perspective. *National Catholic Bioethics Quarterly* 4 (4): 719–38.

Baehr, Ninia. 1990. *Abortion without apology: A radical history for the 1990s*. Cambridge, MA: South End Press.

Baird, Robert D. 1971. *Category formation and the history of religions*. The Hague: Mouton.

Bakken, Kenneth. 1975. *The call to wholeness: Health as a spiritual journey*. New York: Crossroad.

Bandura, A. 1986. *Social foundation of thought and action*. Englewood Cliffs, NJ: Prentice Hall.

Barber, Bernard, Daniel Sullivan, John J. Lally, and Julia L. Makarushka. 1973. *Research on human subjects: Problems of social control in medical experimentation.* New York: Russell Sage Foundation.

Barna Research Group. 2004. Christians more likely to experience divorce than non-Christians. www.Barna.org

Barnhill, M. 1989. The rise and fall of the IUD. *Journal of Gynecological Health* 3 (May–June): 3, 6–10.

Barr, Paul. 2005. Blessings from above. *Modern Healthcare* 16 (April): 6–7.

Bartoli, Elenor. 2003. Psychoanalytic practice and the religious patient. *Bulletin of the Menninger Clinic* 67:4.

Battista, John R., and Justin McCabe. 2005. The case for single prayer, universal health care for the United States. http://cthealth.server101.com/the_case_for_universal_health_care_in_the_united_states.htm

Bayer, Edward. 1985. *Rape within marriage: A moral analysis delayed.* Lanham, MD: University Press of America.

Bayer, Ronald. 1987. *Homosexuality and American psychiatry: The politics of diagnosis.* Princeton, NJ: Princeton University Press.

Beauchamp, Tom L., and James F. Childress. 2001. *Principles of biomedical ethics.* 5th ed. New York: Oxford University Press.

Beck, Aaron T. 2004. Home page. http://mail.med.upenn.edu/~abeck

Beck, John, and Michael Young. 2005. The assault on the professions and academic and professional identities. *British Journal of Sociology of Education* 26:2.

Becker, Ernest. 1973. *The denial of death.* New York: Free Press.

Becker, Howard. 1960. The nature of profession. In *Education for the professions,* ed. Nelson B. Henry, 27–46. Chicago: University of Chicago Press.

Beckwith, Francis J. 1993. *Politically correct death: Answering the arguments for abortion rights.* Grand Rapids, MI: Baker.

———. 2004. The explanatory power of the substance view of persons. *Christian Bioethics* 10: 33–54. http://homepage.mac.com/francis.beckwith/ChristianBioethics.pdf

Bedate, C. A., and R. C. Cefalo. 1989. The zygote: To be or not to be a person. *Journal of Medicine and Philosophy* 14:641–45.

Beitman, Bernard D., and Gerald L. Klerman, eds. 1991. *Integrating pharmacotherapy and psychotherapy.* Arlington, VA: American Psychiatric Association.

Bellah, Robert M. 1986. *Habits of the heart: Individualism and commitment in American life.* Berkeley: University of California Press.

———. 1991. *The good society.* New York: Random House.

Belmont Report. 1978. *The Belmont report: Ethical principles and guidelines for the protection of human subjects of research.* The National Commission for the Protection of Human Subjects of Biomedical and Behavioral Research. Bethesda, MD: U.S. Government Printing Office.

Benedict XVI, Homily for the funeral mass of Pope John Paul II. *Origins* (April 21, 2005): 34, 44, 705–7.

Bennet, Michael. 2001. *The emphatic healer: An endangered species?* San Diego, CA: Academic Press.

Bennett, Belinda. 2001. Prenatal diagnosis, genetics and reproductive decision-making. *Journal of Law and Medicine* 9 (August): 28–40.

Berg, Thomas. 2005. Seeking an ethical option to embryonic stem cell research. Interview, Zenit News Agency, June 13. http://www.catholiceducation.org/articles/medical_ethics/me0082.html

Bernadine, Joseph, Cardinal. 1995. *Signs of hope IV.* St. Louis: Catholic Health Association.

Bernat, James L. 2001. Philosophical and ethical aspects of brain death. In *Brain death,* ed. Eelco F. M. Wijdicks, 13. Philadelphia: Lippincott, Williams and Wilkins.

Beurton, Peter J., Raphael Falk, and Hans-Jorg Rheinberger, eds. 2000. *The concept of the gene in development and evolution: Historical and epistemological perspectives*. New York: Cambridge University Press.

Bezchlibnyk-Butler, Kalyna Z., and J. Joel Jeffries. 2003. *Clinical handbook of psychotropic drugs*. 3rd ed. Cambridge, MA: Hogrefe and Huber.

Bicknell, G. R., S. T. Williams, J. A. Shaw, J. H. Pringle, P. N. Furness, and M. L. Nicholson. 2000. Differential effects of cyclosporin. *British Journal of Surgery* 87:1569–75.

Bidwell, Duane R. 2004. *Short-term spiritual guidance*. Minneapolis, MN: Fortress Press.

Billings, Evelyn L. 2003. Natural family planning and conjugal relationship. www.lifeissues.net/ writers/bil/bil_10mrsconjugalrelation1.html

Birch, Bruce C. 1991. *Let justice roll on down: The Old Testament, ethics and Christian life*. Louisville, KY: Westminster/John Knox.

Bissell, LeClair, and James Royce. 1987. *Ethics for addiction professionals*. Center City, MN: Hazelden Foundation.

Black, Peter, and Thomas Szasz. 1977. The ethics of psychosurgery: Pro and con. *The Humanist* 37:6–11.

Blackless, Melanie, Anthony Charuvastra, Amanda Derryck, Anne Fausto-Sterling, Karl Lauzanne, and Ellen Lee. 2000. How sexually dimorphic are we? Review and synthesis. *American Journal of Human Biology* 12:151–66.

Blankenhorn, David, and Don S. Browning. 2004. *Does Christianity teach male headship? The equal-regard marriage and its critics*. Grand Rapids, MI: Eerdmans.

Block, Sidney, Paul Chodoff, and Stephen Green, eds. 1999. *Psychiatric ethics*. New York: Oxford University Press. (Originally published 1981.)

Bloom, Alan. 1987. *The closing of the American mind: Education and the crisis of reason*. New York: Simon and Schuster.

Blum, Henrik L. 1983. *Expanding health care horizons: From general systems concept of health care to a national policy*. Oakland, CA: Third Party Publications.

Bockting, Walter, and Eli Coleman. 1993. *Gender dysphoria: Interdisciplinary approaches in clinical management*. Binghamton, NY: Haworth Press.

Bodlung, O., et al. 1993. Personality traits and disorders among transsexuals. *Acta Psychiatrica Scandinavia* 88 (November): 322–27.

Boeree, George. 2004. Personality theories: Introduction www.ship.edu/%7Ecgboeree/ persintro.html

Boff, Leonardo. 1987. *Introducing liberation theology*, Trans. Paul Burns. Maryknoll, NY: Orbis.

———. 1992. *Faith on the edge: Religion and marginalized existence*. Trans. Barr. Maryknoll, New York: Orbis Books.

Bole, Thomas. 1992. The licitness of inducing the non-viable anencephalic fetus. *HCE Forum* 4 (2): 121–33.

Boonin, D. 2002. *A defense of abortion*. New York: Cambridge University Press.

Booth, J. V., D. Grossman, J. Moore, C. Lineberger, J. D. Reynolds, J. G. Reves, and D. Sheffield. 2002. Substance abuse among physicians: A survey of academic anesthesiology programs. *Anesthesia & Analgesia* 95 (4): 1024–30.

Boros, Ladislaus. 1965. *The mystery of death*. New York: Herder and Herder.

Bouwsma, William J. 1988. *John Calvin: A sixteenth century portrait*. New York: Oxford University Press.

Bowman, Marcus. 2000. *The significance of psychoanalysis in modern thought*. London: British Psychoanalytical Society.

Boyd, K. 1992. HIV infection and AIDS: The ethics of medical confidentiality. *Journal of Medical Ethics* 18 (4): 173–79.

Boyle, Mary. 2002. *Schizophrenia: A scientific delusion*. 2nd ed. London: Routledge.

Boyle, Philip, and Kevin O'Rourke. 1986. Presumed consent for organ donation. *America* 155 (November 22): 326–32.

Braine, David. 1992. *The human person: Animal and spirit*. Notre Dame, IN: University of Notre Dame Press.

Breedlove, Marc. 2005. The chicken-and-egg argument as it applies to the brains of transsexuals: Does it matter? www.genderpsychology.org/psychology/BSTc.html

Breggin, Peter. 1972. New information in the debate over psychosurgery. *Congressional Record* (March 30): E3380–86.

———. 1979. *Electroshock: Its brain-disabling effects*. New York: Springer.

Brennan, Carl. 1994. Restoring intimacy to the physician-patient relationship. *Health Progress* 72 (2): 79–80.

Brennan, William. 1995. *Dehumanizing the vulnerable: When word games take lives*. Chicago: Loyola University Press.

Brint, Steven. 1994. *In an age of exgens: The changing role of the professional in politics and public life*. Princeton, NJ: Princeton University Press.

Brock, Dan. 1997. Death and dying. In *Medical ethics*, 2nd ed., ed. Robert Veatch. Boston: Jones & Bartlett.

———. 2001. Panel says ethics allows compensation for organ donations. *Los Angeles Times*, December 4.

Brodeur, Dennis. 1984. Toward a clear definition of ethics committees. *Linacre Quarterly* 51(3): 233–47.

Brody, Baruch A. 2002. Freedom and responsibility in genetic testing. In *Bioethics*, ed. Ellen Frankel Paul, Fred D. Miller, and Jeffrey Paul, 343–88. New York: Cambridge University Press.

Brody, Baruch, and Tristam H. Engelhardt Jr., eds. 1980. Mental illness: Law and public policy. In *Philosophy and medicine*. Vol. 5. Boston: Reidel.

Brody, Howard. 1981. *Ethical decisions in medicine*. 2nd ed. Boston: Little, Brown.

Browning, Don. 1973. *Generative man: Psychoanalytic perspectives*. Philadelphia: Westminster Press.

Browning, Don S., and Terry D. Cooper. 2004. *Religious thought and the modern psychologies*. 2nd ed. Minneapolis, MN: Augsburg Fortress.

Brownlee, Shannon. 2002. Designer babies. *Washington Monthly* (March 1).

Brumbaugh, Richard. 2002. The Oregon Death with Dignity Act. *Saint Louis University Law Review* 21 (2): 377–94.

Bruskewitz, Fabian, Robert F. Vasa, Walt F. Weaver, Paul A. Byrne, Richard G. Nilges, and Joseph Seifert. 2001. Are organ transplants ever morally licit? *The Catholic World Report* 2 (March): 50—56.

Buratovich, Michael. 2003. The explanatory power of the substance view of persons: Personal email correspondence from Michael Buratovich to Francis J. Beckwith, June 12.

Burge, Frederick, P. McIntyre, D. Kaufman, I. Cummings, G. Frager, and A. Pollett. 2000. Family medicine residents' knowledge and attitudes about end-of-life care. *Journal of Palliative Care* 16 (Autumn): 8.

Burley, J. 1999. The ethics of therapeutic and reproductive cloning. *Cell and Developmental Biology* 10 (June): 287–94.

Byk, C. 1996. Living organ donation: European perspectives. In *Living organ donation in the nineties: European medico-legal perspectives*, ed. David Price and Hans Akveld, 53–62. Leicester, UK: EUROTOLD Project, University of Leicester, Leicester General Hospital.

Byock, Ira. 2003. Rediscovering community at the core of the human condition and social covenant. *Hastings Center Report* 33 (March–April): 33.

Byrne, Paul. 2005. Vatican organs. Reported by Carol Glatz. *Catholic News Service*, February 4.

Byrne, Paul, Sean O'Reilly, Paul M. Quay, and Peter W. Salsich. 2000. Brain death: The patient, the physician, and society. In *Beyond brain death: The case against brain based criteria for human death,* ed. Michael Potts, Paul A. Byrne, and Richard G. Nilges, 21–89. Boston: Kluwer Academic.

Callahan, Daniel. 1981. Arguing the morality of genetic engineering. In *Medical ethics and the law: Implications for public policy,* ed. Marc Hiller, 441–49. Cambridge, MA: Ballinger.

———. 1988. *Setting limits: Medical goals in an aging society.* New York: Simon and Schuster.

Callahan, Sydney. 1993. Ethical issues in professional life. *Health Progress* 74 (7): 42–43.

Campbell, Courtney. 1994. Gifts and caring duties in medicine. In *Duties to others,* ed. Courtney Campbell, S. Lutwig, and B. Andrew, 181–97. Boston: Kluwer Academic.

Camus, Albert. 1956. Preface. *The rebel.* New York: Vintage Books.

———. 1969. *The myth of Sisyphus and other essays.* New York: Knopf.

Canada Law Reform Commission. 1981. *Criteria for the determination of death.* Ottawa: The Commission.

Capizzi, Joseph E. 2003. The influence of bioethics on moral theology. *Josephinum Journal of Theology* 10 (2): 285–99.

Capps, Donald. 1990. *Reframing: A new method in pastoral care.* Minneapolis, MN: Fortress Press.

———. 1995. *Agents of hope: A pastoral psychology.* Minneapolis, MN: Fortress Augsburg Press.

Capron, Alexander M. 1984. Current issues in genetic screening. In *Biomedical ethics review,* ed. James Humber and Robert F. Almeder, 121–49. Clifton, NJ: Humana Press.

———. 1993. Duty, truth and whole human beings. *Hastings Center Report* 23 (4): 13–14.

Carey, Benedict. 2005. Inside the injured brain: Many kinds of awareness. *New York Times:* Science Times; Late edition final; sec. F; page 1, col. 3.

Carr, D. B., and L. C. Goudas. 1999. Acute pain. *The Lancet* 353 (June 12): 2053.

Carroll, Douglas, and Mark O'Callaghan. 1984. Regulating psychosurgery: Ethical, social, and scientific considerations. *Medicine and Law* 3 (2): 193–203.

Carson, Rachel. 1994. *Silent spring.* Boston: Houghton Mifflin. (Originally published 1962.)

Cassell, Eric. 1976. *The healer's art.* New York: Lippincott.

Cassem, Ned. 2003. Comments from the optimum care committee consultant. *Journal of Clinical Ethics* 14 (Fall): 199–200.

Cataldo, Peter J. 1995. The principle of the double effect. *Ethics & Medics* 20:1–3.

———. 1996. Reproductive technologies. *Ethics and Medics* 21 (January): 1–3.

———. 2004. Compliance with contraceptive insurance mandates: Licit or illicit cooperation in evil? *The National Catholic Bioethics Quarterly* 4 (Spring): 103–30.

Cataldo, Peter J., and A. Moraczewski. 2001. *A moral analysis of pregnancy prevention after sexual assault: A manual for ethics. Ethics committees in Catholic hospitals.* Boston: National Catholic Bioethics Center.

Catholic Answers. 2004. Library: *Contraception and sterilization.* www.catholic.com

Catholic Medical Association. 2004. Homosexuality and hope. www.catholiceducation.org/articles/homosexuality/ho0039.html

Catholic Pages Directory. 2004. www.catholic-pages.com/dir/papal.asp

CCBI (Canadian Catholic Bioethics Institute). 2004. Reflections on artificial nutrition and hydration. Colloquium of the Canadian Catholic Bioethics Institute. *NCBQ* 4 (Winter): 773–82.

CCC. 2000. *Catechism of the Catholic Church.* 2nd ed. Vatican City: Libreria Vaticana.

CDF (Congregation for the Doctrine of the Faith). 1963. Cremation. In *Canon Law Digest,* 6. Milwaukee, WI: Bruce Books.

———. 1974. Declaration on procured abortion. In Vatican Council II, *More Post Conciliar Documents,* Vol. 2, ed. A. Flannery, 476–82. Northport, NY: Costello 1982.

———. 1975. Statement on sterilization. *Commentary of National Conference on Catholic Bishops.* Washington, DC.

————. 1979. The reality of life after death. In Vatican Council II, *More Post Conciliar Documents*, Vol. 2, ed. A. Flannery. Northport, NY: Costello 1982.

————. 1980. Declaration on euthanasia. In Vatican Council II, *More Post Conciliar Documents*, Vol. 2, ed. A. Flannery. Northport, NY: Costello 1982.

————. 1984. Instruction on certain aspects of "The theology of liberation." *Libertatis Nuntius*, AAS 76, 867–77. Boston: St. Paul Editions.

————. 1986. *Instruction on Christian freedom and liberation*, AAS 79. Boston: St. Paul Editions.

————. 1987. Instruction on respect for human life. *Donum vitae. Origins* 40: 697–709.

————. 1989. The moral norms of *Humanae vitae* (February 16). *Origins* 18 (38): 110–12.

————. 1990. Instruction on the ecclesial vocation of the theologian. *Origins* 20 (8): 117–26.

————. 1998. Commentary on *Tuen duca fibem. Origins* 28 (8): 116–19.

————. 2004. On collaboration of men and women in church and world. *Origins* 34 (11): 169–76.

Center for Naturalism. 2005. *Spirituality*. www.naturalism.org/spirtua.html

Cessario, Romanus. 1997. Infallible teaching and the gift of divine truth. www.catholic.net/rcc/Periodicals/Dossier/2000–5-6/article.html

CHA (Catholic Health Association). 1994. Leaders for the new reality. In *Perspectives* 3. St. Louis: Catholic Health Association.

————. 2004. Persistent vegetative state and artificial nutrition and hydration: Questions and answers; resources for understanding the Pope's *Allocution on Persons in a Persistent Vegetative State*.

————. 2005. Statement of shared identity. www.chausa.org

Chalmers, David J. 1996. *The conscious mind: In search of a fundamental theory*. Oxford: Oxford University Press.

Chassin, Mark, and Glavin, Robert. 1998. The urgent need to improve health care quality. *JAMA* 280:1000–1005.

Cherry, Mark J. 2000. Body parts and the market place: Insights from Thomistic philosophy. *Christian Bioethics* 6 (August): 171–93.

Cholbi, Michael. 2004. Suicide. *The Stanford encyclopedia of philosophy*, ed. Edward N. Zalta. http://plato.stanford.edu/entries/suicide/

Chollet, Deborah. 2005. Insuring the uninsured: Finding the road to success. *Frontiers of Health Services Management* 21 (4): 17–28.

Church of England, Board of Social Responsibility. 1975. *On dying well: An Anglican contribution to the debate on euthanasia*. London: Church Information Service.

Ciarrocchi, Joseph W. 1993. *A minister's handbook of mental disorders*. New York: Paulist Press.

————. 1995. *The doubting disease, help for scrupulosity and religious compulsions*. New York: Paulist Press.

CIC (Code of Canon Law). 2000. Latin–English ed. Commentary. Canon Law Society of America. Ed. John Beal, James Coriden, Thomas Green. Mahwah, NJ: Paulist Press.

Claire, Miriam. 1995. *The abortion dilemma: Personal views on a public issue*. New York: Insight Books.

Clark, Henry. 1987. *Altering behavior: The ethics of controlled experience*. Newbury Park, CA: Sage.

Cleary, John. 1999. The secularity of religion. *The religion report*, June 6. www.abc.net.au/rn/talks/8.30/relrpt/stories/s27641.htm

Clements, Colleen. 1983. Common psychiatric problems and uncommon ethical solutions. *Psychiatric Annals* 13 (April): 289–301.

Clinebell, Howard. 1995. *Counseling for spiritually empowered wholeness: A hope-centered approach*. Binghamton, NY: Haworth Press.

Coberly, Margaret. 2003. *Sacred passage: How to provide fearless, compassionate care for the dying*. Boston: Shambhala.

Cohen-Almagor, Raphael. 2001. *The right to die with dignity: An argument in ethics, medicine, and law*. New Brunswick, NJ: Rutgers University Press.

Cohen-Kettemis, P. T., and L. J. Gooren. 1999. Transsexualism: A review of etiology, diagnosis and treatment. *Journal of Psychosoma Research* 46 (April): 315–33.

Cole-Turner, Ronald. 2000. Genes and Genesis: Religion and genetic testing. *Park Ridge Center Bulletin* 13 (January–February): 5–7.

Collinge, William. 1996. *The American holistic health association complete guide to alternative medicine*. New York: Warner Books.

Cone, James H. 2000. *The risks of faith: The emergence of a black theology of liberation, 1968–1988*. Boston: Beacon Press.

Conn, Walter E. 1998. *The desiring self: Rooting pastoral counseling and spiritual direction in self-transcendence*. New York: Paulist Press.

Connor, Paul. 2002. The indignity of human cloning. *National Catholics Bioethics Quarterly* 2 (Winter): 635–58.

Connors, Russell, and Patrick McCormick. 1998. *Character, choices, and community*. New York: Paulist Press.

Connery, John. 1977. *Abortion: The development of the Roman Catholic perspective*. Chicago: Loyola University Press.

———. 1980. Prolonging life: The duty and its limits. *Catholic Mind* (October 11): 43–57.

———. 1981. Catholic ethics: Has the norm for rule making changed? *Theological Studies* 42:232–50.

———. 1986. The ethical standards for withholding and withdrawing nutrition and hydration. *Issues in Law and Medicine* 2 (September): 89.

Conrad, Peter, and Rochelle Kern, eds. 1981. *The sociology of health and illness*. New York: St. Martin's Press.

Conway, Pierre. 1960. *Principles of education*. Washington, DC: Thomist Press.

Cooper, David, and Robert P. Lanza. 2000. *Xeno: The promise of transplanting animal organs into humans*. New York: Oxford University Press.

Corr, Charles A., Clyde M. Nabe, and Donna M. Corr. 2000. *Death and dying, life and living*. Belmont, CA: Wadsworth.

Council of Collaboration. 2004. *Common standards for pastoral educators/supervisors, Council of Collaboration*. www.professionalchaplains.org/pdf/common-standards-professional-chaplaincy.pdf

Courage. 1999. The response of Courage to the decision of the Sacred Congregation of the Doctrine of the Faith concerning the Nugent-Gramick matter. http://www.catholic-pages.com/dir/homosexuality

Cozzens, D. 2000. *The changing face of the priesthood*. Collegeville, MN: Liturgical Press.

Crawshaw, R., D. E. Rogers, E. D. Pellegrino, R. J. Bulger, G. D. Lundberg, L. R. Bristow, C. K. Cassel, and J. A. Barondess. 1996. Patient-physician covenant. *JAMA* 273:1553.

Cremins, Dick. 2005. Consequences of contraception: Prophecy of Fr. Lestaphis. www.geocities.com/Heartland/Meadows/2879/lestapis.html

Crissman, Susan, and Linda Betz. 1987. Education and image: Critical issues confronting the nursing profession. *Journal of Contemporary Health Law & Policy* 3 (Spring): 174–84.

Criticisms of Psychoanalysis: Bibliography. 1999. www.angelfire.com/ny/metapsychology/analcrit.html

Cronin, Daniel. 1989. The moral law in regard to ordinary and extraordinary means of conserving life. In *Conserving human life*, ed. Russell Smith, 235–75. Braintree, MA: Pope John XXIII Medical Moral Research Center.

Cronin, John. 1950. *Catholic social principles*. Milwaukee, WI: Bruce Books.

Cross, F. L., and E. A. Livingstone. 1997. *The Oxford dictionary of the Christian Church*. New York: Oxford University Press.

Croxatto, H. B. 2005. Emergency contraception prevents fertilization not implantation. www.religiousconsultation.org/News_Tracker/emergency_contraception_prevents_fertilization_not_implantation.htm

Cunningham, Bert. 1944. *The morality of organic transplantation.* Washington, DC: Catholic University of America Press.

Cunningham, P., and C. Forsythe. 1992. Is abortion the first right for women: Some consequences of legal abortion. In *Abortion, medicine and the law*, ed. J. D. Butler and D. F. Walbert. 4th ed. New York: Facts on File.

Curran, Charles, E. 1979. *Moral norms and the Catholic tradition: Readings in moral theology.* New York: Paulist Press.

———. 1984. *Critical concerns in moral theology.* Notre Dame, IN: University of Notre Dame Press.

Curran, Charles E., Margaret Farley, and Richard A. McCormick, eds. 1996. *Feminist ethic and the Catholic moral tradition: Readings in moral theology.* No. 9. New York: Paulist Press.

Curran, Charles E., and Richard A. McCormick, eds. 1980. *The distinctiveness of Christian ethics: Readings in moral theology.* No. 2. New York: Paulist Press.

Curran, Charles E., and Richard A. McCormick. 1986. *Official Catholic social teaching.* Mahwah, NJ: Paulist Press.

Daar, Abdallah, and A. Binsumeit Khitamy. 2000. Bioethics for clinicians: Islamic bioethics. *Canadian Medical Association Journal* 164 (1): 60–63.

Daly, Tom. 1987. When does human life begin? The search for a marker event. In *Proceedings of the Conference: IVF. The current debate*, ed. Karen Dawson and Jill Hudson, 79. Clayton, Victoria, Australia: Monash Center for Human Bioethics.

Darley, John M., Israela Loeb, and Jane Hunter. 1999. Community attitudes on the family of issues surrounding the death of terminal patients. *Journal of Social Issues* 52 (Summer): 85–104.

Davis, D. 2001. *Genetic dilemmas: Reproductive technology, parental choices, and children's futures.* New York: Routledge.

Davis, Ronald M. 1999. Meeting the demand for donor organs in the U.S.: It's time for bold public policy, such as mandated choice or presumed consent (editorial). *British Medical Journal* 319 (November 27): 1382–83.

Dawkins, Richard. 1990. *The selfish gene.* 2nd ed. New York: Oxford University Press.

Dayringer, Richard. 1998. *The heart of pastoral counseling: Healing through relationship.* Binghamton, NY: Haworth Pastoral Press.

de Castro, L. D. 2003. Human organs from prisoners: Kidneys for life. *Journal of Medical Ethics* 29 (June): 171–75.

DeGrazia, David. 2005. Biology, consciousness, and a definition of death. *Report of the Institute of Philosophy and Public Policy* 18 (Winter–Spring): 18–22.

DeHullu, James. 1989. Bibliography on abortion. http://users.telerama.com/~jdehullu/abortion/abbiog.htm

Dekkers, Wim J. M. 2001. Images of death and dying. In *Bioethics in a European Perspective*, ed. Henk ten Have and Bert Gordijn, 411–31. Boston: Kluwer Academic.

DeKoninck, Charles. 1945. In defense of St. Thomas. *Laval Theologique et Philosophique* 1 (2): 1–103.

DeKraai, Mark, and Braaj Sales. 1984. Confidential communications of psychotherapists. *Psychotherapy* 21 (Fall): 293–318.

DeMarco, Donald. 1999. Not making the genetic cut. *Human Life Review* 25 (Fall): 57–61.

———. 2000. The zygote and personhood. *Human Life Review* 26 (Spring/Summer): 91–98.

DeMets, David L. 1999. Statistics and ethics in medical research. *Science and Engineering Ethics* 5 (January): 97–117.

Diamond, Eugene. 1996. *The large family: A blessing and a challenge.* San Francisco: Ignatius Press.

Didache. 1991. *Teaching of the twelve apostles: The Apostolic Fathers.* Vol. 1. Loeb Classics. Trans. K. Lake. Cambridge, MA: Harvard University Press.

Dietrich, William F. 2001. The origin and implications of the Human Genome Project: Scientific overview. *National Catholic Bioethics Quarterly* 1 (Winter): 489–95.

DiNoia, J. A. 1988. Authority, public dissent and the nature of theological thinking. *The Thomist* 52 (2): 185–207.

Doerflinger, Richard. 2001. Testimony before the House Sub-Committee on labor, health and human affairs. *National Catholic Bioethics Quarterly* 3 (Winter): 767–86.

———. 2004. John Paul II on the vegetative state. *Ethics and Medics* 29 (June): 2–4.

Doka, Kenneth, Cindy Hylton Rushton, and Timothy A. Thorstenson. 1994. A Health Care Ethics Forum '94: Caregivers distress: "If it is so ethical, why does it feel so bad?" *AACN Clinical Issues in Critical Care Nursing* 5 (August): 346-52.

Dombrowski, Daniel, and Robert Deltere. 2000. *A brief, liberal, Catholic defense of abortion.* Champaign-Urbana: University of Illinois Press.

Doms, Herbert. 1939 *The meaning of marriage.* New York: Sheed and Ward.

Donceel, Joseph. 1970. Immediate animation and delayed hominization. *Theological Studies* 31:75–105.

Donchin, Anne, and Laura M. Purdy, eds. 1999. *Embodying bioethics: Recent feminist advances.* Lanham, MD: Rowman and Littlefield.

Doeser, M. C., and J. N. Kray, eds. 1986. *Facts and values: Philosophical reflections from western and non-western perspectives.* Dordrecht: Martinus Nijhoff.

Dossey, Barbara Montgomery, Louise C. Selanders, Deva-Marie Beck, and Alex Attewell. 2005. *Florence Nightingale today: Healing, leadership, global action.* Silver Spring, MD: American Nurses Association.

Dougherty, C. J. 1995. Institutional ethics committees. In *Encyclopedia of bioethics,* rev. ed., ed. Warren Reich, 402–12. New York: Simon and Schuster.

Doyle, John. 1997. *On homicide and commentary on Summa Theologiae I & II,* q. 64. Milwaukee, WI: Marquette University Press.

Drane, James. 1992. Anencephaly and the interruption of pregnancy: Policy proposals for hospital ethics committees. *HEC Forum* 4 (February): 103–19.

DuBois, James M. 1999a. Ethical assessments of brain death and organ procurement policies: A survey of transplant personnel in the United States. *Journal of Transplant Coordination* 9 (December): 210–18.

———. 1999b. Non-heart-beating donors: A defense of the required determination of death. *Journal of Law, Medicine and Ethics* 27:126–36.

———. 2001. Non-heart-beating organ donation: Designing an ethically acceptable protocol. *Health Progress* (January–February): 18–21.

———. 2002. Organ transplantation: An ethical road map. *National Catholic Bioethics Quarterly* 2 (Autumn): 413–53.

Duggan, Miriam. 2002. Combatting the spread of AIDS. In *Culture of life, culture of death,* ed. Luke Gormally, 257–69. London: Linacre Center.

Duke, Leela. 1983. Amniocentesis debate continued. *Economic and Political Weekly* 18 (September 17): 1633–35.

Dulles, Avery. 1991. The magisterium, theology and dissent. *Origins* 20 (42): 692–96.

Dupont, Jacques. 1969. *Les Béatitudes.* Paris: J. Gabalda.

Durkheim, Emile. 1951. *Suicide.* Glencoe, IL: Free Press.

Dworkin, R. 1993. *Life's dominion: An argument about abortion, euthanasia and individual freedom.* New York: Knopf.

Dyck, Arthur. 2002. *Life's worth: The case against assisted suicide.* Grand Rapids, MI: William B. Eerdmans.

Eaton, John. 2002. Psychotherapy and moral inquiry. *Theory and Psychology* 12 (June): 367–86.

Edelstein, Ludwig. 1943. *The Hippocratic oath: Text, translation, and interpretation.* Baltimore: Johns Hopkins University Press.

———. 1967. *Ancient medicine: Selected papers.* Ed. O. Tembia and C. Tembia. Baltimore: Johns Hopkins University Press.

Edleman, Gerald. 1995. *The remembered present: A biological theory of consciousness.* New York: Basic Books.

Edwards, R. G. 1981. Mental health as rational autonomy. *Journal of Medicine and Philosophy* 6:3.

Edwards, R., and Helen K. Beard. 1997. Destruction of cryopreserved embryos. *Human Reproduction* 12:3.

Ehrman, Lee et. al. 1980. *The Supreme Court and patenting life.* Hastings Center Report 10:1–15.

Eisenberg, Daniel. 2003. Professional confidentiality in Jewish law. www.aish.com/societyWork/work/

Eisenberg, Jon B. 2005. *Using Terri: The religious rights conspiracy to take away our rights.* San Francisco: Harper.

Eldredge, Nils. 2004 *Why do we do it? Rethinking sex and the selfish gene.* New York: W. W. Norton.

Elger, B. S., and T. W. Harding. 2002. Should cancer patients be informed about their diagnosis and prognosis? Future doctors and lawyers differ. *Journal of Medical Ethics* 28 (August): 258–65.

El-Hai, Jack. 2001. The lobotomist. *The Washington Post.* February 4, W17.

Elliot, C. 2003. *Better than well: American medicine meets the American dream.* New York: W. W. Norton.

Ellul, Jacques. 1980. *The technological system.* New York: Continuum.

Emanuel, Ezekiel J., Robert A. Crouch, John D. Arras, and Jonathan D. Moreno, eds. 2003. *Ethical and regulatory aspects of clinical research: Readings and commentary.* Baltimore, MD: Johns Hopkins University Press.

Emanuel, Ezekiel J., Anne Wood, Alan Fleischman, Angela Bowen, Kenneth A. Getz, Christine Grady, Carol Levine, Dale E. Hammerschmidt, Ruth Faden, Lisa Eckenwiler, Carianne Tucker Muse, and Jeremy Sugarman. 2004. Oversight of human participants research: Identifying problems to evaluate reform proposals. *Annals of Internal Medicine* 141 (4): 282–91.

Engel, G. L. 1981. The clinical application of the biopsychosocial model. *Journal of Medicine and Philosophy* 6:2.

Engelhardt, H. Tristram, Jr. 1977. Some persons are humans, some humans are persons, and the world is what we persons make it. In *Philosophical medical ethics,* ed. Stuart F. Spicker and H. Tristram Engelhardt Jr., 183–94. Boston: Reidel.

———. 1986. Endings and beginnings of persons' death and beginning of persons: Death, abortion, and infanticide. In *The foundations of bioethics,* 202–49. New York: Oxford University Press.

———. 1991. *Bioethics and secular humanism: The search for a common morality.* Harrisburg, PA: Trinity Press International.

———. 1995. *The foundations of bioethics.* 2nd ed. New York: Oxford University Press.

———. 2001. The deChristianization of Christian health care institutions, or, how the pursuit of social justice and excellence can obscure the pursuit of happiness. *Christian Bioethics* 7 (1): 151–61.

Engelhardt, H. Tristam, and Mark Cherry, eds. 2002. *Allocating scarce medical resources: Roman Catholic perspectives.* Washington, DC: Georgetown University Press.

England, M. J. 1993. *New directions for mental health services.* San Francisco: Jossey-Bass.

English, Veronica, and Ann Sommerville. 2003. Presumed consent for transplantation: A dead issue after Alder Hey? *Journal of Medical Ethics* 29 (June): 147–52.

ERD. 2001. *Ethical and religious directives for Catholic health facilities.* Washington, DC: U.S. Conference of Catholic Bishops. www.usccb.org/bishops/directives.shtml

Erikson, Erik. 1978. *Identity: Youth and crisis.* New York: W. W. Norton (Originally published 1968.)

Erwin, Richard. 1978. *Behavior therapy: Scientific, philosophical and moral foundations.* New York: Cambridge University Press.

Estadt, Barry K., Melvin C. Blanchette, and John R. Compton, eds. 1991. *Pastoral counseling/ Loyola College pastoral counseling faculty.* 2nd ed. Englewood Cliffs, NJ: Prentice Hall.

Eth, Spencer, Martin Levine, and Martha Lyon-Levine. 1984. Ethical conflicts at the interface of advocacy and psychiatry. *Hospital and Community Psychiatry* 35 (July): 665–66.

Etzioni, Amitai. 2003. Organ donation: A communitarian approach. *Kennedy Institute of Ethics Journal* 13 (March): 1–18.

European Group on Ethics in Science and New Technologies, European Commission (EGE). 1998. Ethical aspects of research involving the use of human embryo in the context of the 5th framework program. Opinion No. 12 of the European Group on Ethics in Science and New Technologies to the European Commission. Brussels, Belgium: European Group on Ethics in Science and New Technologies, November 12.

Evans, J. 2000. A sociologic account of the growth of principlism. *Hastings Center Report* 3:1–38.

Fainsinger, Robin L., Juan M. Nunez-Olarte, and Donna M. Demoissac. 2003. The cultural differences in perceived value of disclosure and cognition: Spain and Canada. *Journal of Palliative Care* 19 (Spring): 43–48.

Families USA: The voice for health care consumers. 2005. The uninsured. www.familiesusa.org

Farley, Margaret A., and Lisa A. Cahill, eds. 1995. *Embodiment, morality and medicine.* New York: Kluwer Academic.

Farris, James R., ed. 2002. *International perspectives on pastoral counseling.* Binghamton, NY: Haworth Pastoral Press.

Faststats. 2004. Drug abuse. www.cdc.gov/nchs/fastats/druguse.htm

Fehlow, P. 2002. On the causes and relevance of fetishism. *Pediatrics and Related Topics* 3 (January): 221–25.

Fehring, Richard D. 2005. An analysis of the majority report: Responsible parenthood and its recommendations on abortion, sterilization and contraception. www.uffl.org/vol13/fehring03.pdf

Feldman, Rabbi David. 1986. *Health and medicine in the Jewish tradition.* New York: Crossroads.

FIAMC (World Federation of Catholic Medical Association). 2004. Considerations of the scientific and ethical problems related to the vegetative state. *National Catholic Bioethics Quarterly* 5 (Autumn): 579–81.

Fine, Perry G. 2002. The ethical imperative to relieve pain at life's end [opinion]. *Journal of Pain and Symptom Management* 25 (April): S53–S62.

Finnis, John. 1980. *Natural law and natural rights.* Oxford: Clarendon Press.

Fins, Joseph J. 2005. Rethinking disorders of consciousness: New research and its implications. *Hastings Center Review* 35 (March–April): 11–12.

Fisher, Anthony. 1991a. Individuogenesis and a recent book by Fr. Norman Ford. *Anthropotes* 7:199–244.

———. 1991b. When did I begin? Revisited. *Linacre Quarterly* (England) 58:59–68.

———. 1996. Patient care. *Proceedings: Medical Ethics Conference.* Manila: University of San Tomas.

———. 2005. Abortion and the Catholic conscience. www.ewtn.com/library/PROLIFE/ PROLIF.TXT

Fitzgerald, Kevin T. 2002. Knowledge without wisdom: Human genetic engineering without religious insight. *Christian Bioethics* 8 (August): 147–62.

Flanelly, J., A. Weaver, and G. Handzo. 2003. A three year study of chaplains' activities. *Psycho-Oncology* 12 (8): 760–68.

Fletcher, A. 1972. New beginnings of life. In *The new genetics and the future of man,* ed. Michael Hamilton. Grand Rapids, MI: Eerdmans.

Fletcher, Joseph. 1954. *Morals and medicine.* Princeton, NJ: Princeton University Press.

———. 1960. The patient's right to die. *Harpers,* October, 138–43.

Foley, Kathleen, and Herbert Hendin, eds. 2002. *The case against assisted suicide: For the right to end-of-life care.* Baltimore, MD: Johns Hopkins University Press.

Ford, Norman F. 1988. *When did I begin? Conception of the human individual in history, philosophy and science.* Cambridge: Cambridge University Press.

———. 2002. *The prenatal person: Ethics from conception to birth.* Oxford: Blackwell.

Foucault, Michel. 1973. *The birth of the clinic.* New York: Pantheon Books.

Fox, Michael W. 2001. *Bringing life to ethics: Global bioethics for a humane society.* Albany: State University of New York Press.

Fox, Renee, and Judith P. Swazy. 1978. *The courage to fail: A social view of organ transplant and dialysis.* 2nd ed. Chicago: University of Chicago Press.

———. 1992. Leaving the field. *Hastings Center Report* 22(5): 9–15.

Francis, Richard, and John Franklin. 1988. Alcohol and other psychoactive substance use disorders. In *Textbook of psychiatry,* ed. John Talbott et al., 313–56. Washington, DC: American Psychiatric Press.

Francoeur, Robert. 1972. We can—we must: Reflections on the technological imperative. *Theological Studies* 33:428–39.

Freedman, D. 1991. The search: Body, mind and human purpose. *American Journal of Psychiatry* 149:858–66.

Freeman, M. 1999. Does surrogacy have a future after Brazier? *Medical Law Review* 7 (1): 1–20.

Freidson, Elliot. 1971. *The profession of medicine: A study of the sociology of applied knowledge.* New York: Dodd, Mead and Co.

Freud, Sigmund. 1900. *The interpretation of dreams.* Reprint, New York: Modern Library, 1994.

———. 1901. *The psychopathology of everyday life.* Reprint, New York: Modern Library, 1971.

———. 1913. *Totem and taboo: Some points of agreement between the mental lives of savages and neurotics.* Reprint, New York: W. W. Norton, 1962.

———. 1930. *Civilization and its discontents.* London: Hogarth.

Freymann, John Gordon. 1974. *The American health care system: Its genesis and trajectory.* New York: Medcom.

Friedman, Milton. 2001. How to cure health care. www.hooverdigest.org/013/friedman.html

Friedmann, Theodore. 2000. Principles for human gene therapy studies. *Science* 287 (March 24): 2163–63.

Fromm, Erich. 1975. *Crisis of psychoanalysis.* New York: Fawcett World Library.

Fuhrman, Mark. 2005. *Silent witness: The untold story of Terri Schiavo's death.* New York: Harper Collins.

Fukuyama, F. 2002. *Our posthuman future: Consequences of the biotechnology revolution.* New York: Farrar, Straus and Giroux.

Furniss, George M. 2004. *The social context of pastoral care: Defining the life situation.* Louisville, KY: Westminster/John Knox Press.

Furton, Edward. 2002. Brain death, the soul, and organ life. *National Catholic Bioethics Quarterly* 2 (Autumn): 455–72.

———. 2003. Bioethics, evolution, and atheism. *National Catholic Bioethics Quarterly* 3 (Autumn): 3.

———. 2005. A defense of oocyte assistant reprogramming. *National Catholic Bioethics Quarterly* 5 (3): 465–68.

Gaillardetz, Richard. 2003. *By what authority.* Collegeville, MN: Liturgical Press.

Gajer, Simon. 2005. Reforming Germany's health care system: The question of keeping solidarity. http://tiss.zdv.uni-tuebingen.de/webroot/sp/spsba01_W98_1/germany5.htm

Gallagher, Christine M., and Eelco F. M. Wijdicks. 2001. Religious and cultural aspects of brain death. In *Brain death*, ed. Eelco F. M. Wijdicks, 135–49. Philadelphia: Lippincott, Williams and Wilkins.

Gallant, D. 1983. The right to refuse psychotropic medications. *Progress in Clinical Biological Research* 139:31–38.

Gamble, Vanessa Northington. 1997. Under the shadow of Tuskegee: African Americans and health care. *American Journal of Public Health* 87 (November): 1773–78.

Garrison, Fielding H. 1960. *An introduction to the history of medicine.* 4th ed. Philadelphia: W. D. Saunders.

Gartrell, Nanette. 1986. Psychiatrist-patient sexual contact: Results of a national survey. *American Journal of Psychiatry* 153 (September): 1126–31.

Gavrilova, L. A., and N. S. Gavrilova. 1991. *The biology of life span: A quantitative approach.* New York: Harwood Academic.

———. 2001. The reliability theory of aging and longevity. *Journal of Theoretical Biology* 213 (December 21): 527–45.

Gaylin, Willard. 1973. Skinner redux. *Harpers,* October, 48–56.

Gender Trust. 2005. Transsexualism: A guide for employers. www.gendertrust.org.uk/php/showarticle.php?aid=21

German Culture. 2005. Health care in German society. www.germanculture.com.ua/library/facts/bl_health_care.htm

Gert, Bernard, Charles M. Culver, and K. Donner Clauser. 1997. *Bioethics: A return to fundamentals.* New York: Oxford University Press.

Geyman, John P. 2005. The politics of policy: Myths and memes about single-payer health insurance in the United States. *International Journal of Health Services,* 35(1): 63–90. http://pnhp.org/facts/myths_memes.pdf

Giacino, J. T., S. Aswal, N. Childs, and R. Cranford. 2002. The minimally conscious state: Definition and diagnostic criteria. *Neurology* 58(3): 349–53.

Giesen, Dieter.1993. The patient's right to know: A comparative law perspective. *Medicine and Law* 12 (6/7/8): 553–65.

Gilbert, Daniel. 1981. Shock therapy and informed consent. *Illinois Bar Journal* 69 (January): 272–87.

Gilbert, Scott F. 2003. *Developmental Biology.* 7th ed. Sunderland, MA: Sinauer Associates.

Gillespie, Michael. 2001. Saving what we love at any cost: The rhetoric of heroic medicine as diversion. *Journal of Medical Humanities* 23 (Spring): 73–86.

Gilson, Étienne. 1955. *History of Christian philosophy in the middle ages.* New York: Random House.

Gladding, S. 2004. *Counseling: A comprehensive profession.* Upper Saddle River, NJ: Pearson/Merrill/Prentice Hall.

Glendon, Mary Ann. 1987. *Abortion and divorce in western law: American failures, European challenges.* Cambridge, MA: Harvard University Press.

———. 1991. *Rights talk: The impoverishment of political discourse.* New York: Free Press.

Glymour, Clark, and Douglas Stalker. 1983. Engineers, cranks, physicians, magicians. *New England Journal of Medicine* 16 (April 21): 308.

Goffman, Erving. 1962. *Asylums: Essays on the social situation of mental patients and other inmates.* Chicago: Aldine.

Goldstein, Robert. 1993. Tarasoff and the practice of psychotherapy. *American Journal of Psychiatry* 150 (August): 1278.

Goode, Erich. 1997. *Between politics and reason: The drug legalization debate.* New York: St. Martin's Press.

Gordon, Elisa J., and Christopher K. Daugherty. 2003. Hitting you over the head: Oncologists' disclosure of prognosis to advanced cancer patients. *Bioethics* 17 (April): 142–68.

Görres, Ida Friederike. 2003. (1901–71). *The hidden face: A Study of St. Thérèse of Lisieux.* Trans. Richard and Clara Winston. San Francisco, CA: Ignatius Press.

Gorsuch, Nancy J. 2001. *Introducing feminist pastoral care and counseling.* Cleveland, OH: Pilgrim Press.

Grabowski, John S. 1996. *Evangelium vitae: A tale of two encyclicals.* www.catholic.net/RCC/ Periodicals/Homiletic/11-96/1/1.html

Graham, Judith. 2005. Hospitals ignore rape victim law. *Chicago Tribune*, May 11, Metro.

Gratzer, Walter Bruno. 2000. Nature and nurtured: The rise and fall of eugenics. In *The undergrowth of science: Delusion, self-deception, and human frailty*, 281–303. New York: Oxford University Press.

Graumann, Charles V. 2002. Bishop of Dallas, Pastoral letter on the Church's care for the sick and dying. www.cathdal.org/Pastoral%20Letter%20Care%20of%20Sick%20Dying%20012121802.htm

Gregorek, Joseph. 1988. Guide for treating rape victims emphasizes compassion, respect. *Health Progress* 69 (September): 71–72.

Grezon, Frederick, and Rudolph de Jong. 2000. Fatal outcomes from liposuction: Census survey of cosmetic surgeons. *Plastic and Reconstructive Surgery* 105 (January): 1.

Grisez, Germain. 1964. *Contraception and the natural law.* Milwaukee, WI: Bruce.

———. 1970. *Abortion: The myths, the realities and the arguments.* New York: Corpus Books.

———. 1983. *Christian moral principles: The way of the Lord Jesus.* Vol. 1. Chicago: Franciscan Herald Press.

———. 1989. When do people begin? Proceedings of the *American Catholic Philosophical Association* 63:27–47.

———. 1993. *Living a Christian life: The way of the Lord Jesus.* Vol. 2. Chicago: Franciscan Herald Press.

———. 1997. *Difficult moral questions: The way of the Lord Jesus.* Vol. 3. Chicago: Franciscan Herald Press.

Grisez, Germain, Joseph Boyle, and John Finnis. 1987. Practical principles: Moral truth and ultimate ends. *American Journal of Jurisprudence* 32:99–151.

Grobstein, Clifford. 1983. A biological perspective on the origin of human life and personhood. In *Defining human life*, ed. M. W. Shaw and A. E. Doudera. Washington, DC: Association of University Programs in Health Administration.

———. 1988. *Science and the unborn: Choosing human futures.* New York: Basic Books.

Gross, Barry R. 1980. *Analytic philosophy: An historical introduction.* Indianapolis: Bobbs-Merrill.

Gubermatis, G., and H. Kliemet. 2000. A superior approach to organ allocation and donation. *Transplantation* 70:699–762.

Guevin, B. 2005. Sex reassignment surgery for transsexuals. *Catholic Bioethics Quarterly* 5 (Winter): 719–34.

Guild of Catholic Doctors. 1998. *Advance directives or living wills.* London: St. Pauls. 32.

Guinan, Patrick. 1999. Catholic healthcare: We are losing the identity battle. www.catholic.net/ rcc/Periodicals/Homiletic/May1999/healthcare.html

———. 2001. Where has catholic medical ethics gone? *Catholic Medical Quarterly* (November). www.catholicdoctors.org.uk/CMQ/Nov_2001/where_has_catholic_medical_ethic.htm

Gustafson, James. 1984. *Ethics from a theocentric perspective.* Vol. 1. Chicago: University of Chicago Press.

Gutiérrez, Gustavo. 1988. *The theology of liberation: History, politics, and salvation.* Trans. Inda Caridad and John Eagleston. Maryknoll, NY: Orbis.

Guydish, J., and J. J. Kramer. 1982. Behavior modification: Doing battle in the ethical arena. *Journal of Behavior Therapy and Experimental Psychiatry* 4 (December): 315–20.

Guyer, Paul, ed. 1992. *Cambridge companion to Kant.* Cambridge: Cambridge University Press.

Haafhems, J., G. Nijhof, and E. Vander Pool. 1986. Mental health care and the opposition movement in The Netherlands. *Social Science and Medicine* 22(2): 185–92.

Haas, John. 2003. Moral absolutes. In *Introduction to moral theology.* International Catholic University. http://icu.catholicity.com/c00505.htm

Haas, John, and Peter Cataldo. 2002. Institutional cooperation: The ERDs. *Health Progress* (November–December): 49–57, 60.

Habermas, Jürgen. 1984. *The theory of communicative action.* Vol. 1, *Reason and the rationalization of society: The theory of communicative action.* Boston: Beacon Press.

———. 1987. *The theory of communicative action.* Vol. 2, *The critique of functionalist reason.* Boston: Beacon Press.

Hall, Charles E. 1992. *Head and heart: The story of the clinical pastoral education movement.* Decatur, GA: Journal of Pastoral Care Publications.

Hall, Jack. 1995. *Affective competence in counseling.* Lanham, MD: University Press of America.

Halvey, Amir, and Baruch Brody. 1993. Brain death: Reconciling definitions, criteria and tests. *Annals of Internal Medicine* 19 (September 15): 727–32.

Hamel, Ron. 2002. Preserving integrity in partnerships directives requires an objective moral analysis of cooperative arrangements. *Health Progress* 83(6): 37–39, 59.

Hamel, Ron, and Michael Panicola. 2002. Emergency contraception and sexual assault. *Health Progress* 83 (September–October): 5, 12–14.

———. 2003. Low risks and moral certitude. *Ethics and Medics* 28 (December): 3.

Hansen, Michelle, J. J. Kurinczuk, C. Bower, and S. Webb. 2002. The risk of major birth defects after intracytoplasmic sperm infection and in vitro fertilization. *New England Journal of Medicine* 346 (10): 725–30.

Haque, A. K. 1996. High autopsy rates at a university medical center. What went right. *Archives Pathological Lab Medicine* 19 (September 15): 519–25.

Hardin, Elizabeth. 1997. *Venus envy: A history of cosmetic surgery.* Baltimore: John Hopkins University Press.

Hardin, Garret. 1993. *Living within limits: Ecology, economics, and population taboos.* New York: Oxford University Press.

Harding, Susan Friend. 2000. *The book of Jerry Falwell: Fundamentalist language and politics.* Princeton, NJ: Princeton University Press.

Hare, Richard M. 1988. When does potentiality count? A comment on Lockwood. *Bioethics* 2 (3): 214.

———. 1991. *The language of morals.* Oxford: Clarendon Press. (Originally published 1952.)

Häring, Bernard, C. 1963. *The law of Christ: Moral theology for priests and laity.* Trans. Edwin Kaiser. Cork: Mercier Press.

———. 1976. New dimensions of responsible parenthood. *Theological Studies* 37:120.

Harper, Robert A. 1959. *Psychoanalysis and psychotherapy: 36 systems.* Englewood Cliffs, NJ: Prentice Hall.

Harper, Terry, et al. 2004. Use of material plasma for noninvasive determination of fetal status. *Journal of Obstetrics and Gynecology* 191:1730–32.

Harrelson, Walter. 1980. *The ten commandments and human rights.* Minneapolis, MN: Fortress Press.

Harris, John, and Soren Holm. 2003. Should we presume moral turpitude in our children? Small children and consent to medical research. *Theoretical Medicine and Bioethics* 24 (2): 121–29.

Hartman, Megan. 1998. *Humanae vitae:* Thirty years of discord and dissent. *Conscience* (Autumn): 8–16.

Hausman, Bernice L. 1995. *Changing sex: Transsexualism, technology, and the idea of gender.* Durham, NC: Duke University Press.

Hays, Charlotte. 2001. Solving the puzzle of natural family planning. *Crisis* (December). www.crisismagazine.com/december2001/cover.htm.

Healy, Edwin. 1956. *Medical ethics: On cooperation.* Chicago: Loyola University Press.

Helmeniak, Daniel A. 2005. FAQ's: Catholicism, homosexuality, and dignity. Dignity USA. www.dignityusa.org/faq.html

Hendren, Hardy, and Craig Lillehi. 1988. Pediatric surgery. *New England Journal of Medicine* 319 (July 14): 89–96.

Hilgers, Thomas W. 1995. *The scientific foundations of the ovulation method.* Omaha, NE: Pope Paul II Institute Press.

Hilgers, Thomas W., and J. B. Stanford. 1998. Creighton model napro-education technology for avoiding pregnancy: Use effectiveness. *Journal of Reproductive Medicine* 43 (June): 6.

Holifield, E. Brooks. 1983. *A history of pastoral care in America from salvation to self-realization.* Nashville, TN: Abingdon Press.

Hollander, Rachelle D. 2000. Scientific research, ethics, values in science. In *Encyclopedia of ethical, legal, and policy issues in biotechnology*, ed. Thomas H. Murray and Maxwell J. Mehlman, 1041–47. New York: John Wiley and Sons.

Holmes, Helen Bequaert, and Laura M. Purdy, eds. 1992. *Feminist directions in medical ethics.* Bloomington: Indiana University Press.

Holt, Robert R. 1980. Freud's impact on modern morality. *Hastings Center Report* 10:38–45.

Holzgreve, W. 1987. Kidney transplantation from anencephalic donors. *New England Journal of Medicine* 316 (April 23): 1069–70.

Hoopes, Tom. 2004. Breaking vows: When faithful Catholics divorce. www.godspy.com/life/Breaking-Vows-When-Faithful-Catholics-Divorce-Tom-Hoopes.cfm

Howe, Leroy T. 2003. *Comforting the fearful: Listening skills for caregivers.* New York: Paulist Press.

Howlett, M. J., Denise Avard, and Bartha Maria Knoppers. 2002. Physicians and genetic malpractice. *Medicine and Law: World Association for Medical Law* 21(4): 661–80.

Hoyt, Robert, ed. 1969. *The birth control debate.* Kansas City, MO: National Catholic Reporter.

Huang, T. T. 1995. Twenty years of experience in managing gender dysphoric patients. *Plastic and Reconstructive Surgery* 96 (September): 921–30.

Hui, E. C. 2002. *At the beginning of life: Dilemmas in theological ethics.* Downers Grove, IL: InterVarsity Press.

Human Body Adventure. 2003. http://vilenski.org/science/humanbody/index.html

Human Genome Project. 2005. www.ornl.gov/sci/techresources

Humphreys, K. 2000. Community narratives and personnel stories in A.A. *Journal of Community Psychology* 28(5): 495–506.

Humphry, Derek. 2002. *Final exit: The practicalities of self-deliverance and assisted suicide for the dying.* 3rd ed. New York: Dell/Random House.

Hurlbut, William B., MD. 2005. Publications. http://www.stanford.edu/~ethics/WBH.htm

Iglesias, Teresa. 1987. What kind of being is the human embryo? In *Embryo and ethics: The Warnock report in debate*, ed. N. C. de S. Cameron, 58–73. Edinburgh: Rutherford House.

Iles, Susan, and Dennis Gath. 1993. Psychiatric outcome of termination of pregnancy for fetal abnormality. *Psychological Medicine* 23:407–14.

Illich, Ivan. 1972. Technology and conviviality. In *To create a different future: Religious hope and technology*, ed. Kenneth Vaux, 40–66. New York: Friendship Press.

Illich, Ivan, Irving K. Zola, and John McKnight. 1978. *Disabling professions.* Boston: Marion Boyars.

Incandela, Joseph M. 2005. *The Catholic Church and surrogate motherhood.* www.saintmarys.edu/~incandel/cst.html

Ingleby, Daniel, ed. 1980. *Critical psychiatry: The politics of mental health*. New York: Pantheon Books.

Institute for Theological Encounter with Science and Technology (ITEST). 1975. *Brain research: Human consciousness*. St. Louis: ITEST Publications.

Institute of Medicine. 1996. *The nation's physician workforce*. Washington, DC: National Academy Press.

———. 2000. *Committee on non-heart-beating transplantation II: The scientific and ethical basis for practice and protocols. Non-heart beating organ transplantation: practice and protocols*. Washington, DC: National Academies Press.

———. 2003. Committee on assessing the system for protecting human research participants. *Responsible research: A systems approach to protecting research participants*, ed. Daniel D. Federman, Kathi E. Hanna, and Laura Lyman Rodriguez, 290. Washington, DC: National Academies Press.

"Integrating cultures." 1999. In supplement to *Health Progress* 80 (March–April): 2. http://findarticles.com/p/articles/mi_qa3859/is_199903/ai_n8845457

Irving, Dianne Nutwell. 1991. Philosophical and scientific analysis of the nature of the early human embryo. Ph.D. diss., Department of Philosophy, Georgetown University, Washington, DC.

———. 1993. Scientific and philosophical expertise: An evaluation of the arguments on personhood. *Linacre Quarterly* 60 (February): 18–46.

———. 1994a. Academic fraud and conceptual transfer in bioethics: Abortion, human embryo research, and psychiatric research. In *Life and learning IV: Proceedings of the fourth university faculty for life conference*, ed. J. W. Koterski, 193–215. Washington, DC: University Faculty for Life.

———. 1994b. New age embryology textbooks: Pre-embryo, pregnancy and abortion counseling. Implications for fetal research. *Linacre Quarterly* 61 (2): 42–62.

———. 2002. The woman and the physician facing abortion. Extensive bibliography. www.catholicculture.org/docs/doc_view.cfm?recnum=2773

Isaacs, Stephen L., and James R. Knickman, eds. 2002. *To improve health and health care*. Vol. 5, *The Robert Wood Johnson Foundation Anthology*. San Francisco: Jossey-Bass/John Wiley and Sons.

Jackson, Timothy P. 2002. *The priority of love: Christian charity and social justice*. Princeton, NJ: Princeton University Press.

Jacobs, Seth. 1980. Determination of medical necessity: Medicaid funding for sex reassignment surgery. *Case Western Reserve Law Review* 31:179.

Jaenisch R., and Ian Wilmut. 2001. Don't clone humans. *Science* 291 (March 30): 5513.

Jaki, Stanley L. 1989. *God and the cosmologists*. Edinburgh: Scottish Academic Press.

Jansen, Lynn A. 2003. A moral irrelevance of proximity to death. *Journal of Clinical Ethics* 14 (Spring–Summer): 49–58.

Janssen, Andre. 2002. The new regulation of voluntary euthanasia and medically assisted suicide in The Netherlands. *International Journal of Law, Policy and the Family* 16 (August): 260–69.

Jansson, B. 2004. Controversial psychosurgery resulted in a Nobel prize. www.nobel.se/medicine/articles/moniz/#8

Janzen, Waldemar. 1994. *Old Testament ethics*. Louisville, KT: Westminster/John Knox.

JCAHO (Joint Commission for Accreditation of Health Care Organizations). 1993. *Manual for hospitals*. Chicago: American Hospital Association.

Jecker, Nancy, and Donnie Self. 1991. Separating care and cure: An analysis of historical contemporary images of nursing and medicine. *Journal of Medicine and Philosophy* 16:285–306.

Jennett, Bryan. 2002. *The vegetative state*. Cambridge: Cambridge University Press.

Johansen, Bruce E. 2000. Stolen wombs, indigenous women most at risk. *Native Americans*, www.ratical.org/ratville/stolenWombs.html

John Paul II. 1979. On the redemption of man (*Redemptor hominis*). March 4, www.TheHolySee/TheHolyFather/JohnPaulII/Encyclicals

———. 1980. Lust and personal dignity. *Origins* 10 (19): 303.

———. 1981. On the human family (*Familiaris consortio*). *Origins* 11 (28–29): December 24.

———. 1983. Charter of rights of the family. Article 3. *Origins* 12: 42–47.

———. 1984. On reconciliation and penance. *Origins* 74 (27): 442.

———. 1986. Medicines at the service of man. *Health Progress* (October 24).

———. 1987. On social development (*Sollicituda rei socialis*). *Origins* 17(33): 279.

———. 1991. The 100th year (*Centesimus annus*). *Origins* 6 (23): 363–87.

———. 1993. The splendor of truth (*Veritatis splendor*). *Origins* 23 (18): 298–336.

———. 1994. *Crossing the threshold of hope*, ed. V. Messori. New York: Alfred Knopf.

———. 1995. Gospel of life (*Evangelium vitae*). *Origins* 24 (42): 689–731.

———. 1997. *The theology of the body, human love, and the divine plan*. Boston: Pauline Books.

———. 1998a. Address of John Paul II to the Bishops of the Episcopal Conference of the United States of America (California, Nevada, and Hawaii). October 2, www.vatican.va/holy_father/john_paul_ii/speeches/1998/october/documents/hf_jp-ii_spe_19981002_ad-limina-usa_en.html

———. 1998b. *Ad tuendum fidem, Mofu proprio*. *Origins* 28 (8): 113–15.

———. 1998c. Faith and reason (*Fides et ratio*). *Origins* 28 (19): 317–48.

———. 1998d. Why natural family planning differs from contraception. *Origins* 27 (40): 680–82.

———. 1999. Message from World Day of Peace. www.vatican.va/holyfather/johnpaulII/audiences/1999/documentshfjpIIand2909/1999en.html

———. 2000. Address to international transplantation society. *National Catholic Bioethics Quarterly* 1 (Spring): 89–92.

———. 2003. Eucharist: Heart of the Church. April 3. www.theholysee/theholyfather/johnpaulii.encyclicals

———. 2004a. Care for patients in a permanent vegetative state. *Origins* 33 (43): 737–40.

———. 2004b. To participants of the Pontifical Council for Pastoral Care. *National Catholic Bioethics Quarterly* 5 (Spring): 153–55.

Johnson, Christopher, and Michael Sheringham. 1993. *System and writing in the philosophy of Jacques Derrida*. Cambridge: Cambridge University Press.

Johnson, Mark. 1995. Quaestio Disputata: Delayed hominization. Reflections on some recent Catholic claims for delayed hominization. *Theological Studies* 56:743–63.

Johnston, George F. 2003. *Abortion from the religious and moral perspective: An annotated bibliography*. Westport, CT: Greenwood.

Johnstone, M. 2004. *Bioethics: A nursing perspective*. London: Churchill Livingstone.

Jonas, Hans. 1979. Toward a philosophy of technology. *Hastings Center Report* 9:34–43.

———. 1984. *The importance of responsibility: In search of an ethics for the technological age*. Chicago: Chicago University Press.

Jones, James 1982. *Bad blood: The Tuskegee syphilis experiment*. New York: Free Press.

Jones, Steve. 2000. *Genetics in medicine, real promises and unreal expectations*. New York: Milbank Memorial Fund Report.

Jung, Carl, ed. 1984. *Man and his symbols*. London: Aldus Books. (Originally published 1964.)

Kahn, Eva. 1987. *Clinical genetics handbook*. Orabell, NJ: National Genetics Foundation.

Kaiser, Walter C., Jr. 1983. *Toward Old Testament ethics*. Grand Rapids, MI: Zondervan.

Kant, Immanuel. 1999. *Kant's practical philosophy*. Trans. and ed. Mary J. Gregor. Cambridge: Cambridge University Press.

Karakatsanis, K. G., and J. N. Tsanakas. 2002. A critique on the concept of brain death. *Issues in Law and Medicine* 18 (Fall): 127–41.

Karasu, Toksoz. 1982. Psychotherapy and pharmacotherapy: Toward an integrative model. *American Journal of Psychiatry* 139:106–12.

Kaserman, David L., and A. H. Barnett. 2002. *The U.S. organ procurement system: A prescription for reform.* Washington, DC: American Enterprise Institute Press.

Kass, Leon. 1985. *Toward a more natural science, biology and human affairs.* New York: Free Press.

———. 2002. Statement on human cloning. In *Human cloning and human dignity: A report by the President's Council on Bioethics.* New York: Public Affairs (Perseus Books Group).

———. 2003. Biotechnology and the pursuit of human improvement. In *Beyond therapy: Biotechnology and the pursuit of happiness.* Paper prepared for the President's Council on Bioethics. Washington, DC: U.S. Government Printing Office.

Kass, Leon R., and Nelson Lund. 1996. Physician-assisted suicide, medical ethics, and the future of the medical profession. *Duquesne Law Review* 35 (Fall): 395–425.

Kass, Leon, and James Wilson. 1998. *The ethics of human cloning.* Washington, DC: American Enterprise Institute Press.

Katz, Jay. 2002. *The silent world of doctor and patient.* Baltimore: Johns Hopkins University Press.

Katz, Jay, Alexander M. Capron, and Elenor Swift-Glass. 1972. *Experimentation with human beings.* New York: Russell Sage Foundation.

Kauffman, Christopher. 1976. *Tamers of death.* New York: Crossroads.

———. 1978. *The ministry of healing.* New York: Crossroads.

Keenan, James F. 1999. Whose perfection is it anyway? A virtuous consideration of enhancement. *Christian Bioethics* 5 (August): 104–20.

Keenan, James, and Kathy Kaveny. 1995. Ethical issues in health care restructuring. *Theological Studies* 5 (6): 136–50.

Keenan, James, and Thomas R. Kopfensteiner. 1995. The principle of cooperation. *Hospital Progress* (April): 26.

Kelly, David F. 1979. *The emergence of Roman Catholic medical ethics in North America.* New York: Mellen Press.

Kelly, Gerald. 1950. The duty of using artificial means to prolong life. *Theological Studies* 11:214–16.

———. 1956. The morality of mutilation: Toward a revision of the treatise. *Theological Studies* 17:322–44.

———. 1958. *Medico-moral problems.* St. Louis, MO: Catholic Hospital Association.

Kenny, Joseph. 1997. *A comparative perspective of bio-ethics: Catholic, Protestant, Muslim views.* UCH conference on medical ethics with help from Benedict Faneye, O.P. Ibadan. February 18.

Kerlanger, Fred. 1986. *Foundations of behavioral research.* New York: CBS College.

Kesey, Ken. 1962. *One flew over the cuckoo's nest.* New York: Viking Penguin.

Khantzian, E. J. 1985. The self-medication hypotheses of addiction disorders: Focus on heroin and cocaine dependence. *American Journal of Psychiatry* 142:1259–64.

Kippley, John. 2004. The effectiveness of natural family planning. www.ccli.org/nfp/effect1.shtml

Kippley, John, and Sheila K. Kippley. 1996. *The art of natural family planning.* 4th ed. Cincinnati, OH: Couple to Couple League International.

Kirk, Katherine M., Simon P. Blomberg, David L. Duffy, Andrew C. Heath, Ian P. F. Owens, and Nick G. Martin. 2001. Natural selection and quantitative genetics of life history traits in Western women: A twins study. *Evolution* 55 (2): 423–35.

Kirkwood, Neville A. 1995. *Pastoral care in hospitals.* Alexandria, Australia: E. J. Dwyer.

Kischer, C. Ward. 1992. In defense of human development. *Linacre Quarterly* 59:68–75.

———. 1993. Human development and reconsideration of ensoulment. *Linacre Quarterly* 60 (1): 57–63.

———. 1994. A new-wave dialectic: The reinvention of human embryology. *Linacre Quarterly* 61:66–81.

———. 2005. The third holocaust: The war against the human embryo and fetus. www.lifeissues.net/writers/kisc/kisc_15thirdholocaust.html

Kischer, E. 1996. The beginning of life and the establishment of the continuum. *Linacre Quarterly* 63 (August): 73–78.

Kissling, Francis, president, Catholics for a Free Choice. 2005. Taking on the hard questions. www.ms4c.org/update/400lead.htm

Klaus, Hanna. 1995. *Natural family planning: A review.* 2nd ed. Bethesda, MD: NFP Center of Washington, DC.

Kleinig, John I. 1985. *Ethical issues in psychosurgery.* Boston: Allen and Unwin.

Klerman, Gerald L. 1991. Ideological conflicts in integrating pharmacotherapy and psychotherapy. In *Integrating pharmacotherapy and psychotherapy*, ed. G. Klerman and G. Beitman, 2–20. Washington, DC: American Psychiatric Press.

Klimon, William. 2004. Contraception: Early church teaching. http://ic.net/~erasmus/RAZ274.HTM

Knauer, Peter. 1967. The hermeneutic function of the principle of double effect. *National Law Forum* 12:132–62.

Koch, Jean Holt. 1997. *Robert Guthrie: The PKU story. A crusade against mental retardation.* Pasadena, CA: Hope.

Kolata, Gina. 1998. *Clone: The road to Dolly, and the path ahead.* New York: William Morrow and Company.

Kolb, Lawrence, and Keith Brodie. 1982. *Modern clinical psychiatry.* Philadelphia: W. B. Saunders.

Kopfensteiner, Thomas. 2005. A summary of the development of the *Ethical and Religious Directives for Catholic Health Care Services.* www.findarticles.com/p/articles/mi_qa3859/is_200111/ai_n9007144

Korbling, M., and Z. Estrov. 2003. Adult stem cells for tissue repair: A new therapeutic concept. *New England Journal of Medicine* 349 (August 7): 570–82.

Kosnick, Anthony R., et al. 1977. *Human sexuality: New directions in American Catholic thought.* New York: Paulist Press.

Kosten, T. R., B. J. Rounsaville, and H. D. Kleber. 1985. Comparison of clinical ratings to self reports of curing detoxification. *American Journal of Alcohol Abuse* 11:1–10.

Kraemer, David. 2000. *The meanings of death in Rabbinic Judaism.* London: Routledge.

Kreeft, Peter, and Ronald K. Tacelli. 1994. *Handbook of Christian apologetics.* Downers Grove, IL: Intervarsity.

Kroll, J., and B. Bachrach. 1984. Sin and mental illness in the middle ages. *Psychological Medicine* 14 (August): 507–14.

Kubler-Ross, Elisabeth. 1969. *On death and dying.* New York: Macmillan.

Kucinich, Dennis. 2005. On universal health care. www.kucinich.us/issues/universalhealth.php

Kuliev, A., L. Jackson, U. Froster, B. Brambati, J. L. Simpson, Y. Verlinsky, N. Ginsberg, S. Smidt-Jenson, and H. Zakut. 1996. Chorionic villi safety: Report of W.H.O. *American Journal of Obstetrics and Gynecology* 174:807–11.

Kung, Hans. 1984. *Eternal life: Life after death as a medical, philosophical, and theological program.* Garden City, NY: Doubleday.

Ladd, Everett C., and Karlyn H. Bowman. 1999. *Public opinion about abortion: Twenty-five years after* Roe v. Wade. Washington, DC: AEI Press.

Laing, R. D. 1976. *The politics of experience.* New York: Ballantine Books.

Lamberg, Lynne. 1998. Gay is okay with APA (American Psychiatric Association). *JAMA* 280:497–99.

Larsen, William J., Lawrence S. Sherman, Steven Potter, and William J. Scott. 2001. *Human embryology.* London: Churchill Livingston.

Lartey, Emmanuel Yartekwei. 2003. *In living color: An intercultural approach to pastoral care and counseling.* Foreword by James N. Poling. London: Jessica Kingsley.

Lawler, Ronald, Joseph Boyle, and William E. May. 1985. *Catholic sexual ethics.* Huntington, IN: Our Sunday Visitor.

Lawrence, Anne A. 2003. Factors associated with satisfaction or regret following male to female sex reassignment surgery. *Archive of Sexual Research* 32 (August): 299–315.

Lawrence, Paul, and Nitin Nohria. 2001. *Driven: How human nature shapes our choices.* Foreword by Edward Osborn. San Francisco: Jossey-Bass.

Lebacqz, Karen. 1999. *Sexuality, A reader.* Cleveland, OH: Pilgrim Press.

Lebacqz, Karen, and Joseph Driskill. 2000. *Ethics and spiritual care: A guide for pastors, chaplains, and spiritual directors.* Nashville, TN: Abingdon.

Lee, Patrick. 1996. *Abortion and unborn human life.* Washington, DC: Catholic University of America Press.

———. 2004. A Christian philosopher's view of recent directions in the abortion debate. *Christian Bioethics* 10:7–31.

Lee, Simon J. Craddock. 2002. In a secular spirit: Strategies of clinical pastoral education. *Health Care Analysis* 10:339–56. www.lib.berkeley.edu/ANTH/pdfs/In_a_secular_spirit_s.lee.pdf

Lehmann, H. E. 1979. Problems with ethical aspects of psychotropic drug use. *Prog. Neuropsychopharmacol.* 3 (1–3): 271–75.

Lehrman, Dorothy, ed. 1988. *Fetal research and fetal tissue research.* Washington, DC: Association of American Medical Colleges.

Lehrman, Sally. 1995. Genetic testing needs more checks. *Nature* 378 (November): 120.

Lejeune, Jrome. 1989. Testimony in *Davis v. Davis,* Circuit Court for Blount County, State of Tennessee at Maryville, Tennessee. In *A symphony of the pre-born child*: Part II, 9–10. Hagerstown, MD: National Association for the Advancement of Preborn Children.

Leo XIII. 1891. Rights and duties of capital and labor (*Rerum novarum*). See Misner, Paul. *Social Catholicism in Europe.* New York: Crossroads (ch. 11).

Lester, Andrew D. 2003. *The angry Christian: A theology for care and counseling.* Louisville, KY: Westminster/John Knox Press.

Levey, R. E. 2001. Sources of stress for residents and recommendations for programs to assist them. *Academic Medicine* 76 (2): 142–50. www.ncbi.nlm.nih.gov/entrez/query.fcgi?cmd=Retrieve&db=PubMed&list_uids=11158832&dopt=Citation

Levine, Robert. 1983. Informed consent in research and practice: Similarities and differences. *Archives of Internal Medicine* 143 (June): 1229–31.

Lewis, C. S. 1943. *The problem of pain.* New York: Macmillan.

Lezak, Anne, and Elizabeth Edgar. 1998. *Preventing homelessness among people with serious mental illness: A guide for states.* Delmar, NY: National Resource Center on Homelessness and Mental Illness.

Lifshitz, Samuel. 1999. Rape. In *Principles and practice of emergency medicine*, ed. George Schwartz, Barbara K. Hanke, Thomas A. Mayer, James S. Cohen, John Dale Dunn, and Joseph C. Howton. Baltimore: Lippincott, Williams & Wilkens. (Originally published 1986.)

Lifton, Robert Jay. 1986. *The Nazi doctors.* New York: New York Press.

Light, Donald. 1980. *Becoming psychiatrists.* New York: W. W. Norton.

Linn, Dennis, Sheila Fabricant Linn, and Matthew Linn. 1993. *Belonging: Bonds of healing and recovery.* New York: Paulist Press.

Lockwood, Michael. 1988. *Warnock v Powell* (and Harradine): When does potentiality count? *Bioethics* 2:187–213.

Lofton, Kevin. 2005. The difficult realities of healthcare in our country. *Frontiers of Health Care Services Management* 21 (4): 29–33.

Lohse, Bernhard. 1999. *Martin Luther's theology: Its historical and systematic development*, Trans. and ed. Roy A. Harrisville, 28–34, 145–50. Minneapolis, MN: Fortress Press.

London, Perry. 1979. *Behavior control.* New York: Harper and Row.

Lothstein, Leslie M. 1982. Sex reassignment surgery: Historical, bioethical, and theoretical issues. *American Journal of Psychiatry* 139:417–26.

Luciano, A., G. Roy, and E. Solima. 2001. Ectopic pregnancy: Surgical emergency to medical management. *Annals of New York Academy of Science* 943:235–54.

Lynch, Peter. 2005. *The church's story: A history of pastoral care and vision.* Boston, MA: Pauline Books and Media.

Lynn, Joanne. 2001. Serving patients who may die soon and their families: The role of hospice and other services. *JAMA* 185 (February 21): 925–32.

Lysaught, M. Therese. 2006. Vulnerability within the body of Christ. In *Health and human flourishing: Religion, medicine, and moral anthropology,* ed. Carol Taylor and Roberto Dell'Oro, 159–82. Washington, DC: Georgetown University Press.

MacCrae, Melissa. 2005. Reclaiming Eve: Toward a pro-choice ethic for Catholic women. www.fawi.net/ezine/vol3nof/ReclaimingEve.html

MacCulloch, Diarmaid. 2003. *The reformation, a history.* New York: Viking Press.

MacGillivray, Ian K. 1988. *Twinning and twins.* New York: John Wiley and Sons.

Machan, Tibor R. 1974. *The pseudo-science of B. F. Skinner.* New York: Arlington House.

MacIntyre, Alisdair. 1979. Seven traits for designing our descendants. *Hastings Center Report* 9:5–17.

Macklin, Ruth. 1983. Philosophical conceptions of rationality and psychiatric notions of competency. *Synthese* 57 (November): 205–25.

———. 1985. Mapping the human genome: Problems of privacy and free choice. In *Genetics and the law,* ed. Aubrey Milunsky and George Annas, 107–14. New York: Plenum Press.

———. 2003. Bioethics, vulnerability, and protection. *Bioethics* 17 (October): 472–86.

Maddi, Salvatore R. 1996. *Personality theories: A community analysis.* 6th ed. Pacific Grove, CA: Brook/Cole.

Mahkorn, S., and W. Dolan. 1981. Sexual assault and pregnancy. In *New perspectives in human abortion,* ed. T. Hilgers, D. Horan, and D. Mall, 182–99. Frederick, MD: University Publications of America.

Malony, H. Newton. 2001. *Pastoral care and counseling in sexual diversity.* New York: Haworth Pastoral Press.

Mangan, J. 1949. An historical analysis of the principle of double effect. *Theological Studies* 10:40–61.

Marks, Lara V. 2004. *Sexual chemistry: A history of the contraceptive pill.* New Haven, CT: Yale University Press.

Marmer, Stephen. 1988. *Theories of mind and psychopathology in textbook of psychiatry,* ed. J. Talbot, 129–41. Washington, DC: American Psychiatric Press.

Marquis, D. B. 1991. Four versions of double effect. *Journal of Medicine and Philosophy* 16:515–44.

———. 1995. Fetuses, futures, and values: A reply to Shirley. *Southwest Philosophy Review* 6 (2): 263–65.

———. 1998a. A future like ours and the concept of a person: A reply to McInerny and Paske. In *The abortion controversy 25 years after* Roe v Wade: *A reader,* ed. L. P. Pojman and F. J. Beckwith, 354–69. Belmont, CA: Wadsworth.

———. 1998b. Why abortion is immoral. In *The abortion controversy 25 years after* Roe v. Wade: *A reader,* ed. L. P. Pojman and F. J. Beckwith, 320–37. Belmont, CA: Wadsworth.

Martin, J., M. Lloyd, and S. Sough. 2002. Professional attitudes: Can they be taught in medical education? *Clinical Medicine* 2 (3): 217–27.

Maslow, Abraham H. 1970. *Motivation and personality.* 2nd ed. New York: Harper and Row.

———. 1994. *Religions, values, and peak experiences.* New York: Viking.

Masters, William H., and Virginia Johnson. 1976. *The pleasure bond.* New York: Bantam Books.

Masters, William H., Virginia Johnson, and Robert Kolodny. 1986. *Masters and Johnson on sex and human loving.* Boston: Little, Brown.

Mathis, Stephen. 1997. *Reconstructive surgery: Principles, anatomy and techniques.* New York: Quality Medical Publications.

Maurer, Armand A. 1999. *The philosophy of William of Ockham in the light of its principles.* Toronto: Pontifical Institute of Medieval Studies.

May, Rollo. 1983. *Freedom and destiny.* New York: Dell Books.

May, William E. 1994. The management of ectopic pregnancies: A moral analysis. In *The fetal tissue issue: Medical and ethical aspects,* ed. Peter Cataldo and Albert Moraczewski, 121–48. Braintree, MA: Pope John XXIII Center.

———. 1995. *Introduction to moral theology.* Rev. ed. Huntington, IN: Our Sunday Visitor.

McArthur, John F., Jr., and Wayne A. Mack. 1997. *Introduction to biblical counseling: A basic guide to the principles and practice of counseling.* Dallas, TX: Word Pub.

McCarrick, Theodore. 2004. Interim reflections on the task force on Catholic politicians. *Origins* 34:7.

McCarthy, E. P., R. S. Phillips, Z. Zhong, and J. Lynn. 2000. Dying with cancer: Patient's function, symptoms, and care preferences as death approaches. *American Journal of Geriatric Society* 48 (5 suppl): S110–21.

McClory, Robert. 1995. *Turning point: The inside story of the papal birth control commission, and how* Humanae vitae *changed the life of Patty Crowley and the future of the church.* New York: Crossroad.

McCloskey, Elizabeth. 1991. The patient self determination act. *Kennedy Institute of Ethics Journal* 1 (2): 163–69.

McCormick, Richard A. 1973. *Ambiguity in moral choice.* Pere Marquette Theology Lecture. Milwaukee, WI: Marquette University.

———. 1990. The embryo debate 3: The first 14 days. *The Tablet,* March 10, 301.

———. 1991a. The pre-embryo as potential: A reply to John A Robertson. *Kennedy Institute of Ethics Journal* 1 (4): 303–5.

———. 1991b. Who or what is the pre-embryo? *Kennedy Institute of Ethics Journal* 1:1–15.

McCuen, Gary E., ed. 1998. *Human experimentation: When research is evil.* Hudson, WI: Gem Publications.

McDonald, J. C. 1988. The national organ procurement and transplantation network. *JAMA* 259: 725–26.

McFadden, Charles J. 1976. *Medical ethics.* 6th ed. Philadelphia: Davis.

McHugh, Paul. 1992. Psychiatric misadventures. *The American Scholar* 60–61: 497–510.

McInerny, Ralph. 1987. Fundamental option. In *Persona Verita Morale,* 427–34. Rome: Citta Nuova Editrice.

McMahon, Kevin, T. 2003. Emergency contraception in the treatment of rape victims. Consultation conducted by the Doctrine Committee of the USCCB, Pope John Paul II Cultural Center, Washington, DC, February 12. www.scs.edu/faculty/faculty_docs/mcmahon_rev_monsignor_kevin_t.htm

McManamy, John. (2005) Father of the lobotomy. www.mcmanweb.com/article-122.htm

McMinn, Mark R. 1991. *Cognitive therapy techniques in Christian counseling.* Nashville, TN: Thomas Nelson.

Medvedev, Roy A., and Zhores A. Medvedev. 1971. *A question of madness.* New York: Knopf.

Meier, Levi, ed. 1986. *Jewish values in bioethics.* New York: Human Services Press.

Melina, Livio. 2002. Faith in the incarnation, death, and resurrection of Jesus, and the culture of life. In *Culture of life, culture of death,* ed. Luke Gormally. London: Linacre Center for Health Care Ethics.

Menart, Teresa C. 2005. Morning after pill. www.omsoul.com/item329.html

Menninger, Karl. 1938. *Man against himself.* New York: Harcourt Brace.

———. 1958. *Theory of psychoanalytic technique: On transference.* New York: Basic Books.

Merkelbach, Benedictus. 1949. On cooperation. *Summa Theologiae Moralis.* 10th ed. Vol. 1, 487–92. Burge, Belgium: Desclee de Brouwer.

Merton, Robert. 1960. Some thoughts on the professions in American society. Presidential address, Brown University.

Meyer, J. K. et al. 1979. Sex reassignment: Follow up. *Archives of General Psychiatry* 36 (August): 1010–15.

Migliore, Archbishop Celestino. 2003. Creation of human beings for the purpose of destroying them. October 27. www.zenit.org/english/visualizza.phtml?sid=43521

Miller, D. F., and L. X. Aubin. 1940. *Saint Alphonsus Mary De' Liguori: Founder, Bishop, and Doctor (1696–1787). Saint Anne de Beaupre.* Quebec: Saint Alphonsus' Bookstore.

Miller, J. D. 1983. *National survey on drug abuse: Main findings.* Rockville, MD: National Institute of Drug Abuse.

Minogue, Brendon. 1996. *Bioethics: A committee approach.* Sudbury, MA: Jones & Bartlett.

Minois, G. 1999. *History of suicide.* Baltimore, MD: Johns Hopkins University Press.

Mitchell, T. M., 1997. *Machine learning.* New York: McGraw-Hill.

Mitford, Jessica. 2000. *The American way of death revisited.* New York: Vintage Books/Random House.

Moline, Jon. 1986. Professionals and professions: A philosophical examination of an ideal. *Social Science and Medicine* 22 (5): 501–8.

Monte, Christopher F. 1999. *Beneath the mask: An introduction to theories of personality.* 6th ed. New York: Harcourt Brace.

Monteleone, James A. 1981. The physiological aspects of sex. In *Human sexuality and personhood,* 71–85. St. Louis: Pope John XXIII Medical-Moral Research and Education Center.

Moore, Keith L. 1988. *The developing human: Clinically oriented embryology.* 4th ed. Philadelphia: Saunders.

Moore, Keith L., and T. V. N. Persaud. 2003. *Before we are born: Essentials of embryology and birth defects.* 6th ed. Philadelphia: W. B. Saunders.

Moore, Max. 1995. The diachronic self: Identity, continuity, transformation, a dissertation. www.maxmore.com/disscont.htm

Moore, Robert L. 1978. Ethics in the practice of psychiatry: Update on the results of enforcement of the code. *American Journal of Psychiatry* 142 (September): 1043–46.

Moraczewski, Albert. 1996. Managing tubal pregnancy: Part II. *Ethics and Medics* 21 (August): 8.

Moran, Frances M. 1997. *Listening: A pastoral style.* Alexandria, New South Wales, Australia: E. J. Dwyer.

Moreland, J. P. 1995. Humanness, personhood, and the right to die. *Faith and Philosophy* 12 (1): 95–112.

Moreland, J. P., and S. Rae. 2000. *Body and soul: Human nature and the crisis in ethics.* Downers Grove, IL: InterVarsity.

Moreno, Jonathan D. 1999. Ethics of research design. *Accountability in Research* 7 (2–4): 175–82.

Morowitz, Harold J., and James S. Trefil. 1992. *The facts of life: Science and the abortion controversy.* New York: Oxford University Press.

Morrison, James K., Bruce D. Layton, and Joan Newman. 1982. Ethical conflict among clinical psychologists and other mental health workers. *Psychological Reports* 51 (December): 703–15.

Mosgofian, Peter, and George Ohlschlager. 1995. *Sexual misconduct in counseling and ministry* Dallas, TX: Word Pub.

Moyers, Bill. 1993. *Healing and the mind.* New York: Doubleday.

Mullady, Brian. 1986. *The meaning of the term "moral" in St. Thomas Aquinas.* Rome: Libreria Editrice Vaticana.

Murnion, Philip. 1984. A sacramental church in a sacramental world. *Origins* 14 (6): 81–90.

Murphy, Ronald E. 1990. The tree of life: An exploration of biblical wisdom literature. New York: Anchor Bible Reference Library.

Murray, Joseph E. 1986. Decisions on the frontlines of surgery. *Harvard Medical Journal*, Boston: Harvard Medical School: 18–24.

Murray, J., and R. A. Pagon. 1984. Informed consent for research publication of patient related data. *Clinical Research* 32 (October): 404–8.

Naam, Ramez. 1995. *More than human: Embracing the promise of biological enhancement*. New York: Random House/Broadway Books.

NACC (National Association of Catholic Chaplains). 1993. Sacraments for the dying in the absence of a priest: Viaticum. *Ritual for laypersons: Rites for Holy Communion and the pastoral care of the sick and dying*, 7–8. Collegeville: Liturgical Press.

———. 1995. Shared statement of identity for the catholic health ministry. www.nacc.org/

———. 1996. Report of NCCB Subcommittee on Lay Ministry. *Lay ecclesial ministry: The state of the question*. www.usccb.org/laity/laymin/updates/01summer.shtml

Nakken, Craig. 1997. *The addictive personality: Understanding the addictive process and compulsive behavior*. Rev. ed. Center City, MN: Hazelden Publishing and Educational Services.

NaPro Technology. 2005. www.fertilitycare.org/nptech.html

Nash, George. 1976. *The Conservative Intellectual Movement in America since 1945*. New York: Basic Books.

National Institute of Drug Abuse. 1986. *Drug use among American high school students and other young adults*. Washington, DC: U.S. Department of Health and Human Services.

National Organization of Mothers of Twins Clubs. 2005. Is the incidence of multiple births increasing? www.nomotc.org/newsroom_pdf/increasing_incidence_of_multiple_births_release. pdf

Natural Death Center. 2003. *The natural death handbook*. London: National Death Center. www.growthhouse.org/links.html

Natural Family Planning Site. 2004. www.bygpub.com/natural/natural-family-planning.htm

NBAC (National Bioethics Advisory Commission). 2001. *Ethical and policy issues in research involving human participants*. Vol. II, Commissioned papers, J1–J33. Federal agency survey on policies and procedures for the protection of human subjects in research.

NCBC (National Catholic Bioethics Center). 2004. Statement on Pope John Paul's address on nutrition and hydration. April 23, 2004, Philadelphia. www.ncbcenter.org

NCCB (National Conference of Catholic Bishops). 1992. *Nutrition and hydration: Moral and pastoral reflections*. Committee for Pro-Life Activities. www.usccb.org/prolife/issues/euthanas/nutindex.htm

———. 1996. Committee on doctine. Moral principles concerning infants with anencephaly. *Origins* 26 (17): 276.

———. 2001. *Ethical and Religious Directives for Catholic Health Care Services*. 4th ed. www.usccb.org/bishops/directives.shtml

Neuger, Christie Cozad. 2001. *Counseling women: A narrative, pastoral approach*. New York: Haworth Pastoral Press.

Nevin, Norman C. 1999. Ethical issues in gene therapy. In *Understanding gene therapy*, ed. N. R. Lemoine, 155–62. Oxford: BIOS Scientific Publishers.

Nichols, Aidan. 1990. *From Newman to Congar*. London: T & T Clark.

NIH (National Institutes of Health). 1985. Consensus conference: Electroconvulsive therapy. *JAMA* 254 (October 18): 2105–8.

———. 1987. *Human somatic cell gene therapy prospects for treating inherited diseases*. Washington, DC: National Institutes of Health.

———. 1994. *Report of the human embryo research panel*. Bethesda, MD: National Institutes of Health.

———. 1999. Repetitive transcranial stimulation. *Journal ECT* 1 (March): 39–59.

———. 2000. *Stem cells: A primer.* Bethesda, MD: National Institutes of Health.

Noonan, John T. 1965. *Contraception: A history of its treatment by the Catholic theologians and canonists.* New York: Harvard University Press.

———. 1970. An almost absolute value in history. In *The morality of abortion*, ed. J. T. Noonan Jr., 59. Cambridge, MA: Harvard University Press.

Nouwen, Henri M. J. 1979. *The wounded healer.* New York: Image Books.

Oates, Wayne E. 1985. *Grief, transition, and loss: A pastor's practical guide.* Philadelphia: Westminster Press.

———. 1997. *Behind the masks: Personality disorders in religious behavior.* Minneapolis, MN: Fortress Press.

O'Brien, Mary Ellen. 2001. *Living well and dying well: A sacramental view of life and death.* Franklin, WI: Sheed and Ward.

O'Connor, P. G., and A. Spickard. 1997. Physician impairment by substance abuse. *Medical Clinics of North America* 81(4): 1037–52.

O'Donnell, James J., and Allan Fitzgerald. 1999. *St. Augustine through the ages: An encyclopedia.* Grand Rapids, MI: Eerdmans.

O'Donnell, T. J. 1957. *Medicine and Christian morality.* Boston: St. Paul Press. (Reprint 1996.)

O'Donnell, Thomas. 1987. Fatal pathology, not removal of life support. *Medical Moral Newsletter,* February.

OHSR (Office of Human Services Research). 2002. Protection of human subjects. www.hhs.gov/ohrp/humansubjects/guidance/45cfr46.htm

Oldham, L. H. 1999. Attitude change in response to information that male homosexuality has a biological cause. *Journal of Sex and Marital Therapy* 2 (2): 12–124.

Olick, Robert S. 2001. *Taking advance directives seriously: Prospective autonomy and decisions near the end of life.* Washington, DC: Georgetown University Press.

O'Meara, Thomas. 1997. *Thomas Aquinas, theologian.* Notre Dame, IN: University of Notre Dame Press.

———. 2000. *Theology of ministry.* 2nd ed. New York: Paulist Press.

OPTN. (Organ Procurement Transplantation Network). 2005. Data. www.optn.org/data

O'Rahilly, Ronan, and Fabiola Muller. 1994. *Human embryology and teratology.* New York: John Wiley and Sons.

Ordanoz, Teofilo, ed. 1960. *Francisco de Vitoria OP, Relictio de temperant a obres: Reflectiones Theologiae.* Vol. 3. Madrid: Biblioteca de Autores Christianos.

Ornstein, Paul, and Jerald Kay. 1985. Ethical problems in the psychotherapy of the suicidal patient. *Psychiatric Annals* 13 (April): 332–40.

O'Rourke, Kevin. 1988. Physician competency: Whose responsibility? June, IX: 10. St. Louis, MO: St. Louis University Medical Center. www.op.org.DomCentral/study/kor/index.htm

———. 1996a. Health care models: New and old. Op. ed. *St. Louis Post Dispatch,* February 16, 6C.

———. 1996b. Ethical opinions in regard to early delivery of anencephalic infants. *Linacre Quarterly,* August, 55–59.

———. 2002. Catholic health care and sterilization. *Health Progress* (November–December): 43–48.

———. 2003. Catholic health care and sterilization. *Health Progress* (November–December): 43.

———. 2004. Stem cell research: Prospects and problems. *National Catholic Bioethics Quarterly* 4 (Summer): 289–99.

———. 2006. The embryo as person. *National Catholic Bioethics Quarterly* 6 (Summer): 1–12.

Panicola, Michael. 2003. Organ retrieval after cardiac death. Unpublished essay in response to editorial in St. Louis Review May 23. *St. Louis Review,* June.

Parens, Erik. 1998. *Enhancing human traits: Ethical and social implications.* Washington, DC: Georgetown Press.

Parfit, Derek. 1984. *Reasons and persons.* Oxford: Oxford University Press.

Parker, Michael, and Anneke Lucassen. 2002. Working towards ethical management of genetic testing. *Lancet* 360 (November 23): 1685–88.

Paul VI. 1968. *Humanae vitae: Encyclical letter on the regulation of births.* Washington, DC: USCC.

———. 1972. *Apostolic constitution on anointing the sick.* November 30. *Catechism of the Catholic Church,* 1512. Vatican City: Liberia Vaticana.

PCB (President's Council on Bioethics). 2002. *Human cloning and human dignity, an ethical inquiry.* Washington, DC: U.S. Government Printing Office.

———. 2003. *Beyond therapy: Biotechnology and the pursuit of happiness.* Washington, DC: U.S. Government Printing Office.

———. 2004a. *Monitoring stem cell research.* Washington, DC: U.S. Government Printing Office.

———. 2004b. *Reproduction and responsibility.* Washington, DC: U.S. Government Printing Office.

———. 2005. *Taking care: Ethical caring in our aging society.* Washington, DC: U.S. Government Printing Office.

PCEMR (President's Commission for the Study of Ethical Problems in Medicine and Biomedical and Behavioral Research). 1981. *Report on the definition of death legislation.* Washington, DC: U.S. Government Printing Office.

Pellegrino, Edmund D. 1987. Altruism, self-interest and medical ethics. *JAMA* 258 (14): 1139–40.

———. 1989. Character, virtue and self-interest in the ethics of the professions. *Journal of Contemporary Health Law and Policy* 5 (Spring): 53–73.

———. 1991. Trust and distrust in professional ethics. In *Ethics, trust and the professions,* ed. E. D. Pellegrino, R. Veatch, and J. Langan, 69–85. Washington, DC: Georgetown University Press.

———. 1992. Character and the ethical conduct of research. *Accountability in Research* 2(1): 1–11.

———. 2002. The physician's conscience, conscience clauses, and religious belief: A Catholic perspective. *Fordham Urban Law Journal* 30 (1): 221–44.

Pellegrino, Edmund D., and David C. Thomasma. 1981. *What is medicine? A philosophical basis of medical practice.* New York: Oxford University Press.

———. 1988. *For the patient's good: The restoration of beneficence in health care.* New York: Oxford University Press.

Pemico, Giacomo. 1993. La civilta Catolica (July 3). *Davenport and Catholic Messenger,* July 10, 1.

Penrose, Roger. 1995. *Shadows of the mind: A search for the missing science of consciousness.* New York: Oxford University Press.

Percival, Thomas. [1803] 1927. *Percival's medical ethics.* Ed. Chauncey D. Leake. Baltimore: Williams and Wilkins.

Perez-Carceles, M. D., M. A. Esteban, E. Osuna, and A. Luna. 1999. Medical personnel and death. *Medicine and Law: World Association for Medical Law* 18 (4): 497–504.

Perl, Mark, and Earl Shelp. 1982. Psychiatric consultation: Masking moral dilemmas in medicine. *New England Journal of Medicine* 307 (14): 618–21.

Pernick, Martin S. 1997. Eugenics and public health in American history. *American Journal of Public Health* 87 (November): 1767–72.

Perry, David L. 2005. Abortion and personhood: History and comparative notes. home.earthlink.net/~davidperry/abortion.htm

Perry, Joshua, Larry R. Churchill, and Howard S. Kirshner. 2005. The Terri Schiavo case: Legal, ethical, and medical perspectives. *Annals of Internal Medicine* 143 (10): 744–48.

Perry, Ralph. 1980. *General theory of value.* Cambridge, MA: Harvard University Press.

Persson, Ingmar. 2002. Human death: A view from the beginning. *Bioethics* 16 (February): 20–32.

Peterson, James C. 2001. *Genetic turning points: The ethics of human genetic intervention.* Grand Rapids, MI: Eerdmans.

Pew Commission. 1993. *Contemporary issues in health professions education and workforce reform.* San Francisco: Center for Health Professions, University of California.

———. 1995. *Critical challenges: Revitalizing the health professions for the 21st century.* San Francisco: Center for Health Profession, University of California.

Philosophers' Brief. 1997. *New York Review of Books,* May 21.

Pieper, Josef. 1966. *Four cardinal virtues.* Notre Dame, IN: University of Notre Dame Press.

Pierce v. Swan Point Cemetery. 1872. 10 Rhode Island 227.

Pinckaers, Servais. 1995. *The sources of Christian ethics.* 3rd ed. Washington, DC: Catholic University of America Press.

———. 2002. *Morality: The Catholic view.* South Bend, IN: St. Augustine Press.

Pincus, H. A., T. L. Tanielian, and S. C. Marcus. 1998. Prescribing Trends in Psychotropic Medications. *JAMA* 279 (February): 526–31.

Pinker, Steven. 2002. *The blank slate: The modern denial of human nature.* New York: Viking Press.

Pius XI. 1930. Quadregesimo anno, no. 184. www.vatican.va/holy_father/pius_xi/encyclicals/documents/hf_p-xi_enc_19310515_quadragesimo-anno_en.html

Pius XII. 1944. Allocution to the Italian medical-biological union of St. Luke. (Nov 12). *The human body: Papal teachings.* Boston: St Paul Editions. 1979 [1960], nos. 165–79.

———. 1952. Allocution to the first international congress of histopatholory. (September 14). *The human body: Papal teachings.* Boston: St. Paul Editions.

———. 1956. Allocution to a group of eye specialists, May 14. *The human body: Papal teachings.* Boston: St. Paul Editions [1960], nos. 637–49.

———. 1958. Prolongation of life (November 24, 1957). *The Pope speaks* 4 (4): 395–96. Reprinted in *Origins,* 2004, 33(43).

Plomp, Karen. 2000. Large families FAQ. www.plomp.com/largefam/comebacks.htm

Poddimatam, Feliz. 1986. *Fundamental option and mortal sin.* Bangalore: Asian Trading Corp.

Ponnuru, Ramesh. 2005. Learning from teratomas, II. www.techcentralstation.com/121004C.html

Pontifical Academy of Life. 2001. *Prospects for xenotransplantation: Scientific aspects and ethical considerations.* Vatican City: Lebreria Editrice Vaticana.

Pontifical Academy of Sciences. 1985. Clinical determination of death. *Origins* (February): 3.

Pontifical Council for Pastoral Assistance to Health Care Workers. 1995. Charter for Health Care Workers. www.wf-f.org/healthcarecharter.html

Porter, Jean. 1990. *The recovery of virtue: The relevance of Aquinas for Christian ethics.* Louisville, KY: Westminster/John Knox Press.

———. 1995a. *Moral action: Christian ethics.* New York: Cambridge University Press.

———. 1995b. Individuality, personal identity, and the moral status of the preembryo: A response to Mark Johnson. *Theological Studies* 56:763–70.

———. 2002. Is the embryo a person? Arguing with the Catholic traditions. *Commonwealth,* 8. www.pfaith.org/catholic.htm

Porter, Roy, ed. 2001. *The Cambridge illustrated history of medicine.* Cambridge: Cambridge University Press.

Potter, Van Rensselaer. 1971. *Bioethics: Bridge to the future.* Englewood Cliffs, NJ: Prentice Hall.

Powell, Robert C. 2000. *Whatever happened to CPE?* Princeton, NJ: Princeton University Press. www.pastoralreport.com/the_archives/1999/03/whatever_happen.html

Prentice, Ernest D., and Bruce G. Gordon. 2001. Institutional review board assessment of risks and benefits associated with research. In *National Bioethics Advisory Commission. Ethical and policy issues in research involving human participants.* Vol. II: Commissioned papers. Rockville, MD: National Bioethics Advisory Commission. L1–L16.

Prummer, Dominicus M. 1958. *Manuale Theologiae Moralis.* 14th ed. Vol. 1. Barcelona: Herder.

Quill, Timothy E. 2000. Initiating end-of-life discussions with seriously ill patients: Addressing the "elephant in the room." *JAMA* 284 (November 15): 2502–27.

Quinlan, John. 2002. *Pastoral relatedness: The essence of pastoral care.* Lanham, MD: University Press of America.

Quitkin, Frederic M., ed. 1998. *Current psychiatric drugs.* 2nd ed. Arlington, VA: American Psychiatric.

———. 1999. Placebos, drug effects, and study design: A clinician's guide. *American Journal of Psychiatry* 156 (June): 829–36.

Rachels, James. 1986. *The elements of moral philosophy.* New York: Random House.

Radical Academy. 2000. The human person. www.radicalacademy.com/adiphilcritperson1.htm

Rahner, Karl. 1963. The church and the sacraments. In *Questiones Disputatae,* no. 9. New York: Herder and Herder.

———. 1965. *On the theology of death.* New York: Herder and Herder.

———. 1972. The problem of genetic manipulation. In *Theological investigations.* New York: Sabor Press.

Ramsay, Sarah. 1996. *Transsexuals: Candid answers to private questions.* Dalinghurst, Australia: Crossing Press.

———. 2000. Enforced sterilization in Sweden confirmed. *Lancet* 355 (April 8): 1232.

Ramsey, Paul. 1970. *The patient as person: Explorations in medical ethics.* New Haven: Yale University Press.

Rawls, John. 1971. *A theory of justice.* Cambridge, MA: Belknap Press of Harvard University Press.

Ray, Oakley, and Charles Ksir. 2003. *Drugs, society, and human behavior.* New York: McGraw-Hill.

Reardon, Donald C. 1994. Informed consent: The abortion industry's Achilles heel. *The Post Abortion Review* 2 (Spring/Summer): 2.

Reilly, Phillip R. 1991. *The surgical solution: A history of involuntary sterilization in the United States.* Baltimore, MD: John Hopkins University Press.

Reiner, William G. 1996. Sex reassignment on a teenage girl. *Journal of the American Academy of Child and Adolescent Psychiatry* 35 (June): 799–803.

Reiner, William G., and John P. Geaarhart. 2004. Discordant sexual identity in some genetic males with cloacal exstrophy assigned to female sex at birth. *New England Journal of Medicine* 350 (January): 333–41.

Reiser, Stanley. 1993. The era of the patient: Using the experience of illness in shaping the mission of health care. *JAMA* 269 (8): 1012–17.

Reiss, Michael J. 1999. What sort of people do we want: The ethics of changing people through genetic engineering. *Notre Dame Journal of Law, Ethics and Public Policy* 13 (1): 63–92.

Resnik, David B. 2003. Exploitation in biomedical research. *Theoretical Medicine and Bioethics* 24 (3): 233–59.

Restak, Richard M. 1975. *Pre-meditated man: Bioethics and the control of future human life.* New York: Viking Press.

Revel, Michel. 2000. Research on animal cloning technologies and their implications in medical ethics: An update. *Medicine and Law: World Association for Medical Law* 19 (3): 527–43.

Rice, Charles E. 1999. Abortion, euthanasia, and the need to build a new "culture of life." *Notre Dame Journal of Law, Ethics and Public Policy* 12 (2): 497–528.

Rich, Warren Thomas, ed. 1995. *Encyclopedia of bioethics,* rev. ed. New York: Simon and Schuster Macmillan.

Rieff, Philip. 1968. *The triumph of the therapeutic: Uses of faith after Freud.* New York: Harper and Rowe.

Rigali, Justin. 2003. Organ donation and definition of death. Editorial: *St. Louis Review.* May 23.

Roberts, Celia. 2000. Biological behavior? Hormones, psychology, and sex. *National Women's Studies Association Journal* 12 (3): 1–20. http://muse.jhu.edu/journals/nwsa_journal/v012/12.3roberts.html

Roberts, Judy C. 1997. The myth of confidentiality. www.academyprojects.org/lerobe1.htm

Robertson, John A. 2002. Sex selection: Final word from the ASRM ethics committee on the use of PGD. *Hastings Center Report* 32 (March–April): 6.

Robinson, James. 2001. The end of managed care. *JAMA* 285(20): 2622–28.

Roe v. Wade. 1973. www.tourolaw.edu/patch/Roe

Rokeach, Milton. 1973. *The nature of human values.* New York: Free Press.

Rosenfield, Israel. 1995. *The strange, familiar, and forgotten: An anatomy of consciousness.* New York: Vintage.

Rosner, Fred. 2001. *Biomedical ethics and Jewish law.* NY: Ktav Publishing House.

Ross, Judith Wilson. 1994. Spirit, emotion, and meaning: The many voices of bioethics—Literature, bioethics and the priestly physician. *Hastings Center Report* 24 (3): 25–26.

Ross, Sarah. 2005. *Doctors, drink and drugs. Christian medical fellowship booklet.* London. www.cmf.org.uk/literature/doctors_drink_and_drugs.htm

Rothman, David J. 1980. *Conscience and convenience: The asylum and its alternatives in progressive America.* Boston: Little, Brown.

———. 1998. The international organ traffic. *New York Review of Books* 45 (March 26): 14–17.

Rowland, Christopher, ed. 1999. *The Cambridge companion to liberation theology.* Cambridge: Cambridge University Press.

Royal Society (Great Britain). 2000. *Therapeutic cloning: A submission by the Royal Society to the Chief Medical Officer's expert group.* London: Royal Society.

———. 2002. *Human reproductive cloning: A statement by the Royal society.* London: Royal Society. December 2. www.royalsoc.ac.uk

Rubenstein, R. E. 2003. *Aristotle's children.* Orlando, FL: Harcourt.

Ruzek, Sheryl Burt, Virginia L. Olesen, and Adele E. Clarke, eds. 1997. *Women's health: Complexities and differences.* Columbus, OH: Ohio State University Press.

Sabbatini, Renato. 2004. The history of psychosurgery. www.nobel.se/medicine/articles/moniz/#8

Sadler, Alfred, Jr., B. L. Sadler, and E. B. Stason. 1968. The uniform anatomical gift act. *JAMA* 206:2501–6.

SAMHSA. *Results from the 2001 national household survey on drug abuse: Emergency department trends from the drug abuse warning network, preliminary estimates January to June 2001, with revised estimates, 1994–2000, 2002.* National Institute on Drug Abuse, Prescription Drug Abuse and Addiction, 2001. U.S. Department of Health and Human Services and National Clearinghouse for Alcohol and Drug Information. http://ncadi.samhsa.gov/govpubs/prevalert/v7/4.aspxC

Sande, Ken. 2004. *Peacemaker: A biblical guide to resolving personal conflict.* 3rd ed. Grand Rapids, MI: Baker.

Santamaria, B.A. 1988. *Humanae vitae* twenty years later. www.ad2000.com.au/articles/1988/jul1988p3_563.html

Satinover, Jeffry. 1996. *Homosexuality and the politics of truth.* Grand Rapids, MI: Baker Books.

Schiavo, Michael, with Michael Hirsch. 2006. *Terri: The truth.* New York: Dutton.

Schiff, Nicolas, and Joseph Fins. 2003. Hope for "comatose" patients. *Cerebrum* 5 (Fall): 7–24.

Schmid, Donald, P. S. Appelbaum, L. H. Roth, and C. Lidz. 1983. Confidentiality in psychiatry: A study of the patient's views. *Hospital and Community Psychiatry* 34 (April): 353–55.

Schnackenburg, Rudolf. 1973. *The moral teaching of the New Testament.* New York: Seabury.

Schrage, Wolfgang. 1988. *The ethics of the New Testament.* Philadelphia: Fortress Press.

Schwartz, Stephen D. 1990. *The moral question of abortion.* Chicago: Loyola University Press.

Schwartz, Stephen D., and R. K. Tacelli. 1989. Abortion and some philosophers: A critical examination. *Public Affairs Quarterly* 3:81–98.

Selling, Joseph A., and Jan Jans. 1995. The splendor of accuracy: An examination of the assertions made by *Veritatis Splendor.* Grand Rapids, MI: Eerdmans.

Settlage, Diane S., M. Motoshima, and D. R. Tredway. 1973. Sperm transport from the external cervical to the fallopian tubes in woman: A time and quantitation study. *Fertility and Sterility* 24 (September): 655–61.

Seyfer, Tina L. 2003. Medical and ethical concerns over I.V.F. *Ethics and Medics* 28 (August): 8.

Sgreccia, Elio, Don Maurizio Calipari, and Marialuisa Lavitrano. 2001. Church backing depends on ethical use of animals (letter). *Nature* (December 13): 687.

Shaller, D.V., R. S. Sharpe, and R. D. Rubin. 1998. A national action plan to meet health care quality information needs in the age of managed care. *JAMA* 279:1254–58.

Shannon, Thomas A., and James J. Walter. 2004. Implications of the Papal allocution on feeding tubes. *Hastings Center Report* 34 (July–August): 4.

Shannon, Thomas, and Alan Wolter. 1990. Reflections on the moral status of the pre-embryo. *Theological Studies* 51:603–26.

Shapiro, Larry, D. E. Comings, O. W. Jones, and D. L. Rimoin. 1986. New frontiers in genetic medicine. *Annals of Internal Medicine* 104 (April): 527–39.

Sharp, Leslie A. 1995. Organ transplantation as transformative experience. *Medical Anthropology Quarterly* 9:357–89.

Sharpe-Stimac, Monica, Ying Wang, Charlotte M. Druschel, and Philip K. Cross. 2004. Follow-up survey of parents of children with major birth defects in New York State. In *Birth defects research: From surveillance to epidemiology to prevention,* ed. Russell E. Kirby and Robert E. Meyer. Special issue of *Clinical and Molecular Teratology* 70 (9): 597–602.

Shea, J. B. 2004. The morning after pill. http://catholicinsight.com/online/bioethics/printer_mornpill.shtml

Sheehan, Myles N. 2000. On dying well: How does one live spiritually in the hope of dying well? *America* 183 (July 29–August 5): 12–15.

———. 2005. Catholic health care and physicians: Who are we? An audio presentation. www.nacc.org/

Shelton, Deborah L. 2005. Series on organ donation. *St. Louis Post-Dispatch,* May 6–12. www.STLtoday.com/organs

Shewmon, Alan. 2001. The brain and somatic interaction. *Journal of Medicine and Philosophy* 26 (5): 457–78.

Shivanandan, Marie. 1997. *Crossing the threshold of love: Contemporary marriage in the light of John Paul II's anthropology.* Edinburgh: T & T Clark.

Sider, Roger C. 1983. Mental health norms and ethical practice. *Psychiatric Annals* 13 (April): 302–9.

Sieber, Joan E. 2001. Privacy and confidentiality: As related to human research in social and behavioral science. In *National Bioethics Advisory Commission. Ethical and policy issues in research involving human participants.* Vol. 2, Commissioned papers. N1–N50. Rockville, MD: National Bioethics Advisory Commission.

Siegal, Eric, and Robert Orr. 1995. Should religiously oriented health care facilities name members with opposing views? *HEC Forum* 7 (November): 6.

Sigerist, Henry E. 1951. *History of medicine.* New York: Oxford University Press.

Silver, L. 1997. *Remaking Eden: Cloning and beyond in a brave new world.* New York: Avon Books.

Siminoff, Laura A., and Matthew D. Leonard. 1999. Financial incentives: Alternatives to the altruistic model of organ donation. *Journal of Medicine and Philosophy* 9 (December): 250–6.

Simpson, Joe Leigh, and Sandra Ann Carson. 2002. Sex selection. In *Assisted reproductive technologies: Current accomplishments and new horizons,* ed. C. De Jonge and C. Barratt, 384–96. Cambridge: Cambridge University Press.

Singer, Peter. 1975. *Animal liberation.* New York: Avon Books.

———. 2000. *Animal liberation.* Uniondale, NY: Hearst.

Singer, Peter, and Helga Kuhse. 1988. The ethics of embryo research. *Law, Medicine and Health Care* 14:13–14. Answer by Gavin J. Fairbairn. 1988. Kuhse, Singer and slippery slopes. *Journal of Medical Ethics* 14:134.

Skinner, B. F. 1971. *Beyond freedom and dignity.* New York: Alfred A. Knopf.

———. 1976. *About behaviorism.* New York: Random House.

———. 1985. *A matter of consequences.* New York: University Press.

Skocpol, Theda. 1996. *Boomerang: Clinton's health security effort and the turn against government in U.S. politics.* New York: W. W. Norton.

Smart, R. G., and G. F. Murray. 1985. Narcotic drug abuse in 153 countries: Social and economic factors as predictors. *International Journal of Addiction* 20: 737–49.

Smith, Janet E. 1988. Paul VI as prophet: Have *Humanae vitae's* bold predictions come true? www.goodmorals.org

———. 1991. *Humanae vitae: A generation later.* Washington, DC: Catholic University of America Press. http://omsoul.com

———. 1993. *Why Humanae vitae was right: A reader.* San Francisco: Ignatius Press.

Smith, Mickey. 1991. *Social history of the minor tranquilizers: The quest for small comfort in the age of anxiety.* Binghamton, NY: Haworth Press.

Smith, Quentin. 1997. *Ethical and religious thought in analytic philosophy of language.* New Haven, CT: Yale University Press.

Smith, Tom W. 2003. American sexual behavior: Trends, socio-demographic differences, and risk behavior. National Opinion Research Center. Chicago: University of Chicago. www.norc.uchicago.edu/library/sexual.pdf

Snaith, R. 1994. Transsexualism and gender reassignment. *British Journal of Psychiatry* 165 (September): 419–29.

Snow, C. P. 1999. *The two cultures.* 2nd ed. (with an introduction by Stefan Collini). Cambridge: Cambridge University Press. (Originally published 1959.)

Solomon, L., J. Landrogan, C. Flynn, and G. C. Benjamin. 1999. Barriers to HIV testing and confidentiality: The concerns of HIV positive and high risk individuals. *AIDS Public Policy* 14 (4): 147–56.

Sparks, Anne. 1988. Rape crisis programs help restore dignity and control. *Health Progress* 69 (September): 68–72.

Sparks, Richard C. 1997. *Helping Catholic couples conceive.* www.americancatholic.org/Messenger/Apr1997/feature1.asp#F7

Sprague, Robert. 1978. Principles of clinical trials ands social ethical and legal issues of drug use in children. In *Pediatric psychopharmacology: The use of behavior modifying drugs in children,* ed. John S. Werry. New York: Brunner/Mazel.

Stanton, Judith, and Woody Caan. 2003. How many doctors are sick? *British Medical Journal* 326:S97a.

Steinfels, Peter. 1994. Psychiatrist and Pope discuss end to longtime hostility. *New York Times,* January 3.

———. 2003. *A people adrift: The crisis of the Roman Catholic Church in America.* New York: Simon and Schuster.

Steinhoff-Smith, Roy Herndon. 1999. *The mutuality of care.* St. Louis, MO: Chalice Press.

Steinman, Theodore. 2002. A dangerous argument against organ donation. *National Catholic Bioethics Quarterly* 4 (Autumn): 473–78.

Stevens, M. L. Tina. 2000. *Bioethics in America: Origins and cultural politics.* Baltimore, MD: John Hopkins University Press.

Stevens, Rosemary. 2001. Public roles for the medical profession: Beyond theories of decline and fall. *Millbank Quarterly* 7913 (September): 327.

Stevenson-Moessner, Jeanne, ed. 1996. *Through the eyes of women: Insights for pastoral care (The handbook of women care).* Minneapolis, MN: Augsburg Fortress.

Stock, G. 2002. *Redesigning humans: Our inevitable genetic future.* New York: Houghton Mifflin.

Stone, Deborah. 1999. Managed care and the second great transformation. *Journal of Health Politics, Policy and Law* 24:1213–18.

Stone, Howard W. 2001. *Strategies for brief pastoral counseling.* Minneapolis, MN: Fortress Press.

Stover, Eric, and Elena Nightengale, eds. 1985. *The breaking of bodies and minds: Torture, psychiatric abuse, and the health professions.* New York: W. H. Freeman.

Stretton, Dean. 2002. Essential properties and the right to life. *Bioethics* 18 (June): 264–82.

———. 2003. The fallacy of essential moral personhood. www.tip.net.au/~dean/femp.html

Stromberg, B., G. Dahlquist, A. Ericson, O. Finnstrom, M. Koster, and K. Stjernquist. 2002. Neurological sequelae in children born after in-vitro fertilization: A population-based study. *Lancet* 359 (February 9): 461–65.

Suarez, Antoine. 1990. Hydatidiform moles and teratomas confirm the human identity of the pre-implantation embryo. *Journal of Medicine and Philosophy* 15:627–35.

Sugar, M. 1995. A clinical approach to childhood gender identity disorder. *American Journal of Psychotherapy* 49 (Spring): 260–81.

Suits, G. Steven. 2005. Ensoulment and the sacredness of human life. www.palmettofamily.org/bioethic.htm

Sullivan, Francis. 1983. *Magisterium and teaching authority in the Catholic Church.* Dublin: Gill and Macmillan.

Sullivan, Scott. 1995. A brief survey of contemporary Catholic arguments on immediate versus delayed animation. www.vanderbilt.edu/SFL/scott_sullivan.htm

Sulmasy, Daniel P. 2006. End of life care revisited, *Health Progress*, August, 50–56.

Sultan, Charles, et al. 2002a. Ambiguous genitalia in the newborn. *Reproductive Medicine* 20:181–88.

———. 2002b. Ambiguous genitalia in the newborn: Diagnosis, etiology and sex assignment. In *Pediatric and adolescent gynecology: Evidence-based clinical practice,* Vol. 7, ed. Charles Sultan, 23–38. New York: Basel Karger.

Swartz, Katherine. 1999. The death of managed care as we know it. *Journal of Health Politics, Policy and Law* 24:1201–5.

Sytsma, Sharon. 1996. Anencephalics as organ sources. *Theoretical Medicine and Bioethics* 17 (March): 19–32.

Szasz, Thomas. 1974. *The myth of mental illness.* Rev. ed. New York: Harper and Row. (Originally published 1961.)

———. 1982. The psychiatric will: A new mechanism for protecting persons against psychosis and psychiatry. *American Psychologist* 37 (July): 762–70.

———. 1987. *Insanity: The idea and its consequences.* New York: John Wiley and Sons.

———. 1998. The ethics of psychoanalysis. *Society* 35 (January/February): 16–21.

Szubka, T., and R. Warner, eds. 1994. *The mind–body problem: A guide to the current debate.* Oxford: Blackwell.

Tacelli, Ron. 2005. Were you a zygote? www.archindy.org/prolife/zygote.htm

Tauer, Carol. 1985. Personhood and human embryos and fetuses. *Journal of Medicine and Philosophy* 10 (3): 253–66.

Taylor, James Stacey. 2002. Autonomy, constraining options and organ sales. *Journal of Applied Philosophy* 19 (3): 273–85.

Taylor, Michael A. 1982. Human generation in the thought of Thomas Aquinas: A case study on the role of biological fact. *Theological Science*, February, 461–65.

Taylor-Corbett, Shaun. 2000. *Embryo research: Profit vs. ethics?* Washington, DC: Center for Public Integrity. www.publicintegrity.org/genetics/report.aspx?aid=325

Theological Commission (International). 1976. *Thesis on the relationship between the ecclesiastical magisterium and theology.* Washington, DC: U.S. Catholic Conference.

Thomasma, David C. 1994. Telling the truth to patients: A clinical ethics exploration. *Cambridge Quarterly of Healthcare Ethics* 3 (3): 375–82.

Thomasma, David C., and Thomasine Kushner, eds. 1996. *Birth to death: Science and bioethics.* Cambridge: Cambridge University Press.

Thompson, S. Anthony. 2002. My research friend? My friend the researcher? My friend, my researcher? Mis/informed consent and people with developmental disabilities. In *Walking the tightrope: Ethical issues for qualitative researchers*, ed. Will van den Hoonaard, 95–106. Toronto: University of Toronto Press.

Thomson, Judith Jarvis. 1971. A defense of abortion. *Philosophy and Public Affairs* (Fall): 47–66.

Thorup, Oscar, et al. 1985. High tech cardiology-issues and costs: A panel discussion. *Pharos* 48 (Summer): 31–37.

Timmons, Mark. 2002. *Kant's metaphysics of morals: Interpretative essays.* New York: Oxford University Press.

Tong, Rosemarie. 1997. *Feminist approaches to bioethics: Theoretical reflections and practical applications.* Boulder, CO: Westview Press.

Tooley, Michael. 1974. Abortion and infanticide. In *The rights and wrongs of abortions*, ed. Marshall Cohen, Thomas Nagel, and Thomas Scanlon, 59, 64, 94. Princeton, NJ: Princeton University Press.

———. 1983. *Abortion and infanticide.* Oxford: Oxford University Press.

Topper, Charles. 2003. *Spirituality in pastoral counseling and the community helping professions.* New York: Haworth Pastoral Press.

Torrell, J. P. 1996. *St. Thomas Aquinas. Vol. 1, The person and his work.* Washington, DC: Catholic University of America Press.

Torrey, E. Fuller. 1972. *The mind game: Witchdoctors and psychiatrists.* New York: Bantam Books.

Trent, R. J. 1993. *Molecular medicine.* New York: Churchill Livingston.

Trimpey, Jack. 1997. *Rational recovery: The new cure for substance abuse.* New York: Pocket Books.

Turnquist, Arlynne. 1983. The issue of informed consent and the use of neuroleptic medications. *International Journal of Nursing Studies* 20 (3): 181–16.

UDDA. 2005. Uniform definition of death act. Uniform Law Commissioners. 1980. www.ascensionhealth.org/ethics/public/issues/udda.asp

Udry, J. Richard. 1995. Policy and ethical implications of biosocial research. *Population Research and Policy Review* 14 (September): 347–57.

Uniform Anatomical Gift Act. 1968. An act authorizing the gift of all or part of a human body after death for specified purposes. National Conference of Commissioners on Uniform State Laws.

United Nations. 1948. *Universal declaration of human rights.* New York: United Nations Publications.

University of Kansas Medical Center. 2002. *Hospital ethics handbook.* 5th ed. www.kumc.edu/hospital/ethics/ethics.htm

Ursano, Robert, and Robert Silberman. 1988. Individual psychotherapies. In *Textbook of psychiatry*, ed. John Talbott, Robert Hales, and Stuart Yudofsky, 855–91. Washington, DC: American Psychiatric Press.

USCC (United States Catholic Conference). 1979. *The deacon, minister of word and sacrament.* Washington, DC: USCC.

———. 1995. Remarks on the Christian coalition's catholic allegiance. *Origins* 25 (25): 417–30.

———. 1998. Resolution on health care. *Origins* 23 (7): 97–102.

———. 2001. *Ethical and religious directives for Catholic health services.* Washington, DC: USCC. www.usccb.org/bishops/directives.shtml

U.S. General Accounting Office (GAO). 1987. *Medical malpractice: Characteristics of claims closed in 1984.* Washington DC: U.S. General Accounting Office.

U.S. Population Pyramids. 2005. Population of the United States, by age and sex, 1950–2050. www.ac.wwu.edu/~stephan/Animation/pyramid.html

U.S. Supreme Court. 1973. Roe v. Wade. 410 U.S. 113.

———. 1990. *Cruzan v. Director Missouri Department of Health.* 110 S. Ct. 2841.

U.S. Surgeon General. 1999. Overview of etiology. In *Mental health: A report of the surgeon general of the U.S.A.* www.surgeongeneral.gov/library/mentalhealth/chapter2/sec3.html

Vaillant, G. E. 1984. Alcohol abuse and dependence. *American Psychiatric Association Annual Review.* Washington, DC: American Psychiatric Press.

Valenstein, Elliot S. 1987. Great and desperate cures: The rise and decline of psychosurgery and other radical treatments for mental illness. New York: Basic Books.

VandeCreek, Larry, and Laurel Burton, eds. 2005. Professional chaplaincy: Its role and importance in healthcare. www.healthcarechaplaincy.org/publications/publications/white_paper_05.22.01/index.html

Van Kaam, Adrian. 1985. *Human formation.* New York: Crossroad.

———. 1986. *Formation of the human heart.* Formative spirituality, vol 3. New York: Crossroad.

———. 1995. *Transcendence therapy.* Formative spirituality, vol. 7. New York: Crossroad.

Van Spengen, Linda. 1995. *The nature and causes of homosexuality.* Ancaster, Ontario: Redeemer University College.

Vatican Council II. 1964. *The documents of Vatican II,* ed. Walter M. Abbott. New York: Association Press.

———. 1965. Pastoral constitution on the church in the modern world (*Gaudium et spes*). December 7. Part 2, I, nos. 40, 47–52. The dignity of marriage and the family. www.vatican.va/archive/hist_councils/ii_vatican_council/documents/vat-ii_cons_19651207_gaudium-et-spes_en.html

Vaughan, Richard P. 1994. *Pastoral counseling and personality disorders: A manual.* Kansas City, MO: Sheed and Ward.

Veatch, Robert. 1981. *Medical ethics.* 2nd ed. Boston: Jones and Bartlett.

———. 2000. *Transplantation ethics.* Washington, DC: U.S. Government Printing Office.

———. 2003. The dead donor rule: True by definition. *American Journal of Bioethics* 3 (Winter): 10–11.

Vitz, Paul. C. 1994. *Psychology as religion: The cult of self-worship.* 2nd ed. Grand Rapids, MI: Eerdmans.

Viviano, Benedict. 1988. *The kingdom of God in history.* Wilmington, DE: Michael Glazier.

Vladeck, Bruce. 1999. Managed care's fifteen minutes of fame. *Journal of Health Politics, Policy and Law* 24: 1207–11.

Von Hildebrand, Dietrich. 1984. *Marriage: The mystery of faithful love.* Chicago: Franciscan Press.

Wadell, Paul. 1992. *The primacy of love: An introduction to the ethics of Thomas Aquinas.* New York: Paulist Press.

Walker, Adrian J. 2005. A way around cloning objection against ANT: A brief response to the joint statement on the production of pluripotent stem cells by oocyte assisted reprogramming. *Communio* 32:188–94.

Walker, Caroline Bynam. 1987. *Holy feast and holy fast: The religious significance of food to medieval women.* Berkeley and Los Angeles: University of California Press.

Wallace, William. 1989. Nature and human nature as the norm in medical ethics. In *Catholic perspectives on medical morals,* ed. Edmund D. Pellegrino, John Langan, and John Collins Harvey, 23–53. Dordrecht: Kluwer Academic.

————. 1991. *Galileo, the Jesuits, and the medieval Aristotle*. Aldershot, UK: Variorum.

Walters, Jack. 1995. *Jesus: Healer of our inner world*. New York: Crossroad.

Walters, James J. 1999. Uniqueness of Christian morality: An historical and critical analysis of the debate in Roman Catholic ethics. In *Method and Catholic moral theology: The ongoing reconstruction*, ed. Todd A. Salzman. Omaha, NE: Creighton University Press.

Warnock, Mary. 1984. Report of the committee of inquiry into human fertilization and embryology. London: Her Majesty's Stationary Office.

————. 1987. Do human cells have rights? *Bioethics* 1:2.

Watson, J. B. 1913. Psychology as the behaviorist views it. Lecture at Columbia University. *Psychology Review* 20:158–77.

Webster, Richard. 1995. *Why Freud was wrong*. London: Harper Collins.

Weisheipl, James A. 1974. *Friar Thomas D'Aquino: His life, thought and work*. Garden City, NY: Doubleday.

Weschler, Toni. 2001. *Taking charge of your fertility: The definitive guide to natural birth control and pregnancy achievement*. New York: Quill Harper Collins.

Weyers, Wolfgang. 2003. *The abuse of man: An illustrated history of dubious medical experimentation*. New York: Ardor Scribendi.

White, Andrew Dickson. 1896. *A history of the warfare of science with theology in Christendom*. New York: Dover.

Whitehead, Neil, and Brian Whitehead. 1999. *My genes made me do it! A scientific look at sexual orientation*. Lafayette, LA: Huntington House.

Wicks, Robert J., and Barry K. Estadt, eds. 1993. *Pastoral counseling in a global church: Voices from the field*. Maryknoll, NY: Orbis Books.

Wijdicks, Eelco F. M. 2001. The diagnosis of brain death. *New England Journal of Medicine* 344 (April): 1215–21.

Wikipedia. 2005. Roe v. Wade. http://en.wikipedia.org/wiki/Roe_v_wade

Wildes, Kevin. 1996. Ordinary and extraordinary means and the quality of life. *Theological Studies* 57 (September): 510.

————. 2000. *Moral acquaintances: Methodology in bioethics*. Notre Dame, IN: University of Notre Dame Press.

Williams, Earle. 2002. *Spiritually aware pastoral care: An introduction and training program*. New York: Paulist Press.

Williams, Oliver, and John Houck. 1987. *The common good and U.S. capitalism*. Lanham, MD: University Press of America.

Williams, Simon. 2001. Sociological imperialism and the profession of medicine revisited: Where are we now? *Sociology of Health and Illness* 23(2): 135.

Wills, Gary. 2000. *Papal sins: Structures of deceit*. New York: Doubleday.

Wilmut, Ian. 1997. Viable offspring derived from fetal and adult mammalian cells. *Nature* 385 (February): 810–13.

Wilson, Henry S., Takatso Mofokeng, Alice Frazer Evans, Judo Poerwowidagdo, and Robert A. Evans. 1996. *Pastoral theology from a global perspective: A case study approach*. Maryknoll, NY: Orbis Books.

Wimberley, Edward P. 1994. *Using scripture in pastoral counseling*. Nashville, TN: Abingdon Press.

Wisemann, Theresa M., and Mary-Lou Pardue, eds. 2001. *Exploring the biological contributions to human health: Does sex matter?* Institute of Medicine. Washington, DC: National Academies Press.

Wolf, Susan M., ed. 1996. *Feminism and bioethics*. New York: Oxford University Press.

Wolpe, Joseph. 1966. The comparative clinical status of conditioning theories and psychoanalysis. In *The conditioning therapies: The challenge of psychiatry*, ed. Joseph Wolpe, Andrew Slater, and L. J. Reyna, 3–20. New York: Holt, Rinehart and Winston.

Wolter, Alan B. 1997. *Duns Scotus on the will and morality*. Ed. William A. Frank. Washington, DC: Catholic University of America Press.

World Council of Churches. 1994. WCC's intervention at the UN world conference on population and development, September, Cairo.

World Health Organization. 1957. Geneva declaration on human research. *Encyclopedia of bioethics*. Vol. 4. New York: Free Press.

———. 1958. *"Constitution": The first ten years of the World Health Organization*. Geneva: WHO.

———. 1964. Helsinki statement on research on human subjects. *Encyclopedia of bioethics*. Vol. 4. New York: Free Press.

———. 1981. A prospective multi-center trial of the ovulation method of natural family planning: II. The effectiveness phase. *Fertility and Sterility* 36 (5): 591–98.

Wozniak, Robert. 1995. Mind and body: René Descartes to William James. http:// serendip.brynmawr.edu/Mind/ref.html

Wundt, Wilhelm. 1904. *Principles of physiological psychology*. Trans. Edward Bradford Titchener. London: Swan Sonnenschein.

———. 1961. Contributions to the theory of sense perception. In *Classics in psychology*, ed. T. Shipley, 51–78. New York: Philosophical Library.

Yankelovich, Daniel. 1998. How American individualism is evolving. *The Public Perspective*, February/March. www.danyankelovich.com/howamerican.html

Zenit News Agency. 1999. Notification of the Congregation for the Doctrine of the Faith concerning Sr. Jeannine Gramick, SSND, and Fr. Robert Nugent, SDS. www.cin.org/lor/ gramick.html

Zito, J. 2003. Psychotropic practice patterns for youth: A 10 year prospective. *Archives of Pediatric and Adolescent Medicine* 157:17–23.

Zohar, Noam, J. 1997. *Alternatives in Jewish bioethics*. Albany: State University of New York Press.

Zumbach, Clark. 1984. *The transcendent science: Kant's conception of biological methodology*. The Hague: Martinus Nijhoff.

INDEX

AA (Alcoholics Anonymous), 156–57, 160

abortion, 27, 80–81, 90, 101–2, 122

abreaction, 151–52

abstinence, periodic, 75

abstract thought, 71

ACPE (Association for Clinical Pastoral Education), 237

acquired immunodeficiency syndrome (AIDS), 214, 248

action therapy, 138, 139–41, 142

Acts of the Apostles, 220

acute illness, 35

Adderall, 135–36

addiction, 155–60

addictive personality, 155–56

"Address to the Bishops of the Episcopal Conference of the United States of America" (John Paul II), 194–95

ADHD (attention deficit/hyperactivity disorder), 135–46

adjustment disorders, 127

administrative staff, 239–41

adoption, 66

adult stem cells. *See* umbilical cord cells

advance directives, 192

affective drives, 147

agape, 47, 257

Age of Enlightenment, 4

agents, moral, 37

aggressive drives, 49

aggressive treatment, 195. *See also* extraordinary means

aging, 35, 109

AHA (American Hospital Association), 107

AHN (assisted hydration and nutrition), 188, 191, 193, 197

AIDS (acquired immunodeficiency syndrome), 214, 248

alcoholic beverages, 150

Alcoholics Anonymous (AA), 156–57, 160

alcoholism, 36, 149, 155–60

"Allocution to the Participants in the 19th International Conference of the Pontifical Council for Pastoral Care" (John Paul II), 195

allowing to die, 182–83, 198–99

alternative medicine, 206–7

ambiguous genitalia, 109, 112–13

American Hospital Association (AHA), 107

American Medical Association (AMA)

    Code of Medical Ethics, 4

    on determination of death, 172

    Principles of Medical Ethics, 240

American Psychiatric Association (APA). See also
    *Diagnostic and Statistical Manual of Mental
    Disorders*
    on homosexuality, 67–68
    on oppression, 126
    on therapist sexual relations, 151
amniocentesis, 99, 101, 102
anatomical gift, 177. *See also* organ donors
Anatomical Gift Act, 107
anatomical integrity, 104–5
anencephaly, 81–83, 107–8
angiograms, 172
animal–human hybrids, 97
animals, nonhuman
    as organ donors, 107
    personhood of, 39
    research on, 115
    rights of, 37
animate body, 145–47, 146f
annulment, 68
anointing the sick, 250–51
antianxiety drugs, 132
anticommunism, nationalistic, 221
antidepressants, 132, 135
antihistamines, 133
antimanic drugs, 133
antipsychiatry, 126, 152
Antipsychiatry Coalition, 126
antipsychotic drugs, 133
Antonelli, Giuseppe, 9
Antonius of Florence, 9
anxiety disorders, 127, 132, 133
APA. *See* American Psychiatric Association
appearance, 109
appendectomy, elective, 105
appetition, 145, 146f
Aquinas. *See* Thomas Aquinas, Saint
Aristotle
    on continence, 49
    on embryos, 72
    on happiness, 13
    on natural law, 22
    on pleasure, 36
    scientific medicine of, 207
    Thomas Aquinas and, 7
Arraj, James, 74
artificial insemination, 86–87

ART (assisted reproductive technology), 86–
    87
asceticism, 48
Asclepius, 207
Ashley, Benedict, 43
aspirin, 132
assisted hydration and nutrition (AHN), 188,
    191, 193, 197
assisted reproductive technology (ART), 86–87
Association for Clinical Pastoral Education
    (ACPE), 237
attention deficit/hyperactivity disorder (ADHD),
    133, 135–46
attractiveness, 109
Augustine of Hippo, Saint, 7
Australian Bishops' Conference, 197
autonomy
    Beauchamp and Childress on, 12
    definition of, 257
    existentialism and, 12
    informed consent and, 57–58
    in life support decision making, 192
    proxy consent and, 58
    psychotherapy and, 142–43
autopsy, 176–77
average, 34
Averroes, 7
awareness, 38
axiology, 32, 257

Banez, Domingo, 185
baptism, 165, 252–53
bariatric surgery, 108
basic health care, 183–84
basic needs, 32–33, 257
Beauchamp, Tom L., 11–12
Beck, Aaron, 141
Becker, Ernest, 166
Becker, Howard, 205
Beckwith, Francis J., 70
behavior
    abnormal, 129
    defensive, 141
behavior control, 149–51
Behavior Control (London), 138
behaviorist therapies, 137, 141, 143
behavior modification, 132, 135–36

Beitman, Bernard D., 133–34
Belgium, 179
Bellah, Robert, 216
Belmont Report, 116, 225
Benedict XVI (Joseph Ratzinger), 25, 166
beneficence, 12, 257
benefits of life support, 186–87, 188–89
Benefratelli, Hospital of the, 207
Bentham, Jeremy, 15
best interests of the patient, 192
beta-blockers, 133
the Bible, 5–6, 8
Billings method, 74
Bini, Lucio, 131
bioethics. *See also* ethics; health care ethics
    Church teachings on, 29
    current methodologies in, 9–18, 18f
    definition of, 257
    literature on, 4
    multiculturalism and, 19, 20–21
    ordinary teachings and, 29–30
    origins of, 3–4
    sacraments and, 254–55
    secular, 3–5, 19–20, 30, 262
    sexuality and, 68–69
Bioethics (Potter), 3–4
biologism, 35, 257
Biomedical Ethics and Jewish Law (Rosner), 9
biotechnology, 91, 122–23. *See also* technology
bipolar disorder, 127
The Birth of the Clinic (Foucault), 206
birth rate, 79
bisexuality, 67–68
bishops, 23
black liberation, 17
Blackmun, Harry A., 70
blood flow studies, 171, 172
blood transfusions, 105
Bloom, Alan, 153–54
Blum, Henrik, 33
bodily identity, 38
body. *See* human body
body–mind dualism. *See* mind–body dualism
body–soul dualism, 48
Boeree, George, 136–37
Book of Job, 165

Book of Tobit, 175
Boudewyns, Michael, 9
Boyle, Joseph, 12–13
brain
    blood flow studies, 171, 172
    creativity and, 93
    electrical stimulation of, 131
    higher, 108
brain death
    determination of, 103, 107–8, 169–73
    total, 172–73
brainstem, 107–8, 172
breathing, spontaneous, 170, 173
Breggin, Peter, 131
Breuer, Joseph, 137
Brody, Howard, 173
Brophy case, 190
Buchman, Frank, 156
Buddhism, 20
burden of life support, 187–89
burial, 176
Bush, George W., 226
business model, 214, 215, 217–18

cadaver
    care for, 175–77
    organ donors, 103, 171, 177
Calvin, John, 8–9
The Cambridge Illustrated History of Medicine (Porter), 5
Camus, Albert, 180
Capelmann, Karl, 9
capitalism, 153, 218–19, 221, 222–23, 231
capital punishment, 27
capitation, 217, 258
Capron, Alexander M., 113
cardinal virtues, 42–50, 258
caring, 211, 246
Cartesian, 258. *See also* Descartes, René
castration, 110
casuistry, 12–13, 14, 258
The Catechism of the Catholic Church (CCC)
    on baptism, 252–53
    on childless couples, 66
    for decision making, 45
categorical imperative, 10–12, 258
Catherine of Siena, Saint, 148

Catholic Bishops of the United States, 4. See
    also *Ethical and Religious Directives for
    Catholic Health Care Facilities*
Catholic Church. *See also* church teachings
    Christian ethics and, 21–22
    conservative movement and, 221
    human rights and, 29–30
    modern health care ethics and, 19–20
    moral controversies and, 22–26
    on suicide, 179
Catholic Health Association (CHA), 4, 197,
    231–33
Catholic health care facilities
    Catholic identity for, 230–31
    characteristics of, 232
    extent of, 230
    healing ministry of, 232–33
    leadership in, 231–33
    mergers of, 231
    pastoral care in, 237
    rape victims in, 83, 85–86
    responsibilities of, 227–33
    surgical sterilization in, 79–80
Catholic Hospital Association. *See* Catholic
    Health Association
Catholic hospitals. *See* Catholic health care
    facilities
Catholic identity, 230–31
Catholic saints, 148
CCC. See *The Catechism of the Catholic Church*
CDF. *See* Congregation for the Doctrine of the
    Faith
celibacy, 49–50, 64, 66–67
Center for Health Care Ethics, 227
cerebral cortex, 107–8, 172–73
Cerlett, Ugo, 131
certification of death, 171
certitude, moral and physical, 258
CHA (Catholic Health Association), 4, 197,
    231–33
Chakrabarty, Diamond v., 98
chaplains, 237, 241, 249
character, 42–50
charismatic physicians, 209
charity, 47, 104
chemical dependency. *See* addiction
childless couples, 66–67

children
    adoption of, 66
    psychotropic drugs for, 135–36
    sex selection of, 95–96, 98
Childress, James F., 11–12
chimera, 96–97
choice, free, 37, 54–55, 119
chorionic villi sampling, 99
Christianity
    compared to other religions, 20
    on death and suffering, 163–65
    ethics of, 21–22
    mental illness and, 145–48
    politics and, 46
    ritual care of the dead, 175–76
    sexuality and, 49–50
    on suicide, 179–80
Christianity and Social Progress (John XXIII),
    218
Christian physicians, 209–10
chronic illness, 35
The Church in the Modern World (*Gaudium et
    spes*), 77, 218
church, separation from state, 20–21
church teachings
    on bioethics, 29
    changes in, 25, 26, 28–29
    for decision making, 45
    levels of, 23–25
    obedience to, 44–45
    ordinary, 24
    right to dissent from, 25–27, 45
    sensus fidei and, 27–29
CIC. *See* Code of Canon Law
cingulotomy, 130–31
circumstances, 53, 258
Civilization and Its Discontents (Freud), 147
client relationships. *See* professional–client
    relationship
clinical pastoral education (CPE), 237–38
clinical signs of death, 170–72
clinical training, 167
Clinton, Bill, 216, 226
cloning, 97, 98, 120–21, 226
The Closing of the American Mind (Bloom),
    153–54
cocaine, 155

Code of Canon Law (CIC)
  on burial, 176
  on levels of teaching, 23–24
  on marriage, 65–66
Code of Medical Ethics (AMA), 4
codependency, 151–52
codes of ethics, 5
cognition, 145, 146f
cognitive therapy, 125, 139, 140, 141–42,
    157
collective unconsiousness, 147
collectivism, 45–46
college students, 153–54
coma, 131, 170
coministry, 240–41
The Committee on Doctrine and Pastoral
    Practices of the NCCB, 85
common good
  exclusion from, 219–20
  health care policy and, 218–19
  vs. individual good, 46
  innate needs and, 33
  liberationism and, 17
  social responsibility and, 220
  universal coverage and, 216
common sense, 145–47
communication
  with dying patients, 173–74
  of knowledge, 204
  professional, 212–13
communication theory, 59
communion, 251, 253–54
communism, 24, 221, 222
community
  life support withdrawal/withholding and,
    193–94
  responsibility to, 203
  solidarity, 221
community good. See common good
community hospitals, 79–80
compassion, 167–69, 195
competitive individualism, 222
comprehension, 58
conception, 70, 72–73, 83–86
conditioning, 139, 140
confession, 8
confidentiality, 58–60, 150, 213–14

Congregation for the Doctrine of the Faith (CDF)
  on bioethics, 29
  "Declaration on Euthanasia," 181, 183, 185,
    187, 190, 191
  The Declaration on Procured Abortion, 73, 81
  on euthanasia, 180
  on homosexuality, 67
  Instruction on the ecclesial vocation of the
    theologian, 27
  on levels of teaching, 23–24
  on objective and subjective morality, 89
  on suicide, 179
Congressional Biomedical Ethics Advisory
    Board, 226
Connery, John, 55, 188, 193
Conrad, Peter, 34
Conroy case, 190
conscience
  in decision making, 51
  definition of, 258
  formation of, 22
  social, 154
consent
  informed. See informed consent
  proxy. See proxy consent
  vicarious, 117
consequentialism, 14–15
conservatism, 221
The Conservative Intellectual Movement in
    America since 1945 (Nash), 221
consumer participation, 215
continence, 49, 258
contraception, 75–80
  after rape, 83–86
  John Paul II on, 15, 74, 76–77, 84
  vs. natural family planning, 74
  oral contraceptives for, 75–76, 77, 85
  Papal Commission on, 77–78
contrition, 252
controlled research, 115–17
conversion, 243, 248, 252
convulsions, 131
Conyers, John, 223–24
cooperation
  between hospitals, 79–80
  formal vs. material, 55–57
  legitimate, 55–57

coping, 136
corpse. *See* cadaver
Cor Unum, 189
cosmetic surgery, 108–13, 123
costs
    increasing, 215–16
    managed care and, 217
    of uninsured persons, 218
    of universal coverage, 224
Council of Trent, 25
Council on Ethical and Judicial Affairs (AMA), 172
counseling. *See also* pastoral counseling
    crisis, 173
    ethical, 241–44
    genetic, 98–99, 101–3
    by health care professionals, 210–12
    spiritual, 244–49
couples, childless, 66–67
covenant, 211, 212
CPE (clinical pastoral education), 237–38
creation, 93–94
creativity, 93, 94
Creighton Method, 74
cremation, 176
crisis counseling, 173
Cruzan case, 190
cultural relativism, 33
culture
    Catholic, 232
    pluralistic. *See* multiculturalism
curing, 211
Curran, Charles E., 15
curriculum, 215
cyclosporin, 106

DEA (Drug Enforcement Administration), 135
deacons, 237
death
    allowing to die, 182–83, 198–99
    brain, 103, 107–8, 169–73
    certification of, 171
    clinical signs of, 170–72
    criteria for, 169–70
    definition of, 166, 169–71, 172–73
    with dignity, 180
    fear of, 166–69
    future after, 39

    meaning of, 163–65
    personhood and, 175
    sin and, 164
    the soul after, 38
    suffering and, 50
decentralization, 221, 224
deception, 119
decision making
    for allowing to die, 198–99
    character and, 42
    church teachings for, 45
    duty ethics for, 13–14
    by ethics committees, 229
    goals in, 21
    for happiness, 52
    information for, 58, 173–74, 217
    Kant on, 18
    for life support withdrawal/withholding, 188, 189–94, 198–99
    objective and subjective morality in, 242–44
    participation in, 46–47, 215
    physician's role in, 211
    prudent, 50–53
    shared, 222, 224
    social, 221–23
    value systems in, 32
    virtue ethics theory in, 17
"Declaration on Euthanasia" (CDF), 181, 183, 185, 187, 190, 191
"Declaration on Life Support" (Pius XII), 187
The Declaration on Procured Abortion (CDF), 73, 81
defensive behavior, 141
Dekkers, Wim J., 166
delayed hominization, 72–73, 258
Delgado, Jose, 131
demons, 129, 168
denial, 157
deontology, 5–6, 258, 263
Department of Health and Human Services, 106, 225
dependency, 157–58
depersonalization, 204–6
deposit of the faith, 258
Depositum fidei, 26
depression
    in dying patients, 174

electroconvulsive therapy for, 131
  major, 127
  psychotropic drugs for, 132, 133
depressive disorders, 127–28
Derrida, Jacques, 19
Descartes, René, 10, 14, 35, 126, 258
desensitization, 139
De Somniis (Aristotle), 207
developmental individuation, 70–71
development of doctrine, 25–26, 259
de Vitoria, Francisco, 184–85
DHEW (Department of Health, Education,
    and Welfare). *See* Department of Health
    and Human Services
*Diagnostic and Statistical Manual of Mental
    Disorders* (APA)
  on homosexuality, 67–68
  on transsexualism, 109
  on types of disorders, 127–28
Diamond v. Chakrabarty, 98
Didache, 80
dignity, 168, 180
Directive 22, 237
Directive 36, 85, 87
Directive 48, 82
Directive 56, 189
Directive 57, 189
Directive 58, 191, 197
Directive 66, 122
directness, 247
direct sterilization, 78–80
discernment, 246–48
disease. *See also* illness
  medical approaches to, 34, 211
  prevention of, 50, 221, 223, 224
disproportionate life support, 185, 186
dissidents, 126
distributive justice, 45
divine revelation. *See* revelation
divinity, 204
divorce, 78
doctors. *See* physicians
doctrine, development of, 25–26, 259
Doerflinger, Richard M., 197
Dolly (cloned sheep), 120
Dominicans, 8–9
dominion over nature, 92

donors. *See* organ donors
Donum Vitae (CDF), 29
double-blind research, 115–17
double effect, principle of, 54–55
Down syndrome, 189
Driven: How Human Nature Shapes Our Choices
    (Lawrence and Nohria), 32
drug abuse, 150
drug addiction. *See* addiction
Drug Enforcement Administration (DEA), 135
dualism
  body–soul, 35, 48
  health and, 35
  mind–body, 35, 37–38, 72, 126, 207
  suicide and, 179
duty ethics
  in the Bible, 5, 6
  Calvin and, 8
  casuistry, 12–13
  history of, 7–8, 9
  Kantian, 10–12
  strengths and weaknesses of, 13–14
  varieties of, 10–14, 18f
dying
  anointing the sick, 251
  baptism for, 253
  care of the, 167–69
  communication with, 173–74
  health care professionals and, 166–67
  information for, 173–74
  pastoral counseling for, 173

EAB (Ethics Advisory Board), 225
eating disorders, 127
ecclesia semper reformanda, 239
ecology, 98
economic guidelines, 205
ECT (electroconvulsive therapy), 131–32, 150
ectopic pregnancy, 81–82
ecumenism, 22, 259
education
  for decision making, 222
  ethics committees for, 229–30
  health, 225
  higher, 222
  medical, 215, 225
  ministerial, 237

education (*continued*)
　for pastoral care, 237–38
　psychotherapy as, 136
EEG (electroencephalography), 132, 171
ego, 138f, 140, 141
electrical stimulation of the brain (ESB), 131
electroconvulsive therapy (ECT), 131–32, 150
electroencephalography (EEG), 132, 171
elitism, 223
embryos
　Aristotle on, 72
　developmental modification, 92
　personhood of, 69–70, 71–72
　research on, 119–20
　sexual differentiation, 64
emotivism, 11
ends. *See* goals
ends–means ethics
　Dominicans and, 9
　intentions in, 52–53
　natural law and, 22–23
　needs and, 31–32
　proportionalism, 15–16
　strengths and weaknesses of, 18
　teleology and, 6
　Thomas Aquinas and, 7
　varieties of, 14–18, 18f
　virtue ethics, 16–18
Engelhardt, H. Tristram, Jr., 19, 21, 37
English, Joseph, 160–61
Enhanced Medicine for All (H.R. 676), 224
Enlightenment, 208
ensoulment, 72–73
environmental factors
　in health, 224–25
　in mental illness, 129
Epicureans, 179
epieikeia, 15
equality, gender, 68–69
ERD. See *Ethical and Religious Directives for
　　Catholic Health Care Facilities*
Erikson, Erik, 153
ESB (electrical stimulation of the brain), 131
eschatology, 47–48, 259
*Ethical and Religious Directives for Catholic
　　Health Care Facilities* (ERD)
　bioethics teachings, 29
　on communication with the dying, 173

　on cooperation, 57
　definition of, 259
　Directive 22, 237
　Directive 36, 85, 87
　Directive 48, 82
　Directive 56, 189
　Directive 57, 189
　Directive 58, 191, 197
　Directive 66, 122
　on ectopic pregnancy, 82
　for ethics committees, 229
　hospital mergers and, 231
　on life support, 188–89
　on life support decision making, 192, 193
　origins of, 4
　on pain control, 198
　on pastoral care, 236, 238
　on surgical sterilization, 79
ethical counseling, 241–44
ethical norms. *See* moral norms
ethical skills, 43
ethics. *See also* bioethics
　Christian, 21
　duty. *See* duty ethics
　ends–means. *See* ends–means ethics
　feminist, 17, 69
　health care. *See* health care ethics
　heteronomous, 14
　medical, 4
　reason-based, 20–21
　situational, 15, 263
　virtue, 16, 18
Ethics Advisory Board (EAB), 225
ethics committees, 228–30, 239
Eucharist, 253–54
eugenics, 79, 93, 97–98, 100
European Union, 46–47
euthanasia, 27, 180–83
evaluative sense, 147
Evangelium vitae (John Paul II), 29, 191
evil
　consent and, 58
　contraception as, 77
　greater good and, 41
　healing and, 168
　pain as, 198
evolution, 93, 95
exception, lenient, 15

exchange justice, 45
existentialism, 12
exorcism, 129
experience, 27–29, 118
experimentation, human. *See* research
expressive individualism, 153
extraordinary means, 183, 184–86, 195

facts vs. values, 32
faith
   deposit of the, 258
   in health care ethics, 19–30
   reason and, 44
   sense of, 28–29, 262
   virtue of, 42, 43–45, 43f
faithful, opinion of the, 27–29
faith intuition. See *sensus fidei*
false statements, 213–14
Familiaris consortio (John Paul II), 49, 78–79
family
   in addiction therapy, 159–60
   in life support decision making, 192–93
   sexuality and, 50, 65
   size of, 65, 74
family planning, natural, 73–75, 261
family therapy, 144
feeding tubes, 185
fee-for-service plans, 217, 259
Feldman, David, 9
feminist ethics, 17, 69
fertility, periods of, 74
fertilization, 73
fetishism, 109
fever, 131
Fides et ratio (John Paul II), 5, 30
final communion, 251
financial burdens, 188
finis operantis, 36, 259, 261
Finnis, John, 12–13
Fins, Joseph J., 194
fittest, survival of, 95
Fletcher, Joseph, 9, 15, 179
forgoing life support. *See* life support
   withdrawal/withholding
formal cooperation, 55–57
formalism, 217
fortitude, 47–49, 217
Foucault, Michael, 206

Fox, Michael W., 39
free choice
   morality and, 54–55
   nonhuman animals and, 37
   in psychological research, 119
freedom
   alcoholic beverages and, 150
   behavior control and, 149
   in ethical counseling, 241–42
   for informed consent, 58
   intelligent, 36–37, 39
   mental health and, 143–44
   mental illness and, 144–45, 147, 149, 152–53
   misuse of, 164
   natural law and, 94
   psychotropic drugs and, 150
   Thomas Aquinas on, 147
freedom of God, 7–8
Freeman, James Watts, 130
Freeman, William, 130
free will, 39, 143
Freidson, Eliot, 34
French Revolution, 206, 208
Freud, Sigmund
   on neurotic guilt, 148
   psychoanalytic theory of, 136, 137–38, 138f,
      140, 141
   on religion, 160
   on spirituality, 147
   value systems of, 153
Freymann, John Gordon, 206
Fromm, Erich, 153
Fuchs, Josef, 15, 77
function, quality of, 189
functional decision making, 47
functional integrity, 104–5
functionalism, societal, 221–23
fundamental option, 51, 217
funding
   organ transplantation, 106–7
   withholding, 225–26

Galen, 207
Galileo, 25, 26, 29
gamete intrafallopian transfer (GIFT), 87
gastrostomy tubes, 188
gender, definition of, 89
gender dysphoria, 109–13

gender equality, 68–69
gender identity, 64, 111
gender role, 64
general practitioners, 208, 214
gene therapy, 94, 96–97, 98
genetic counseling, 98–99, 101–3
genetic disorders
    counseling for, 98–99, 101–3
    gene therapy for, 98
    homosexuality as, 68
    parental responsibility for, 102–3
    screening for, 98–101
    testing for, 99, 101–2
genetic engineering, 92, 94, 95–96, 97
genetic individuation, 70–71
genetic interventions, 94–98, 122–23, 226
genetic reconstruction, 98
genetic screening, 98–101
Geneva Declaration, 181
genitalia, ambiguous, 109, 112–13
genocide, 11
genotype modification, 97, 217
Germany, 224
germ cell genetic engineering, 94, 97
GIFT (gamete intrafallopian transfer), 87
Glendon, Mary Ann, 216
goals
    in decision making, 21
    health as, 31–32
    ultimate end, 13, 36–37, 51, 217
God
    freedom of, 7–8
    kingdom of, 20
    laws of, 5–6, 8, 14
    truth of, 24
good. *See also* common good
    greater, 41
    individual vs. community, 46
goods
    incommensurable, 13–14, 197, 260
    material, 33, 46
Good Samaritan, 244
Gospel of Life (John Paul II)
    on abortion, 27, 80–81
    on euthanasia, 182
    on stem cell research, 122
grace, 217
"grace perfects nature," 40

greater good, 41
Greco-Roman culture, 5, 179, 207
Grisez, Germain, 12–13
Grobstein, Clifford, 70–71
group therapy, 144–45
guidance, 235–36
guilt, 148, 158, 248

Habermas, Jürgen, 19
habits, 42, 139–40
Hannibal, 137
happiness
    decision making for, 52
    definition of, 38–39
    true, 36–37, 38–40, 41, 48, 60
    ultimate goal of, 13
Häring, Bernard, 15, 56
Harper, Robert A., 142
Harvard criteria, 171
Harvey, John, 68
Harvey, William, 207
Hastings Center, 4, 227
healing
    anointing the sick, 250–51
    celebration of, 249–55
    by Jesus Christ, 40, 41, 232, 235, 248–49
    pastoral care for, 235–37
    prayer for, 168, 249
    specialization and, 204
healing ministry, 232–33
health
    definition of, 33–36
    environmental and social factors in, 224–25
    needs, 31–32, 33–36
    physical, 35, 238
    psychological, 35
    responsibility for, 46, 220–21
    right to, 219
Health and Medicine in the Jewish Tradition
    (Feldman), 9
health care
    basic, 183–84
    business model of, 214, 215, 217–18
    distribution of, 220
    fee-for-service plans, 217, 259
    national, 223–25
    new paradigm for, 214–15
    not-for-profit, 214–15

person-centered, 209, 218
politics of, 215–18
quality of, 217
universal, 216
health care ethics. *See also* bioethics
education for, 4
faith and reason in, 19–30
foundations of, 5–9
government guidelines for, 225–27
natural law in, 21–22
origins of, 3
private centers for, 227
public policy and, 225–27
reason in, 21–22
health care policy
common good and, 218–19
functionalism and, 221–23
health care ethics and, 225–27
principles of, 218–25
private centers for, 227
single-payer systems and, 223–25
subsidiarity and, 219–21
health care professionals. *See also* physicians;
professional–client relationship
addiction and, 159–60
communication with, 212–13
communication with the dying, 173–74
counseling by, 210–12
death and, 166–67
ethical counseling of, 242
paramedical, 208
pastoral care by, 240–41
pastoral care of, 239–40
pastoral care with, 238–39
person-centered, 205–6
health care reform, 216, 224
health care team, 238–39
health education, 225
health insurance, 216–17
health maintenance organizations (HMOs), 205
health promotion, 224
Health Security Act (1993), 216
heart function, spontaneous, 170, 173
Helsinki Statement, 114, 181
Hemingway, Ernest, 132
heretical, 206–7
hermaphroditism, 112
heteronomous ethics, 14

higher education, 222
Hilgers, Thomas, 74
Hippocrates, 207
Hippocratic Oath
on confidentiality, 59
definition of, 217
history of, 5
norms of, 229
on physician-assisted suicide, 181
history of medicine, 206–7, 223
Hitler, Adolf, 11
HMOs (health maintenance organizations), 205
holism, 34, 210, 214–15, 238
hominization, delayed, 72–73, 258
homosexuality, 67–68
hope, 43f, 47–49, 50, 255
hormone therapy, 110
hospice, 198
hospitalization, psychiatric, 129
Hospital of the Benefratelli, 207
hospitals
Catholic. *See* Catholic health care facilities
community, 79–80
cooperation between, 79–80, 260
mergers of, 231
pastoral care in, 236–37
secular, 236–37
H.R. 676 (Enhanced Medicine for All), 224
Humanae vitae (Paul VI)
on contraception, 15, 76–77, 84
on marriage, 65–66
on sexuality, 49
human body. *See also* cadaver
anatomical gift of, 177
animate, 145–47, 146f
in death, 169
inanimate, 145–47, 146f
modifying, 91–94
theology of, 237
Human Genome Project, 94–95
humanism
definition of, 260
secular, 4, 21, 30, 223, 231
humanistic therapies, 137
humanization of medicine, 208–9
human nature, 145, 146f
human needs. *See* needs
human persons. *See* personhood

human potential, 37–38
Human Research Act, 225
human research subjects, 113–22
    categories of, 114
    government guidelines for, 225–26
    norms for, 114–15
    selecting, 116–18
    withdrawal from studies, 117–18
human rights. *See* rights
human vs. personhood, 37
Hume, David, 11, 17
The 100th Year (John Paul II), 218
Hurlbut, William, 122
hybrids, animal–human, 97
hydration. *See* assisted hydration and nutrition
hyperactivity. *See* attention deficit/hyperactivity
    disorder
hypnotics, 133
hysterectomy, 78, 110

id, 137–38, 138f, 141
identical twins, 71
identity
    bodily, 38
    Catholic, 230–31
    gender, 64, 111
    pastoral, 246
    professional, 204
ignorance, veil of, 10
Illich, Ivan, 205
illness
    acute and chronic, 35
    conversion during, 248
    definition of, 34
    dignity in, 168
    as sin, 168
immortality, 176
immunosuppressive drugs, 106
implantation, 85
impulse control, 48
inanimate body, 145–47, 146f
incommensurable goods, 13–14, 197, 260
incompetent persons, 150
indirect abortion, 80
indirect sterilization, 78, 79
individual good, 46
individualism
    common good and, 216
    competitive, 222
    expressive, 153
    justice and, 11
    social justice and, 45–46
individuation, genetic vs. developmental, 70–71
induced abortion, 80–81
industrial model, 205
infanticide, 80–81
information
    for decision making, 217
    for dying patients, 173–74
    for informed consent, 58
informed consent
    for ambiguous genitalia treatment, 112–13
    for behavior control, 150
    freedom and, 57–58
    for genetic screening, 99–100
    living organ donors and, 105
    for research, 114–15, 116–18
inheritance, 99
innate needs, 32–33, 257
Innocent X, 9
insight therapy, 138, 139–45, 151–52
instinct, 147
institutional review board (IRB), 113, 114–15,
    225
Instruction on Respect for Human Life, 73, 87
*Instruction on the Ecclesial Vocation of the
    Theologian* (CDF), 27
insulin coma, 131
integrity, 38, 94, 104–5, 114–15
intellectual skills, 43
intelligence, 94
intelligent freedom, 36–37, 39
intentions, 52–53
Internet, 217
The Interpretation of Dreams (Freud), 137
intersexuality, 112–13
introspection, 142, 145
intubation, 188
in vitro fertilization (IVF), 86–87, 95, 97, 98
involuntary sterilization, 78–79
IRB (institutional review board), 113, 114–
    15, 225
Islam, 20, 179
IVF (in vitro fertilization), 86–87, 95, 97, 98

James, William, 156, 160

Jansen, Lynn A., 166
JCAHO (Joint Commission for the Accreditation
    of Health Care Organizations), 107, 228
Jennett, Bryan, 194
Jeremiah, 141
Jesuits, 8–9
Jesus Christ
    as ethical model, 40–42
    healing by, 40, 41, 232, 235, 248–49
    on the kingdom of God, 220
    on lay ministers, 254
    as model, 6–8
    on moral conversion, 243
    on reconciliation, 251–52
    suffering and death of, 165, 198
    touching by, 250
Jewish Chronic Disease Hospital case, 113
Jewish literature, 9
Job, Book of, 165
John Paul II
    on abortion, 27, 80–81
    "Address to the Bishops of the Episcopal
        Conference of the United States of
        America," 194–95
    "Allocution to the Participants in the 19th
        International Conference of the Pontifical
        Council for Pastoral Care," 195
    on bioethics, 29, 30
    on brain death, 103
    on capital punishment, 27
    on conscience formation, 22
    on contraception, 15, 74, 76, 77, 84
    on crossing the threshold of hope, 255
    on death determination, 172
    on euthanasia, 27, 182
    Evangelium vitae, 29
    Familiaris consortio, 49, 78–79
    Fides et ratio, 5, 30
    on gender equality, 68–69
    Gospel of Life, 27, 80–81, 122, 182
    on involuntary sterilization, 78–79
    on levels of teaching, 23–24, 25
    on life support, 183, 185, 186, 188, 191
    on love, 64
    Lust and Personal Dignity, 83
    on marriage, 65–66
    on mental illness, 161
    on moral conversion, 243

    on multiculturalism, 19–20
    On the Human Family, 78–79
    on organ donors, 177
    on persistent vegetative state (PVS), 185, 189,
        194–97
    on proportionalism, 16
    on rape, 83
    on reconciliation, 252
    on scientism, 5
    on sexuality, 49
    on socialism, 218
    on socialism and capitalism, 218
    on stem cell research, 121–22
    suffering and death of, 166
    on suicide, 179
    The Theology of the Body, 74
    on the theology of the body, 237
    "To the Participants in the International
        Congress on 'Life-Sustaining Treatments
        and Vegetative State': Scientific Advances
        and Ethical Dilemmas," 195–97
    on the ultimate end, 51
    Veritatis splendor, 16, 22, 51, 161
John XXIII, 77, 218
John XXIII Medical-Moral Research and
    Education Center, 4
Joint Commission for the Accreditation of
    Health Care Organizations (JCAHO),
    107, 228
joint ventures, 79–80, 260
Jonas, Hans, 92
Joseph of Arimathea, 175
Judaism
    compared to other religions, 20
    on death and suffering, 163–65
    on natural law, 20
    on resurrection, 175
    ritual care of the dead, 175–76
    on suicide, 179
judgment
    guilt and, 248
    Paul, Saint, on, 168
    prudential, 24–25
    substitute, 192
Jung, Carl Gustav, 138, 147, 156
juridic person, 260
justice
    Beauchamp and Childress on, 12

justice (*continued*)
  definition of, 260
  distributive, 45
  exchange, 45
  legal, 45
  social, 45–46, 59–60
  theory of, 10
  virtue of, 45–47

Kant, Immanuel, 10–12, 14, 18
Katz, Jay, 113
Kelly, Gerald, 104, 105
Kennedy Institute for Ethics, 4, 227
Kern, Rochelle, 34
Kesey, Ken, 126
Kevorkian, Jack, 181
kingdom of God, 220
Klerman, Gerald L., 133–34
Knauer, Peter, 15, 213
knowledge, 27–29, 114, 204
Kubler-Ross, Elisabeth, 173, 236
Kucinich, Dennis, 223–24

labor unions, 222–23
language, pseudo-religious, 247
last rites, 260
Lawrence, Paul, 32
Laws of God, 5–6, 8, 14
lay ministers, 254
leadership, 231–33
learning theory, 140
legalism, 260
legal justice, 45
legal profession, 204
legislation
  health care reform, 216, 224
  organ transplantation, 177
  research, 225–26
legitimate cooperation, 55–57
Leibniz, Gottfried Wilhelm, 14
lenient exception, 15
Leo XIII, 218
lepers, 248–49, 250
liberationism, 17, 221, 222
liberty, 10
life
  beginning of, 69–73
  delayed hominization theory, 72–73

personhood and, 69–70, 71–72
  prolonging, 182–83
  quality of, 189
life forms, new, 96–97, 98
life support
  benefits of, 186–87, 188–89
  burdens of, 187–89
  extraordinary means of, 183, 184–86, 195
  function of, 170–71
  ordinary means of, 184–86
  for persistent vegetative state patients, 195–97
  proportionate and disproportionate, 186
  quality of life and, 189
life support withdrawal/withholding
  allowing to die and, 183
  criteria for, 186–94
  decision making for, 188, 189–94, 198–99
Ligouri, Alphonsus, Saint, 9, 15, 148
limbic system, 130–31
listening, 246–47
literature, 4, 6, 9
living organ donors, 104–6
Living the Truth in Love (Ashley), 43
living wills, 181
lobotomy, 130–31, 149–50
London, Perry, 138
Lothstein, Leslie M., 110
love
  Christian, 7
  contraception and, 75–76
  God's Law and, 8
  Jesus Christ on, 6
  John Paul II on, 64
  living organ donors and, 104
  sexuality and, 64, 66
  situational ethics and, 15
  virtue of, 43f, 45–47
Lust and Personal Dignity (John Paul II), 83
Luther, Martin, 8–9
lying, 118–19, 213–14

MacIntyre, Alisdair, 93
Maddi, Salvatore R., 136, 141
magisterium, 260. *See also* church teachings
magnetic resonance imaging (MRI), stereotactic, 130
Maimonides, 9
major depression, 127

malaria, 131
malpractice, 212
managed care
    definition of, 260
    failure of, 217–18
    history of, 216–17
    physician guidelines of, 205
    trusteeship relationship and, 211
marijuana, 155
Mark, Saint, 235
marriage
    homosexual, 68
    love and, 64
    procreation in, 87
    sexuality and, 49–50
    value of, 65–66
Marx, Karl, 220
Maslow, Abraham, 33
mastectomy, 110
masturbation, 156
material cooperation, 55–57
material goods, 33, 46
mature personality, 142–43
May, Rollo, 153
May, William E., 12–13
McCormick, Richard, 15
McFadden, Charles J., 9
MCS (minimally conscious state), 194
mechanists, 34–35
Medicaid, 106, 111
medical decision making. *See* decision making
medical education, 215, 225
medical ethics. *See* health care ethics
Medical Ethics (McFadden), 9
Medical Ethics (Percival), 4
Medical-Legal Questions (Zacchia), 9
medical model, 34, 211
medical professionals. *See* health care
    professionals; physicians
medical schools. *See* medical education
medical therapy
    vs. basic health care, 183–84
    benefits of, 186–87
    burdens of, 187–89
    extraordinary means of, 183, 184–86, 195
    ordinary means of, 184–86
    vs. research, 114
Medicare, 106

medicine
    depersonalization of, 204–6
    heretical (alternative), 206–7
    historical influences on, 223
    history of, 206–7, 208
    humanization of, 208–9
    orthodox, 206–7
    prescientific, 50, 206–7
    preventive, 221, 223, 224
    priestly aspect of, 207, 208–9
    as a profession, 206–10
    scientific, 206–7, 208, 210
    secularization of, 236
    symbol of, 207
Medicine in the Bible and Talmud (Rosner), 9
Meduna, Lasislaus von, 131
memory, sense, 145
Mendel, Gregor, 99
mental health, 126, 143–44
mental illness
    in Catholic saints, 148
    causes of, 123, 128–29, 145, 160
    Christian model of, 145–48
    definition of, 126
    electroconvulsive therapy for, 131–32
    ethical issues in, 148–60
    freedom and, 144–45, 147, 149, 152–53
    hospitalization for, 129
    psychosurgery for, 130–31
    psychotherapy for, 136–45
    psychotropic drugs for, 132–36
    reality of, 128–29
    sin and, 161
    spirituality and, 147–48
    treatment of, 125–26, 130–45
    types and prevalence of, 127–28
mental retardation, 128
mercy killing. *See* euthanasia
Merton, Robert, 205
methotrexate, 82
Meyer, J. K., 111
Middle Ages, 7–8
middle principles, 260
mind–body dualism
    alternative medicine and, 207
    health and, 35
    human potential and, 37–38
    mental illness and, 126

mind–body dualism (*continued*)
  personhood and, 72
minimally conscious state (MCS), 194
ministerial education, 237
ministers, lay, 254
ministry
  definition of, 261
  healing, 232–33
miscarriage, 80
Moniz, Ega, 130
monopolies, 222
Monte, Christopher, 136, 142
Moral Acquaintances (Wildes), 12–13, 19
moral agents, 37
moral certitude, 258
moral compromise, theory of, 15
moral controversies, 22–26
morality
  free choice and, 54–55
  middle principles of, 260
  objective and subjective, 51–53, 88–89, 242–44, 261
  public opinion as, 11
morality gap, 88
moral norms, 53–60
moral object, 52, 53, 229
  total, 261, 263
Moral Re-Armament, 156
Morals and Medicine (Fletcher), 9
moral systems, 8–9, 21–22
moral virtues. *See* virtues
mortal sins, 52
Mosaic Law, 5–6, 261
mothers, surrogate, 88
motivation, 216
MRI. *See* magnetic resonance imaging, stereotactic
Mullerian ducts, 64
multiculturalism
  bioethics and, 19, 20–21
  Catholic health care facilities and, 231
  innate needs and, 33
multipotent cells, 120
murder, 180–81
muscle relaxants, 132
mysterium tremendum, 248
The Myth of Mental Illness (Szaz), 126

NaPro Education Technology, 74

Nash, George, 221
National Bioethics Advisory Commission (NBAC), 226
National Catholic Bioethics Center (NCBC), 4, 197, 227
National Commission for the Protection of Human Subjects of Biomedical and Behavioral Research, 225
national health care, 223–25
National Institutes of Health, 113
nationalistic anticommunism, 221
National Opinion Research Center, 67
National Organ Transplant Act, 177
National Roundtable on Health Care Quality, 217
natural ethics, 21–22
natural family planning, 73–75, 261
natural law
  contraception and, 76
  definition of, 242–44
  freedom and, 94
  in health care ethics, 21–22
  sexuality and, 65
  Thomas Aquinas on, 7, 21–22
  various religions on, 20
nature. *See also* human nature
  dominion over, 92
  grace perfects, 40
Nazi experimentation, 113
NBAC (National Bioethics Advisory Commission), 226
NCBC (National Catholic Bioethics Center), 4, 197, 227
needs
  ethics based on, 29, 30, 31–40
  health, 31–32, 33–36
  health care for, 214–15, 220
  innate (basic), 32–33, 257
  social, 33–36
negative eugenics, 100
Neiswanger Institute for Bioethics and Public Policy, 227
nervous system, 38
The Netherlands, 179, 181
neuroses, 144
newborns
  ambiguous genitalia in, 109, 112–13
  screening, 100

New Jersey Supreme Court, 228
new life forms, 96–97, 98
New Testament, 243–44
NHBD (non-heart-beating organ donation), 103
Nightingale, Florence, 236
Nohria, Nitin, 32
nominalism, 8, 261
non-heart-beating organ donation (NHBD), 103
nonmalfeasance, 12, 261
nontherapeutic research, 114, 117
normal vs. average, 34
norms, moral, 53–60
not-for-profit health care, 214–15
Nouwen, Henri, 239
Nuremberg Code, 114
nurses, 209, 211, 236
nutrition. *See* assisted hydration and nutrition

OAR (oocyte assisted reprogramming), 122
obesity, 108
objective morality, 51–53, 88–89, 242–44, 261
obsessive-compulsive disorder, 127
O'Donnell, Thomas, 189, 190
Old Testament, 5–6, 248
On Care for PVS Patients (John Paul II), 189
"On Reconciliation and Penance" (John Paul II), 252
On Social Development (John Paul II), 218
On the Human Family (John Paul II), 49, 78–79
One Flew Over the Cuckoo's Nest (Kesey), 126
oocyte assisted reprogramming (OAR), 122
operant conditioning, 139
opinion of the faithful, 27–29
opium, 132
oppression, 126
oral contraceptives, 75–76, 77, 85
ordinary means, 184–86
ordinary teachings, 24
Oregon, 179
organ donors
    cadaver, 103, 171, 177
    death determination for, 171
    living, 104–6
    non-heart-beating, 103
    nonhuman animal, 107
    Uniform Anatomical Gift Act and, 177
    waiting for, 106, 107
organic-based disorders, 128

organism, 261
organ systems, 38
organ transplantation, 103–8, 123, 171
original sin, 164, 261
orthodox medicine, 206–7
outcomes, softer, 215
ovulation, 74
ovum, 70
The Oxford Dictionary of the Christian Church, 8
Oxford Group, 156

pain as evil, 198
pain control, 197–98
pain relievers, 155, 157
palliative care, 179
Papal Commission, 77–78
paradigms, new, 214–15
paralysis, 187, 188
paramedical professionals, 208
parents
    genetic counseling and, 101, 102–3
    sex selection by, 96
participation, 215, 219–21
pastoral care, 232, 235–55
    anointing the sick, 250–51
    baptism in, 252–53
    coministry and, 240–41
    definition of, 261
    education for, 237–38
    ethical counseling and, 241–44
    Eucharist for, 253–54
    goals of, 235–37
    objective and subjective morality in, 242–44
    other health care professions and, 238–39
    sacraments and, 249–55
pastoral counseling, 241–44
    for dying patients, 173
    for gender dysphoria, 112–13
    psychotherapy and, 242
    for sexuality, 88–89
pastoral identity, 246
Pastoral Medicine (Antonelli), 9
Pastoral Medicine (Capelmann), 9
pastoral ministry, 22
patents, 98
paternalism, 221
The Patient as Person (Ramsey), 9
patients, best interests of, 192

Paul, Saint
  on baptism, 165
  on death, 167
  on judgment, 168
  on moral controversy, 23
  on resurrection, 175
  on sin and death, 164
  on slavery, 26
  on suffering, 198
Paul VI
  on contraception, 75, 76–77, 78, 84
  Humanae vitae, 15, 65–66, 76–77, 84
  on marriage, 65–66
  on sexuality, 49
  on socialism and capitalism, 218
Pavlov, Ivan, 137
PCEMR (President's Commission for the
    Study of Ethical Problems in Medicine
    and Biomedical and Behavioral Research),
    108, 225, 228
Peoria Protocol, 85
Percival, Thomas, 4
periodic abstinence, 75
persistent vegetative state (PVS), 185, 189, 190,
    194–97
personalism, prudential, 17, 18, 29–30, 57–58,
    262
personality
  addiction and, 155–56, 157–59
  definition of, 39
  mature, 142–43
  theories of, 142
personality disorders, 128
person-centered health care, 209, 218
person-centered professions, 205–6
personhood
  death and, 170, 175
  definition of, 39
  of embryos, 69–70, 71–72
  vs. human, 37
  intelligent freedom and, 36–37, 39
  life support decision making and, 192
  personality and, 39
  potential for, 37–38
  resurrection and, 175
phenotype modification, 97, 217
phenylketonuria, 100
Philemon, 26

physical certitude, 258
physical health, 35, 238
physicalism, 35, 257
physician-assisted suicide, 178, 179–80, 244
physicians
  charismatic, 209
  Christian, 209–10
  communication with, 212–13
  counseling by, 210–12
  death certification by, 171
  decision making role of, 211
  depersonalization of, 204–6
  historical influences on, 223
  as human research subjects, 115
  in life support decision making, 191–92
  motivation of, 216
  pastoral care and, 238–39
  pastoral care of, 239–41
  as professionals, 206–10
  secularization of, 236
  trust in, 207, 211–12
physiological addiction, 158
physiology, 38
Pierce v. Swan Point Cemetery, 176
Pius XII
  on communism, 24–25
  "Declaration on Life Support," 187
  on freedom, 149
  on human research subjects, 115
  on life support, 185, 187, 192
  on organ donors, 103, 177
placebo, 115–16, 261
Plath, Sylvia, 132
Plato, 35, 221
pleasure
  addiction and, 157
  physical, 36–37
  sexual, 65, 66
pleasure drives, 49
Plum, Fred, 194
pluralistic culture. *See* multiculturalism
plurifinalism, 13, 14, 15
pluriformalism, 262
pluripotential cells, 119–20
point of service plan, 262
policy, health care. *See* health care policy
poliomyelitis, 115
political systems, 20–21

politics
    Christian, 46
    of health care, 215–18
Pontifical Academy of Life, 122
Pontifical Council, *Cor Unum*, 189
Porter, Roy, 5
postmodernism, 262
potential, 37–38
Potter, Van Rensselaer, 3–4
poverty, 231
practice, research vs., 204–5
pragmatism, 15
prayer, 168, 249
pre-embryos, 70
pregnancy, ectopic, 81–82
Pre-Meditated Man (Restak), 126
prenatal diagnosis, 99, 101–2
prescientific medicine, 206–7
President's Commission for the Study of
    Ethical Problems in Medicine and
    Biomedical and Behavioral Research
    (PCEMR), 108, 225, 228
President's Council on Bioethics, 226
preventive medicine, 50, 221, 223, 224
priests, 207, 208–9, 237, 240
primary care practitioners, 208, 214
principalism, 11–12, 14, 57, 262
principle of double effect, 54–55
principle of totality, 104, 114–15
Principles of Bioethics (Beauchamp and
    Childress), 11–12
Principles of Medical Ethics (AMA), 240
Principles of Physiological Psychology (Wundt), 137
privacy, right to, 213–14
probabilism, 9
proceduralism, 19
pro-choice, 80, 81
procreation, 65, 74, 87
productive skills, 43
productivity, 205–6
professional–client relationship
    communication in, 212–13
    communication with the dying, 173–74
    consumer participation in, 215
    trust in, 211–12
    validity of, 205
professionals. *See* health care professionals;
    physicians

professions
    definition of, 205
    depersonalizing trends in, 204–6
    historical influences on, 223
    medicine as, 206–10
    person-centered, 205–6
profit, 214, 215
prohibition, 157
proportionalism, 15–16, 17, 262
proportionate life support, 185, 186
Protection of Human Subjects, 113
Protestants, 8, 20
providers, choice of, 216
proxy consent
    for ambiguous genitalia treatment, 112–13
    autonomy and, 58
    for behavior control, 150
    for life support withdrawal, 192
    for research, 117
prudence, 43–45, 50–53, 262
prudential judgment, 24–25
prudential personalism
    definition of, 262
    informed consent and, 57–58
    multiculturalism and, 29–30
    needs and, 17, 18
pseudo-religious language, 247
psychiatric hospitalization, 129
psychiatry, 160
psychoactive drugs. *See* psychotropic drugs
psychoanalysis
    description of, 136
    ending, 143
    id and, 137–38, 138f, 141
    insight therapy and, 140
    payment for, 142
    value systems of, 153
psychodrama, 152
psychological addiction, 158
psychological health, 35
psychological research, 113, 118–19
The Psychopathology of Everyday Life (Freud), 137
psychoses, 131, 144
psychosurgery, 130–31
psychotherapy
    behavior control, 149–51
    codependency in, 151–52
    confidentiality in, 150

psychotherapy (*continued*)
  current modes of, 125–26, 136–45
  empirical validity of, 141–43
  ending, 143–44
  ethical issues in, 148–60
  for gender dysphoria, 110–11
  habits in, 139–40
  pastoral counseling and, 242
  vs. psychotropic therapy, 133–35
  right to privacy limitations, 213
  vs. spiritual counseling, 245, 246–47
  successful, 140–41
  trust in, 144–45, 151, 154
  value systems in, 152–54
psychotropic drugs, 150
  for behavior modification, 135–36
  freedom and, 150
  for mental illness, 132–36
  side effects of, 160
public opinion, 11
public policy. *See* health care policy
punishment, 165–66
purification, spiritual, 154
PVS. *See* persistent vegetative state
Pythagorean sect, 5

quadriplegia, 188
quality of care, 217
quality of function, 189
quality of life, 189
Quinlan, Karen Ann, 228

racism, 88
Rahner, Karl, 166
Ramsey, Paul, 9
randomized trials, 115–17
rape, 83–86
rationalization, 157
Rational Recovery, 157
Ratzinger, Joseph (Benedict XVI), 25, 166
Rawls, John, 10–12, 19
Reagan, Ronald, 216
reality, perception of, 119
reason
  Age of Enlightenment and, 4–5
  ethics based on, 20–21, 29
  faith and, 44
  good vs. bad, 17–18

  in health care ethics, 19–20, 21–22
  proportionate, 15–16
recombinant DNA, 92, 98
reconciliation, 235–36, 251–52
reconstructive surgery, 108–13, 123
reductionism, 35, 210
reeducation, 136, 139, 140
reenactment, 152
referrals, 212
Regents of University of California, Tarasoff v., 213
relationships, social, 45–46
relativism, cultural, 33
religion
  definition of, 20
  psychiatry and, 160
  separation from state, 20–21
religiosity, 154
reproductive technology, assisted, 86–87
research, 113–22. *See also* human research
    subjects
  on behavior control, 150
  cloning for, 120–21
  controlled, 115–17
  double-blind, 115–17
  on embryos, 119–20
  government guidelines for, 225–27
  informed consent for, 114–15, 116–18
  legislation, 225–26
  nontherapeutic, 114, 117
  outcomes of, 215
  vs. practice, 204–5
  principals for, 114–15
  psychological, 113, 118–19
  social, 118
  stem cell, 119–22
  vs. therapy, 114
  withdrawal from, 117–18
researchers, as research subjects, 115
*Research Involving Human In Vitro Fertilization
    and Embryo Transfer*, 225
respirators, 170, 185, 187, 188
responsibility
  for health, 46, 220–21
  parental, 102–3
  social, 203, 219, 220–21, 233
Restak, Richard M., 126
resurrection, 39, 165, 175
revealed truth, 24, 26

revelation, 20, 26, 27
Rieff, Philip, 148, 153, 154
rights
    in health care ethics, 21–22
    innate needs and, 33
    of nonhuman animals, 37
    sensitivity to, 29–30
Rights and Duties of Capital and Labor (Leo XIII),
    218
right to dissent, 25–27
right to health, 219
right to life
    abortion and, 80–83
    contemporary culture and, 90
    contraception after rape and, 84
    genetic counseling and, 101–2
    when life begins, 69–73
right to privacy, 213–14
rigorism, 262
Ritalin, 135–36
Roe v. Wade, 70
romanticism, 5, 11, 262
Rosner, Fred, 9
Rousseau, Jean-Jacques, 11
Russell, Bertrand, 17

sacraments, 65, 249–55, 262
saints, Catholic, 148
Sakel, Manfred J., 131
Sanger, Margaret, 76
Schiavo, Theresa Marie (Terri), 191
schizophrenia, 127, 131, 133, 148
schizophrenia delusional disorder, 128
Schüller, Bruno, 15
scientific medicine, 206–7, 208, 210
scientism, 4–5
SCNT (somatic cell nuclear transfer), 121
Scotus, John Duns, 7–9
screening, genetic, 98–100
Second Vatican Council
    on abortion, 80–81
    on marriage, 65–66
    on pastoral care education, 238
    right to dissent from, 26–27
    on sexuality, 49
    on socialism, 218
    on universal priesthood, 240
secular bioethics, 3–5, 19–20, 30, 262

secular hospitals, 236–37
secular humanism, 4–5, 21, 30, 223, 231
security, 33
sedatives, 133
self-centeredness, 153–54
self-consciousness, 71, 145
self-control, 143
sense
    common, 145–47
    evaluative, 147
sense memory, 145
sensus fidei, 27–29, 77
sensus fidelium, 27–29, 77, 262
separation of church and state, 20–21
serpents, 207
sex determination, 95–96
sex selection, 95–96, 98
sexual assault, 83–86
sexual differentiation, 63–64
sexual disorders, 128, 144
sexuality
    bioethics and, 68–69
    for childless couples, 66–67
    Christian, 49–50
    contraception and, 75–76
    definition of, 64, 89
    love and, 64, 66
    meaning of, 63–69
    pastoral approach to, 88–89
    in psychotherapy relationships, 151
    values of, 64–66
sexual reassignment, 109–13
shared decision making, 222, 224
sheep, cloned, 120
siblings, 74
sickness. *See* illness
sin
    death and, 164
    definition of, 262–63
    forgiveness of, 8
    illness as, 168
    mental illness and, 161
    mortal vs. venal, 52
    original, 164, 261
    suffering from, 165
Singer, Peter, 37, 39, 69
single-payer systems, 223–25
situational ethics, 15, 263

skills, 43
skin grafts, 105
Skinner, B. F., 137, 141, 143
slavery, 26, 219–20, 221
Smith, Robert, 156
Snow, C. P., 5
social conscience, 154
social construction of illness, 34
social control, 153
social decision making, 221–23
social factors
   in health, 224–25
   in mental illness, 129
socialism, 218–19, 222
social justice, 59–60
social needs, 33
social relationships, 45–46
social research, 118
social responsibility, 203, 219, 220–21, 233
Society of Jesus. *See* Jesuits
society, therapeutic, 153
softer outcomes, 215
solidarity, 46, 221–23, 263
somatic cell genetic engineering, 94
somatic cell nuclear transfer (SCNT), 121
soul
   after death, 38
   conception and, 72–73
   creation of, 40
   separation from the body, 169
specialists, 204, 208, 212, 214
species, survival of, 65
sperm, 70
spiritual care. *See* pastoral care
spiritual counseling, 244–49
spirituality
   definition of, 263
   mental illness and, 147–48
   personhood and, 71–72
spiritual purification, 154
sponsors, 263
spontaneous abortion, 80
spontaneous breathing and heart function, 173,
   170
state, separation from church, 20–21
stem cell research, 119–22
stereotactic magnetic resonance imaging (MRI),
   130

sterilization, surgical, 78–80
stigmatization, 100
Stoics, 22, 179
Stretton, Dean, 69
Suarez, Francesco, 8–9
subjective morality, 51–53, 88–89, 242–44, 261
subjects, human. *See* human research subjects
subsidiarity, 46–47, 219–21, 222, 263
substance abuse disorders, 128
substitute judgment, 192
succinylcholine, 132
suffering
   death and, 50
   of Jesus Christ, 198
   meaning of, 163–65
   pain control and, 197–98
   as punishment, 165–66
suicide, 179–82
   vs. allowing to die and euthanasia, 182–83
   definition of, 178
   electroconvulsive therapy and, 132
   euthanasia as, 181
   physician-assisted, 178, 179–80, 244
Summa Theologiae Moralis (Antonius of Florence),
   9
superego, 148, 152
superior race, 97–98
Supreme Court (United States), 98, 179, 180
surgery
   body modification by, 92
   for human improvement, 94
   reconstructive and cosmetic, 108–13, 123
surgical sterilization, 78–80
surrogate mothers, 88
survival of the fittest, 65, 95
sustenance, 235–36
Swan Point Cemetery, Pierce v., 176
Swift-Glass, Elenore, 113
symptom-thermal method, 74
Szasz, Thomas, 34, 126

Tarasoff v. Regents of University of California,
   213
teaching profession, 204
teachings. *See* church teachings
technological imperative, 92
technology
   biotechnology, 91, 122–23

Catholic health care facilities and, 231
government guidelines for, 225–26
humanization of, 206
professionals and, 204
teleology, 6, 15, 263. *See also* ends–means ethics
temperance
addiction and, 155, 156
virtue of, 47–49
Ten Commandments, 21, 54
teratomas, 122
terminal illness, 173–74, 190–91
theologians, role of, 23
theological virtues, 42, 43f
theology of the body, 47, 237
The Theology of the Body (John Paul II), 74
theory of justice, 10–11
Theory of Sense Perception (Wundt), 137
therapeutic society, 153
therapeutic transference, 151
therapy. *See* medical therapy; psychotherapy
Therese of Lisieux, Saint, 148
Thomas Aquinas, Saint
on bodily identity, 38
on cadavers, 175
on delayed hominization, 72
on freedom, 147
on goals, 13
on "grace perfects nature," 40
on human nature, 145, 146f
on innate needs, 32–33
on love, 47
on natural law, 7, 21–22
proportionalism and, 16
on suicide, 182
theological ethics of, 7
thought, abstract, 71
Timothy, 23
Tobit, Book of, 175
Tooley, Michael, 69
Torah, 5–6, 261
total brain death, 172–73
total institution, 126–27
totality, principle of, 104, 114–15
total moral object, 261, 263
Totem and Taboo (Freud), 147
"To the Participants in the International
Congress on 'Life-Sustaining Treatments
and Vegetative State': Scientific Advances

and Ethical Dilemmas" (John Paul II),
195–97
totipotential cells, 119, 120
touch, 250
traditionalism, 221
training, clinical, 167
tranquilizers, 155
transplantation. *See* organ donors; organ transplantation
transsexualism, 109–13
pastoral counseling for, 112–13
sexual reassignment for, 109–12
transvestism, 109
The Triumph of the Therapeutic (Rieff), 148, 153
true happiness, 36–37, 38–40, 41, 48, 60
trust
for dying patients, 173
in physicians, 207, 211–12
in psychological research, 118–19
in psychotherapy, 144–45, 151, 154
in spiritual counseling, 245–46
trusteeship, 211
truth
classes of, 24–25
consistency definition of, 12
for dying patients, 173–74
God's word, 24
good of, 13
ordinary teachings of, 24
revealed, 24, 26
tubal ligation, 79
tube feeding. *See* assisted hydration and
nutrition
Tuskegee study, 113, 225
Twelve Step Program, 156–57
twins, identical, 71

ultimate end, 51
umbilical cord cells, 120, 121–22
unconsciousness
collective, 147
vs. persistent vegetative state, 193–94
Uniform Anatomical Gift Act, 177
Uniform Declaration of Death Act, 103
uninsured persons, 217, 218
United Nations, *Universal Declaration of Human
Rights*, 33, 46, 219
universal coverage, 223–25

Universal Declaration of Human Rights (United
    Nations), 33, 46, 219
universal health care, 216
universal priesthood, 240
U.S. Bishops' Conference, 192
U.S. Supreme Court, 98, 179, 180
utilitarianism, 14–15

vaccines, 122
value systems
    in decision making, 32
    definition of, 32
    in ethical counseling, 241–42
    vs. facts, 32
    in psychotherapy, 152–54
    as religion, 20
    romanticism and, 5
    sexuality and, 64–66
Varieties of Religious Experience (James), 156
vasectomy, 79
Vatican II. *See* Second Vatican Council
Veatch, Robert M., 12
veil of ignorance, 10
venal sins, 52
Ventilabrum Medico-Theologicum (Boudewyns),
    9
Veritatis splendor (John Paul II), 51, 161
Viaticum, 251
vicarious consent, 117
vices, 42
virtue ethics, 16–18
virtues
    cardinal (moral), 42–50, 43f, 258
    definition of, 42
    theological, 42, 43f
virtue theory, 42
voluntarism, 8, 263. *See also* duty ethics

Wade, Roe v., 70

Wagner-Jauregg, Julius, 131
Warnock Committee, 114
Watson, J. B., 137
Weisman, August, 35
welfare system, 221
WHO. *See* World Health Organization
Wildes, Kevin M., 12–13, 19
will. *See* free will
William of Ockham, 7–8
Willowbrook experiments, 113
will power, 49
wills, living, 181
Wilmut, Ian, 120
Wilson, Bill, 156
wisdom literature, 6
withdrawing life support. *See* life support
    withdrawal/withholding
Wittgenstein, Ludwig, 17
Wolf, Susan, 69
Wolffian ducts, 64
Wolpe, Joseph, 142
women, 68–69
World Federation of Catholic Medical
    Associations, 190
World Health Organization (WHO)
    on family planning, 74–75
    Geneva Declaration, 181
    on health, 35–36
    on human research subjects, 114
worldview, 20
Wundt, Wilhelm, 137, 142

xenotransplantation, 107

Yankelovich, Daniel, 153
Y chromosome, 63–64

Zacchia, Paolo, 9
zygotes, 63–64, 70